Strategies
for
Public Health

Promoting Health and Preventing Disease

Strategies for Public Health

Promoting Health and Preventing Disease

Edited by

LORENZ K.Y. Ng

World Man Fund

and

DEVRA LEE DAVIS

Environmental Law Institute

VNR **VAN NOSTRAND REINHOLD COMPANY**
NEW YORK   CINCINNATI   ATLANTA   DALLAS   SAN FRANCISCO
LONDON   TORONTO   MELBOURNE

Van Nostrand Reinhold Company Regional Offices:
New York   Cincinnati   Atlanta   Dallas   San Francisco

Van Nostrand Reinhold Company International Offices:
London   Toronto   Melbourne

Library of Congress Catalog Card Number: 80-13068
ISBN: 0-442-24428-2

Manufactured in the United States of America

Published by Van Nostrand Reinhold Company
135 West 50th Street, New York, N.Y. 10020

Published simultaneously in Canada by Van Nostrand Reinhold Ltd.

15 14 13 12 11 10 9 8 7 6 5 4 3 2 1

Library of Congress Cataloging in Publication Data

Main entry under title:

Strategies for public health.

    Includes index.
    1. Public health. 2. Medicine, Preventive. 3. Occupational and environmental health.
I. Ng, Lorenz K.Y. II. Davis, Devra Lee.
[DNLM: 1. Health promotion—Methods. 2. Preven-
tive medicine. WA108 S898]
RA425.S74   362.1   80-13068
ISBN 0-442-24428-2

敬以此書

獻給我敬愛的父母

陳寶香　黃錫權

黃慶榮敬獻

Contents

Introduction:
Overview

1

National Policy Issues for Health Promotion and Disease Prevention

Devra Lee Davis, Ph.D.

Lorenz K.Y. Ng, M.D.

World Man Fund and Environmental Law Institute

Assembly of this book began at a time when public expectations about health care reform ran high. Debates explored not *whether* something should be done about the lack of a national health policy, but *what* strategies should be preferred. In 1976, the outgoing Assistant Secretary for Health, Theodore Cooper, introduced the third in a series of reports entitled *Forward Plan for Health (FY 1978-82),* which included a tactical statement outlining prevention and cost containment as two important issues for national health policy.[1] That same year, in a speech to the American Public Health Association, then presidential candidate Jimmy Carter declared that:

First, we must return to the basic focus on the prevention of illness and disease . . . Second, we must have a comprehensive program of national health insurance . . .

In July of 1979, the first *Surgeon General's Report on Health Promotion and Disease Prevention (Healthy People)* was issued, calling for a "public health revolution" aimed at reducing the incidence of heart disease, cancer, and accidents.[2] Buoyed by the promise in such reports, the contributors to this volume confront contemporary health care dilemmas and consider the appropriate roles for government, the private sector, the health care delivery system, and individual health consumers.

The leading causes of premature death and disability in America are no longer infectious diseases but are instead associated with where and how we live. Cardiovascular incidents, heart disease, respiratory illnesses, and cancer kill nearly two million people annually and leave many more disabled and in pain. Table 1-1 illustrates the shift in leading causes of mortality from infectious to chronic degenerative diseases and accidents.

Table 1-1. Age-adjusted death rates per 100,000 for selected causes of death in the United States, 1900–1976.[3]

		Cause of Death			
Year	Malignant Neoplasms	Disease of the Heart	Influenza and Pneumonia	Accidents	Homicides
1900	79.6	167.3	209.5	75.3	1.2
1905	90.9	198.7	175.5	85.4	2.1
1910	97.0	201.7	163.0	88.4	4.5
1915	100.8	206.3	154.7	77.4	6.0
1920	104.9	203.6	213.1	74.0	6.9
1925	112.5	229.6	128.1	81.9	8.5
1930	113.4	252.7	108.2	84.6	9.2
1935	117.5	269.0	109.2	80.7	8.6
1940	120.3	292.7	70.2	73.1	6.3
1945	119.9	282.4	45.6	68.7	5.8
1950	125.4	307.6	26.2	57.5	5.4
1955	125.8	287.5	21.0	54.4	4.8
1960	125.8	286.2	28.0	49.9	5.2
1961	125.4	278.6	22.1	48.1	5.2
1962	125.6	282.7	23.7	49.7	5.4
1963	126.7	285.4	27.7	50.9	5.5
1964	125.7	276.9	22.8	52.1	5.7
1965	127.9	275.6	23.4	53.4	6.2
1966	123.4	275.8	23.8	55.6	6.7
1967	129.1	267.7	20.8	54.8	7.7
1968	130.2	270.0	26.8	55.1	8.2
1969	129.7	262.3	24.6	55.3	8.6
1970	129.9	253.6	22.1	53.7	9.1
1971	130.7	252.0	19.3	52.0	10.0
1972	130.7	249.3	20.8	52.0	10.3
1973	130.7	244.4	20.1	51.7	10.5
1974	131.8	232.7	16.9	46.0	10.8
1975	130.9	220.5	16.6	44.8	10.5
1976	132.3	216.7	17.4	43.2	9.5
1977	132.9	209.8	13.8	44.7	10.1

Sources:

U. S. Dept. of HEW, National Office of Vital Statistics, *Vital Statistics Special Reports,* Vol. 43, Nos. 1–31, October 1956.

U.S. Dept. of HEW, National Center for Health Statistics, *Vital and Health Statistics,* Series 20, No. 16, March 1974.

U.S. Dept. of HEW, *Vital Statistics of the United States,* Vol. 11, Mortality–Part A, 1970–1975.

Monthly Vital Statistics Report, Final Mortality Statistics, 1976, Vol. 26, No. 12, Suppl. 2, March 1978.

Recognizing that much of what determines people's health stems from the environment and the way we live, the responsibility for national health changes. We are all part of the health picture. Environmental protection, occupational health and safety, policies concerning food, and other governmental and private sector actions all constitute parts of the national health effort.

At a working conference, convened by the Health Promotion Project of the World Man Fund in February of 1977, issue papers were developed and debated by some of this volume's contributors in anticipation of a national health policy. Now, some three years later, the immediately relevant problems have changed. Economic considerations dominate, with disease prevention and health promotion playing lesser roles.

This book's contributors seek to redirect discussions about national health to promotion and prevention issues. Only when preventive strategies are in place can public health be improved and costs controlled. Providing catastrophic coverage, without preventing some of the causes of medical catastrophes, will only increase the costs for national health care.

Changing Health Problems and Solutions

Frequently, problems are posed in ways that already constrain their solutions, much in the manner that questions are asked in ways that may limit their answers (Such as: "When will you be leaving?" or "Are you still smoking?"). Recent changes in our thinking about health have serious policy implications both for the choice of appropriate questions about health as well as for the selection of appropriate sectors to bear responsibility for developing answers. A central health problem of the sixties, for example, was described as the "shortage" of trained personnel. The inevitable solution to the problem became the creation of more health professionals. In the early seventies, the problem of inadequately distributed health resources was to be attacked by creating incentives for better distribution of health services (such as the 1970 Amendments to the Public Health Services, which created the National Health Service Corps).

Unfortunately, current questions about health are chiefly and narrowly economic; for example, "How can we control hospital and doctor costs?" We contend that equally important questions should be: "How can the demand for hospitals and interventive medical care be reduced?" and "How can the efficiency and quality of care received be improved?"

Economic Issues. The fact that high health care costs characterize such widely different national health systems as those in Great Britain, Canada, Sweden, and the U.S., strongly suggests that the organization of health care delivery may be only one of several factors affecting costs. Furthermore, the nearly universal lack of success of efforts to reduce the rate of inflation in health care costs in all of these systems bolsters the view that improving delivery system efficiency may not markedly reduce health care costs, particularly if the demand for services increases.

The current exclusionary emphasis on health care inflation represents the symptomatic treatment of our health care problem. By treating primarily the symptoms of inflated costs, we allow the fundamental causes of these symptoms to go unchecked. Despite some recent federal rhetoric about preventive programs, considerably more energy and investment has gone into the question of cost containment than has been allotted to the generation of effective policies to reduce the disease burden, and, in turn, the demand for health care interventions.

Public expectations that something must be done about high health care costs have fueled Congressional interest in cost containment. In all of this, there lies a certain myopia. So long as the questions are posed in economic terms, the answers will be chiefly economic strategies. There is no doubt that serious economic nemeses confront modern health care and that appropriate control policies should be developed. At the same time as these controls are devised, however, equal attention must be paid to those factors that produce sickness and death in our society. Otherwise we will simply become more efficient at processing sick people, rather than more adept at promoting health.

Lifestyle and Environmental Issues. In this book, we question the taken-for-granted assumption of fixed levels of sickness or pathology in our society. We propose that the incidences of the current major causes of death and disease can be significantly reduced by developing social and economic incentives for health. We accept the argument that a substantial portion of major illnesses are controllable or preventable by changes in both lifestyle and the environment. The learning and practice of health promotion behaviors for individuals, corporations, health care providers, and the government could result in reductions in morbidity and mortality. Strategies for producing such changes could effectively produce great economic and social savings by reducing demands for acute and chronic health care, increasing the potential labor force and GNP, and vastly improving the quality of life.*[4]

Of course, sound market and bureaucratic policies will also create savings; but without a collaborative health promotion program giving people the motivation and incentives for health, the numbers of people requiring interventive care will not diminish. With health incentive programs, the savings to all segments of society would be considerable in economic terms and immeasurable in terms of improving the quality of life.

---

*Some have made Swiftian arguments that such policies will disastrously increase the tax burden by enabling people to live longer into social security. This possibility constitutes an unquantifiable risk with which a democratic society ought to proudly live.

Shift from Model for Infectious to Model for Chronic Diseases

American health may be better than ever. However, health is caught in a conceptual shift from a medical model for infectious diseases to a broader model for environmental and lifestyle sources of chronic disease. Without examining the implications of this conceptual shift in depth, some critics hold American medicine responsible for problems over which it has little direct control, such as those involving occupational health and safety, housing, nutrition, and unemployment. For instance, Ivan Illich assumes that most of the responsibility for poor health is due to too much—and faulty—medical care, while failing to realize that the rural areas and some urban inner cities of this country (i.e., where much ill health occurs) remain under-served medically.[5] Following the reasoning of these critics, we are urged to leave people to their natural abilities and suffering, leaving out the presumably defective medical care, much as we excise a diseased appendix. No one can deny the validity of Illich's observations concerning the over-medicalized middle and upper middle class population of this country, where clinical "iatrogenesis," or physician-induced disease, can be found. However, such a view does not address the quite different medical problems of the working class in the cities and rural areas. Rural America's health problems have been likened by some critics to those of developing countries.[6]

It has become commonplace to note the change in leading causes of mortality from infectious diseases at the turn of this century to chronic degenerative diseases and accidents today. What is less commonly recognized is that two very different sets of health problems emerge, given these changes: 1) how best to manage (or, when possible, cure) those who now have degenerative chronic diseases; and 2) how best to prevent these diseases from developing in others. Any national health policy must simultaneously assist the afflicted, while restricting any increase in overall afflictions. To achieve this, a two-phase system will have to be devised, which combines curative and preventive strategies.

Historically, public health has not sustained such a twin focus. More recently, scientific and medical advances in surgery and chemotherapy have transfixed attention on medicine's curative powers. Physicians are glamorized and presented in documentaries of their heroic interventions. Where prevention receives attention at all, it is secondary or tertiary prevention, such as screening procedures for already existing chronic diseases. In short, prevention is less glamorous than curative medicine.

Rediscovery of Prevention's Importance

With the advent of scientific medicine at the turn of this century, emphasis in American public health circles focused on curing diseases rather than on preventing them. The apparent successes of mass immunization and available antibodies in controlling some infectious diseases became the firmament upon which ever more costlier and more complicated medical technologies rested. If medicine in its infancy could wipe out diphtheria, then, in its mature phase, it ought to cure cancer and heart disease. This preoccupation with curing inadvertently obscured questions about the potentially preventable causes of such morbidity. Medicine became oriented to curing rather than preventing disease. Physicians were paid when they treated sick people. Only in old China were medical providers paid when people were healthy. In most other countries, fee-for-service while ill was the norm. However, as the costs of improving curative medicine steadily increased, improvements in health failed to grow as rapidly. As a result, public health interest has returned to its nineteenth century concern with preventive strategies.

As the costs of providing small improvements in curative medicine have mounted, public health interest has returned to its nineteenth century concern with preventive strategies. As first set up in the nineteenth century, public health departments concerned themselves with the control of contagion through environmental sanitation. It seemed self-evident to these early pioneers in public health that dirty air, water, and food; poor working conditions; poor diet; and inadequate housing would affect health.[7] With the demonstration at the end of the nineteenth century that specific microorganisms, or pathogens, produced infectious diseases, this focus on environmental factors gave way to the scientific search for specific pathogenic agents and their control and prevention. The drop in diphtheria morbidity and mortality was taken as evidence of the triumph of scientific medicine derived from the germ theory of disease.[8]

But the decline in diphtheria began before the diphtheria antitoxin was actually in use, and continued progressively even before immunization became widespread Thus, the decline of diphtheria was not an isolated incident, but partly the result of overall improvements in environment and lifestyle. The impact of sanitation and nutrition changes did not become evident until the end of the nineteenth century, at which time all countries showed a decline in death rates.[9]

John B. McKinlay and Sonja M. McKinlay estimate that approximately 3.5% of the decline in mortality in influenza, pneumonia, diphtheria, whooping cough, and poliomyelitis in the U.S. since 1900 can be attributed to specific medical measures.[10] They derive this estimate from comparing mortality trends in these diseases with the times of widespread introduction of their antidotes, and 3.5% of their declines in mortality can be explained by the introduction of medical measures for the above five diseases. Figure 1-1 summarizes their findings. Changes in three of the other previous leading causes of death appear to be completely unrelated to medical measures, as Figure 1-2 indicates.

For all practical purposes, deaths from measles, scarlet fever, and typhoid were eliminated *before* vaccine, penicillin, and chloramphenicol were widely introduced. It may, of course, be argued that the availability of these kinds of medical measures provides the basis for preventive public health strategies. But it could

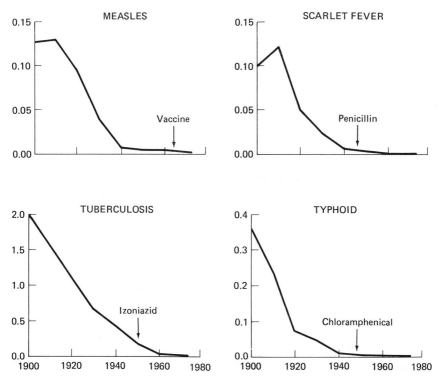

Figure 1-1. The fall in the standardized death rate (per 1,000 population) for four common infectious diseases in relation to specific medical measures, for the United States, 1900-1973.[11]

also be argued that these measures are largely superfluous, since these diseases are no longer leading causes of mortality.

According to medical critics such as Ivan Illich, the infections that prevailed at the onset of the industrial age explain how medicine developed its eminent reputation.[13] On close examination, the incidences of, and death rates from, these diseases had fallen off *before* medical interventions had become widespread. Tuberculosis reached a peak over two generations. In New York in 1812, the death rate was estimated to be higher than 700 deaths per 100,000 persons. By 1882, it had already declined to 370 per 100,000. Although this was the year Robert Koch isolated and cultured the tuberculus bacillus, as McKinlay and McKinlay indicate, widespread use of the drug Izoniazid did not take place in the United States until the late 1940's, when the national mortality rate for tuberculosis was less than 50 deaths per 100,000 persons. Historical epidemiological analysis indicates that much of the decline in cholera, dysentery, and typhoid occurred well before modern therapeutic techniques had become common. The combined death rate from scarlet fever, diphtheria, whooping cough,

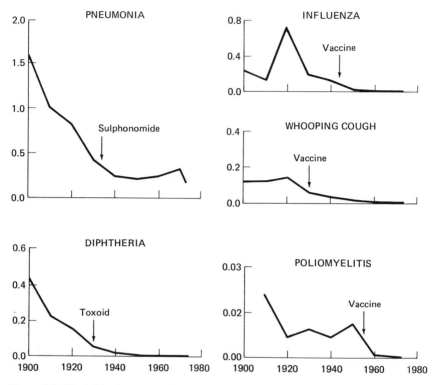

Figure 1-2. The fall in the standardized death rate (per 1,000 population) for four common infectious diseases in relation to specific medical measures, for the United States, 1900-1973.[12]

and measles, among children up to age 15, shows that nearly 90% of the total decline in mortality between 1860 and 1965 occurred before the introduction of antibiotics and extensive immunization.[14]

Environment and Lifestyle Currently Critical for Public Health

The importance of environmental and lifestyle factors as related to illness today cannot be contested, although the exact proportions of illness due to specific agents may be argued. With the exponential growth in chemical production in this country since World War II, larger numbers of people are being exposed to untested, potentially toxic substances. Further, there are numerous toxic compounds to which extensive exposure appears inevitable, either because these substances occur naturally or because of their distribution in the environment. These materials include benzo(a)pyrene, a byproduct of burning fossil fuels and cigarettes; polycyclic aromatic hydrocarbons; aflatoxin, a naturally occurring mold on peanuts, corn, and some milk products; nitrosamines and some nitrogen compounds; asbestos, a naturally occurring, massively produced fiber; and thorium, tritium, radon, and other forms of low level ionizing radiation which occur naturally and are sometimes released in the burning of fossil fuels.[15]

Multiple Exposures to Pollutants and Multiple Effects. Documenting the health effects of pollutants is a complicated task, marked by philosophical controversies concerning causality, inference, and extrapolation from animals to humans. Perhaps the most difficult problem is that few pollutants have one single adverse health effect and few health effects have a single cause. In addition, pollutants never occur naturally in isolation. Thus, people exposed to benzo(a)pyrene are also exposed to other industrial pollutants, such as sulfates, polycyclic organic matter, benzene, and oxides of nitrogen. Moreover, the levels of these pollutants in the air of a city are highly correlated with one another. For these pollutants, the assignment of specific causality to a single suspect substance for a single health effect is impossible. Yet much environmental regulation now rests on determining just such individual risk assessments for single substances and single effects.[16]

Environmental and Occupational Factors Account for Some Diseases. The Clean Air Act Amendments of 1977 mandated the establishment of the National Task Force on Environmental Cancer, and Heart and Lung Diseases as one effort to spur consideration of multiple health problems. In its first *Report to Congress,* this Task Force noted that heart disease morbidity and mortality are greater in areas with more polluted air: 'There is enough evidence of an environmental impact upon heart disease to suggest environmental intervention as a preventive medicine measure."[17]

In an assessment of the fraction of cancer due to occupational exposure in the United States, a recent Health, Education and Welfare report indicated that at least 20% could be associated with occupational exposures.[18]

A further problem with environmental sources of illness is that people display highly varying responses to toxic substances, reflecting their genetic, nutritional, lifestyle, and possibly even personality patterns. George L. Waldbott reports on the idiosyncratic responses to lead poisoning among a family of six:

The father and a 4-year-old boy had had frequent episodes of abdominal colics, simulating bowel obstruction, "intestinal flu", and acute pancreatitis . . . Two other children had had convulsions . . . Another child had a disturbance of the glucose metabolism, simulating diabetes . . . The mother had a brain disease, for which no diagnosis had been made . . . This diagnosis was supported by high lead levels in their food and in body tissues, by lead poisoning encountered in horses near the smelter where they lived and by the fact that most of the vegetables and fruits consumed by the family were raised on their farm.[19]

Table 1-2. Clinical symptoms of certain pollutants.[20]

Pollutant	Symptom
Arsenic	Dark skin, loss of hair
Asbestos	Ferruginous bodies
Barium	Thyroid disease
Boron	Brain damage
Cadmium	Hypertension, emphysema, osteo-porosis
Carbon monoxide	Carboxyhemoglobin
Chromium*	Nasal irritation
Cobalt*	Thyroid disease, asthma
Fluoride	Skin (maculae), dental fluorosis
Iron*	Siderosis
Lead	Anemia, gastrointestinal symp-toms
Hydrogen sulfide	Rotten-egg odor
Manganese*	Ataxia, tremor
Mercury	Tremor
Nickel carbonate	Nasal irritation
Nitrites	Cyanosis
Ozone	Eye irritation
Quartz	Silicosis
Selenium*	Odor of garlic, tooth decay
Tellurium	Garlic-like odor
Titanium	Yellow discoloration of skin
Vanadium	Respiratory symptoms
Zinc*	Fever

*Trace quantities of these elements are essential for life.

To make matters even more problematic, some essential micronutrients, such as selenium, iron, and manganese, are toxic to humans at higher levels. Table 1-2 indicates clinical symptoms produced by some pollutants.

Medical Training on Environmental Health is Inadequate. Most medical training today features little or no information about pollutants and their potential effects.[21] Where pollutant effects are studied, it is primarily with reference to acute episodes rather than to the chronic, low levels of exposure leading to the chronic diseases that most people face. Improving our understanding of the mechanisms of chronic diseases is essential to providing better preventive and curative strategies. For example, workers or their families developed very high fevers following exposure to certain heavy metal fumes such as zinc and manganese.[22] The symptoms included pulmonary complications. By now, these are well documented diseases, and removal of affected workers from exposure is routine. However, until a relationship between exposure and disease was established, patients were diagnosed as hypersusceptible febrile individuals who had weak lungs.

We cannot know how many other disease syndromes which have significant environmental correlates remain to be discovered. It is clear that studies of such potential syndromes are infrequent.

Two public problems of concern that may be associated with exposures to heavy metals can be mentioned in this light: chronic kidney disease and poor school performance. Kidney disease is a serious public health matter. People with chronic renal problems often die of congestive heart failure. Hence, mortality data, limited to single causes of death, understate the magnitude of kidney disease. Kidney dialysis treatment costs about one billion dollars annually. Some research has noted an increase in certain infectious renal disease (glomulero-nephritis) in workers exposed to heavy metals.[23]

Poor school performance, mental retardation, and mental illness also constitute public health topics of grave concern. One of the many troubling areas that require critical study is that of assessing the contribution of environmental pollution to poor school performance of inner city minority children. H.L. Needleman *et al.* suggest in their review of data that exposure to heavy metals such as lead may account for more of this phenomenon than has been recognized in the past.[24]

In light of these studies and the contributions to this volume, it is clear that environmental factors over which people have no control, and lifestyle factors constrained by advertising and other cultural mediations, exert a considerable influence on the status of our health.

National Health Policy Issues

In a world where so many of the bad things that happen to people's health are beyond the immediate reach of medicine, the factors affecting national health policy extend beyond the health care system. The way we think about disease has important social implications.

When disease was understood primarily as a reflection of mechanical processes, the roles of health care providers and patients were clearly delineated. Health care providers treated diseases; patients presented themselves passively for cures. Research was directed to promoting organisms' defenses and providing interventions to attack the causes of diseases. H. Fabrega discusses some of the problems attendant to this person-centered, temporally-bounded, and discontinuous view of disease:

Many of the present problems in health care and its delivery may be traced, at least in part, to problems stemming from the dominating influence of an organismic conception of disease. As implied above, an episodic view of disease underscores the need for only episodic treatment and militates against the comprehensive and continuous evaluation that some patients require. When the disease "appears" as defined by a set of symptoms, the person may then seek help, have his discomfort validated, and pay for it on the basis of a completed service.[25]

In its extreme reduction, this narrow, mechanical model of disease reduces individuals to their medical histories and delimits a set of diagnostic possibilities. This view militates against preventive programs insofar as it stresses the discrete and discontinuous nature of disease. If diseases are distinct events, no systematic supportive programs can be expected to affect their incidence. In this view, patients are rendered passive recipients of diseases and of cures.

This heuristic construction of the mechanical model of disease may never have been dominant in medicine, but variants of it can be noted in patients' expectations and insurance reimbursement policies. Drugs represent ideal, outside, discrete intervenors against disease. People commonly go to their physicians seeking "something" for their discomfort. Drugs, as the discrete evidence that confirms their illness, become the proof that patients are genuinely in need of physicians.

Changes in Medical Practice. When physicians hand out non-discrete care such as dietary advice, or suggestions of lifestyle or environmental changes, some of the resistance they encounter can be attributed to the fact that these "prescriptions" are not what people have come to expect from physicians. This expectation also affects medical reimbursement policies in a vexing manner. Physicians who provide behavioral therapy for such chronic problems as drug addiction, alcoholism, depression, or pain management frequently have difficulty receiving reimbursement from insurance companies that classify such therapies as nonmedical. Patients can be reimbursed for drugs purchased, but often cannot be reimbursed for hot packs, home traction devices, or supplies used in monitoring drug reduction.[26]

As disease comes to be understood as a dynamic, interactive, environmental process, the roles and boundaries between health care providers and patients change markedly. Every part of the social fabric has an impact on disease. In a unified view of disease, the expressions and determinations of disease are conceptualized holistically. Health reflects the human's relationship with the physical, social, and psychological environments. Causes are recognized as multifactorial, processes are interdependent, and manifestations are multifaceted:

. . . in a unified or systems view of disease, not only are the *manifestations* or expressions of what we term "disease" seen as interconnected and hierarchically organized . . . In addition, the *determinants* of disease are also conceptualized holistically. Disease is as a natural consequence of man's open relationship with his physical and social environment. Styles of coping are seen as rooted in patterns of neuromuscular and humoral integration, and difficulties in coping (i.e., stress, frustration, etc.) as expressed in altered biological processes that give rise to symptoms or signs of disordered function (i.e., "disease").[27]

Expanding the Health Field

In a pioneering 1974 report, the Canadian government documented the significance of non-medical factors such as environment and lifestyle for the overall health of a modern country. Distressed by no apparent improvement in health despite rapid improvement in the quality and accessibility of health services, the Canadian Ministry of Health studied the principal causes of premature mortality, or early deaths.

Reasoning that deaths before age 70 should be more preventable, they sought the leading causes of mortality for those dying before age 70. They calculated the years of potential life lost due to each cause, measured against a life expectancy of 70, and putting aside causes of infant mortality. Table 1-3 indicates years of life lost by early deaths due to the five main causes in 1971 for Canadians.

Table 1-3. Years of life lost in 1971 to leading causes of death (excluding infant mortality).[28]

Cause	Total Years Lost
Motor vehicle accidents	213,000
Ischaemic heart disease	193,000
All other accidents	179,000
Respiratory diseases and lung cancer	140,000
Suicide	69,000

Environmental and Lifestyle Key Factors

Based on the findings given in Table 1-3, the Canadians concluded that the development of prepaid health insurance over the past 15 years, which had culminated in the introduction of national universal Medicare in 1967, making health services available to all Canadians, had had little impact on mortality and morbidity rates. An analysis of the principal causes of morbidity and mortality revealed that environmental factors and lifestyle contributed so greatly that these factors constituted the keys to effective disease control.

In further analyzing these years lost, the Canadians discovered a profound male mortality problem. For the five main causes of early death given in Table 1-3, males lost almost three years of potential life for every year lost by females.[29] For instance, between the ages of 35 and 70, there were 18,400 men who died of disease of the cardiovascular system, compared to only 7300 women.

The Canadian study conceptualized the health field as comprised of four significant components: environment, lifestyle, health care organization, and human biology. The advantages of thinking about health this way are exemplified in the following statement:

It permits a system of analysis by which any question can be examined under the four elements in order to assess their relative significance and interaction. For example, the underlying causes of death from traffic accidents can be found to be mainly due to risks taken by individuals, with lesser importance given to the design of cars and roads, and to the availability of emergency treatment; human biology has little or no significance in this area. In order of importance, therefore, Lifestyle, Environment and Health Care Organization, contribute to traffic deaths in the proportions of something like 75%, 20% and 5%, respectively. This analysis permits program planners to focus their attention on the most important contributing factors.[30]

While the need to achieve behavioral and environmental changes as a principal means of disease prevention and health promotion is evident, our understanding of the precise means to accomplish this change is less clear. Ironically, the failure to appreciate the role of behavior and institutions in disease prevention and health promotion stems, in no small measure, from the spectacular success of public health efforts in the elimination of infectious diseases. The public health model for infectious disease control (the "vaccination model") encourages the belief that the most active thing people need do is visit a health care professional once for a disease prevention "shot." The inadequacy of this model in dealing with problems of environmental health and lifestyle is starkly obvious. In order to resolve environmental and lifestyle problems, we will need to develop ways to motivate people and institutions to stop doing things that are detrimental to their health, and to engage in alternative behaviors that will increase their health and well-being.[31]

Health Field Model

The schema in Figure 1-3 estimates the proportionate relationship between environment, lifestyle, health care delivery, and human biology as they account for public health patterns today derived from the Canadian report. These proportions are derived from the Canadian epidemiological analysis. The dotted line between "Environment" and "Lifestyle" indicates the indistinct boundary between these two factors.

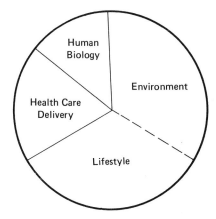

Figure 1-3. Relative effect on public health of environment, lifestyle, health care delivery, and human biology.[31]

The Center for Disease Control supported a more detailed analysis of the four factors by specific disease catagories in the U.S. Using the delphi method of pooling public health experts (which reflects the training and assumptions of those experts), they developed diagrams of these relative relationships within the health field.

Any cursory consideration of health expenditures reveals that spending priorities do not mesh with these factors' importance for public health. Our estimate suggests that budget priorities can be portrayed as in Figure 1-4. In a sense,

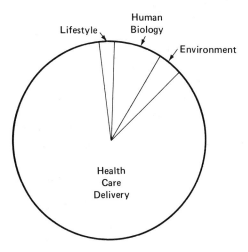

Figure 1-4. Relative proportions of public moneys allocated to environment, lifestyle, health care delivery, and human biology.[32]

incommensurables are being compared in this schema. There will always be significant demands for primary health care. What is key in this schematization, however, is the relative lack of emphasis on the other important components of the health field.

Any overly simplified effort to base the proportion of money allocated on the relative impact these factors have on public health would only increase health care problems. Of course, substantial investment will still have to be made for providing health care delivery, particularly to those millions who already have chronic degenerative diseases. These schema *do* indicate the need for serious rethinking of our relative national investment in other factors of the health field. The National Task Force on Environmental Cancer, Heart and Lung Disease is mandated to recommend comprehensive research programs, preventive strategies, and government coordination appropriate to reducing these degenerative diseases. Given the meager investment in preventing these diseases to date, development of preventive public health strategies should be a key beginning in a needed new direction.

Organization of the Book

As the health field schema makes clear, health policy concerns now include factors traditionally beyond the realm of medicine. This does not in any way mitigate the importance of sound medical practices, such as immunization against childhood diseases. Rather, this expansion of the health field requires comparable attention to nutrition, exposure to toxic substances, social-psychological stress, and health education. The burdens of improving public health will necessarily shift from their traditional locus of the medical professions, to include, in addition to the health professions and health care providers, the research community, the educational system, the public, advertising issues, state and local government, the federal government, the business sector, trade unions, voluntary associations, and the American people as individuals.[32]

The most difficult task will be that of establishing linkages between all the responsible parties, some of whom have conflicting economic interests. An important first step is the acknowledgment that health costs have not yet been adequately assessed, both in economic terms and in terms of their impact on the quality of life.

It may well be the case that we are paying the price now for our neglect of preventive strategies in the past. Particularly in the inner cities, where more than half of all pesticides are used, where most lead pollution from automobile exhaust occurs, where more working class and poor people live, and where the nutritional status is often inadequate and social stress exaggerated, a major part of our so-called welfare and Medicaid problems can be linked to excessive environmental exposures and lifestyle stresses. Certainly, the analysis of the true environmental burden remains to be done for urban America. We can only suggest the obvious: that sick people cannot work as well or as often as well people. Where hypertension, diabetes, obesity, and poor nutrition are from five to seven times more prevalent, as is the case now in the central cities,[33] it is hardly surprising that unemployment sometimes runs more than 50%, that homicide and suicide are important causes of death for males up to age 35, and that health care costs are heavy.[34]

No panaceas can be found here, and anyone suggesting definitive resolutions of our health care problems at this time should be challenged. We need to begin to build demonstrations and tests of preventive strategies along with the more obvious cost containment strategies. Despite the elegance of the Canadian report of 1974, little real advancement or implementation has been affected in that admittedly smaller country. While appealing ideas are important, they have no inherent power. The proof of any national health policy will be that it works.

Individuals and Health. This volume begins with a section exploring holistic and integrative approaches to health enhancement and to the promotion of well-being and wellness as opposed to illness. As Hans Selye points out in his introductory chapter: "Health is largely determined by stable balance—what Walter Cannon called homeostasis." Health is viewed as the problem of the whole person's approach to life. The newly emerging findings in the behavioral and the biomedical sciences can help to elucidate the intimate links that have been shown to exist between the human mind—which is in large measure under the control of the individual—and the human body.

Selye contends that knowledge of the biological stress syndrome and homeostasis will offer insights relevant to both public and private policy in health promotion and disease prevention. He succinctly describes the concept of biological stress that he has helped to develop, pointing out the innumerable hormonal and chemical changes which check and balance the body's functioning and stability, constituting a virtual arsenal of weapons by which the organism defends itself for survival. He notes the influence that can be brought to bear upon the stress response by factors such as heredity, age, previous exposure to stress, nutrition, and many other factors.

Under the influence of such internal or external (endogenous or exogenous) conditioning factors, a normally well-tolerated degree of stress can become pathogenic and cause *diseases of adaption*, selectively affecting those parts of the body that are particularly vulnerable or sensitized both by the conditioning factors and by the specific effect of stressors. Research on stress will be most useful only if it is guided by the principle that to combat stress factors in our lives, we must learn to imitate and, if necessary, to correct and complement the body's own auto-pharmacologic efforts. Today's technology mediates and constrains the quality of life, food, environment, and even behavior, all of which determine health and well-being. And, "just as wars will not be avoided by more sophisticated weaponry, so disease can never be completely eradicated by improvements in pharmacology, immunotherapy, or any other purely medical means." Selye concludes that the goal of medicine should be to understand the patient as a person, and that the modern physician ought to know as much about emotions and thoughts as about disease symptoms and drugs. This approach would appear to hold more promise of cure than anything that medicine has yet developed.

As Lorenz K.Y. Ng, Devra L. Davis, and Ronald W. Manderscheid note: "Health connotes the sense of wholeness or completeness, or the sense of working and functioning well." This generic definition is embodied in the conceptualization by the World Health Organization, which defines health as "a state of complete physical, mental, and social well-being and not merely the absence of disease and infirmity."

Efforts must incorporate the twin concepts of disease prevention and health promotion, including positive strategies for promoting wellness and well-being. Our present view of health is dominated by the biomedical model of disease, where health is often viewed as merely the absence of disease. The development of a biopsychosocial model of wellness and well-being presents a challenge to all of society. From a heuristic standpoint, wellness is conceived as a cumulative process over time, that can be influenced by environmental, physical, behavioral, psychological, and social factors. Thus, illness and wellness are not viewed as mutually exclusive but rather as two independent and intersecting dimensions. From this framework, an ill individual can learn to manage that illness well, so as to reduce stress associated with ill health. People with chronic diseases need to be guided in adapting to these diseases as well as they can. This notion particularly pertains to the estimated million people suffering with chronic pain problems, such as arthritis and low back pain. With appropriate exercise, including relaxation techniques, these people can be eased into more productive lives. As John Bonica and others have noted, this would necessarily reduce the enormous economic drain of the estimated billion dollars now lost when people in pain are unable to work.

Paul Rosch, in his chapter, discusses the need to integrate mind, body, and spirit into a holistic approach for the enhancement of health. He traces the evolution of the holistic health movement, pointing out that holistic medicine is, to a large extent, filling a void that has been created by our own medical technocracy. The doctor-patient relationship, so essential to the healing process, has been steadily disintegrating and becoming more depersonalized, due to factors related to time, cost, specialization, and increasing reliance on technology and machines. In the face of increasing public disenchantment with certain aspects of conventional medicine, the concept of holistic medicine, as well as the closely related subject of the role of stress as a cause of illness, has captured the attention of the public at large in an unprecedented fashion. There is, as a result, a great proliferation of organizations and cults that purport to serve rather lofty aims, but in effect, are dedicated to other goals, or are outright frauds.

We are truly at the crossroads: What should be the response and attitude of the responsible physician and enlightened patient to all of this? We need to strike some kind of balance, says Rosch, that permits us to retain a healthy skepticism until all the facts are in, while, at the same time, we must recognize that our mere inability to explain certain results and observations does not necessarily negate their validity. While it is wise to question and to be discriminative, and to adhere to scientific principles in our evaluation of various modalities of therapy as they arise, it may be imprudent to reject automatically the novel and the innovative, simply because they have no bases in terms of our own training and experience or because we cannot justify their apparent effects. Rosch concludes that allopathic and holistic medicine are neither mutually exclusive nor imcompatible, and that wise physician and patient must choose from the best that both have to offer.

Developing further the positive model of health, Joel Elkes notes that motivation for good health requires awareness of the body and its functions, along with the belief that we are all entitled to live "a good day." The "good day" is a metaphor for our right and potential to pursue the best of health and wellness under all circumstances. The germ of well-being, Elkes maintains, is embedded in the ordinary conduct of the ordinary day. Awareness is the gateway to choice, and to responsibility, shifting control from environment to person. The day (and even periods of the day) are convenient units with which to assess the quality of life as it proceeds. Central to the process of body awareness training is learning to understand the cues the body emits or those the senses convey, and the continuance under which body sensations are experienced. Elkes describes in detail a simple method through which this may be accomplished.

The essence of such a personalized program, which Elkes terms "time out," is to provide an individual with the opportunity to examine the principal forces operating in his or her life. "Time out" affords an individual the opportunity to review the origins, causes, and histories of crises, and allows that person time to develop the skill to listen to his or her own body. The person is able to regard and evaluate the contingencies operating within the immediate day-to-day environment. "Time out" allows an individual to realistically appraise characteristics of his or her own assets and talents, and the degree to which these can be developed, and facilitates identification of any undesirable habits and dependencies which may be at work, eroding day-to-day enjoyment. In short, the person can re-examine the hypotheses governing his or her life, and evaluate alternative hypotheses to acquire simple, easily applicable skills in self-observation, stress reduction, self-regulation, and planning. Such newly developed skills can be monitored through systematic, regular follow-up sessions.

In a slightly different vein, Keith Sehnert outlines the self-care movement, of which he is a leader. He notes that self-care preceded the emergence of the professional physician. Once medicine became a distinct profession, people relegated their care to others. Now, people seldom think of themselves or other non-professionals as appropriate sources of help. Sehnert describes the Course for Activated Patients (CAP) and the Health Activated Person (HAP) program, which have successfully trained people to take more responsibilities for management of common health problems. Such programs reflect the growing interest of health consumers in becoming better informed. They receive a large part of their current impetus from the women's movement, which has consistently stressed the need for access to understandable information about health.

John H. Milsum discusses the concept of health from a systems perspective and makes a case for a health strategy based on active measures to stimulate persons to act on their own behalf. Milsum describes the use of the Health Hazard Appraisal (HHA), which is a self-rating questionnaire designed to elicit information for quantification of a person's individual risk factors. The HHA involves questions about personal and family medical history, and lifestyle practices such as drinking, smoking, and the use of seat belts. It also asks about some occupational factors and a limited number of clinical measures. To date, little occupational, environmental, or nutritional information has been included, although the system is being revised continually. The information from HHA is evaluated in comparison to an idealized norm of life expectancies calculated relative to certain practices and behaviors. The result is a profile of life expectancy as it exists for the individual following his or her practices, and the effect of specific changes in lifestyle and behavior on the expectancy. The intent of the HHA is to motivate individuals to change their lifestyles early enough to avoid risks of contracting diseases known to be affected by imprudent health habits.

There is as yet no convincing long-term evidence that the HHA can persuade individuals to embark on more healthy lifestyles, but preliminary evidence is encouraging. Its primary long-term importance may be in the fact that it creates a "teachable moment" when a health professional and a client/patient can come together and discuss the person's health condition, and the risks to which he or she is exposed. Possible changes in lifestyle can then be discussed in regard to their potential effects, with due respect for the client's present beliefs, reservations, and prejudices. In this way, the decision to change is fundamentally reserved for the client. Although the HHA is not presently as comprehensive in its estimation of risks and stimulation for behavioral change as we would like, it does, as Milsum points out, have the potential to include within its framework new knowledge, and to stimulate the acquisition of such new knowledge. The underlying philosophy behind HHA is to encourage individuals to take more responsibility for their own health. Of necessity, the HHA cannot address institutional responsibilities.

Stephen M. Weiss and Gary E. Schwartz discuss recent developments in the field of behavioral medicine and point to the need to integrate behavioral concepts into our biomedical model of disease. In a sense, the field of behavioral medicine bears testimony to the shift of medical interest from acute infectious diseases to chronic illness, emphasizing the multifactorial nature of the disease process. The search for *the* pathogenic agent failed to come to terms with such health concerns as hypertension, coronary heart disease, cardiac arrhythmias, cancer, etc. Clearly, a more comprehensive approach to disease prevention and control is required to comprehend the multifaceted nature of these serious health problems. As Weiss and Schwartz have noted, within the past ten years, new breakthroughs on the theoretical, conceptual, and technological levels (e.g., biofeedback, the role of the central nervous system in autonomic system mediation, physiologic response to environmental stress) have dramatized the necessity for reconceptualizing the nature of biological and behavioral relationships.

The promise and challenge of behavioral medicine is to establish the value of interactive research designs, methods, and theories. Research designs which actively integrate the behavioral and biomedical sciences represent a central component of behavioral medicine as it is supported by the key resource for the nation's biomedical research effort—the National Institute of Health. The final judgment concerning behavioral medicine will be made if those adopting this model contribute more effectively to solutions of the highly complex issues surrounding the prevention and control of chronic disease.

Risks and Prevention. The importance of assessing risks in order to create effective prevention strategies is recognized by the contributors to this section of the book. Devra Lee Davis and David P. Rall point out that successful disease prevention strategies may be developed before the basic mechanisms of diseases are fully elucidated. They describe the difficulties in forging systematic risk evaluations, particularly problems of inference, research scale, and design. The need for prevention strategies is receiving widespread attention, although specific recommendations remain to be promoted.

Given its relative prominence as a public health concern, cancer becomes a key target for preventive actions. Data suggest that many cancers can be linked with our patterns of industrial activity and lifestyle practices. Besides being the second largest cause of death of Americans today, cancer can strike anyone, regardless of age. For the total U.S. population between the ages of 1 and 64, cancer is the leading cause of potential life loss.

Davis and Rall report on a recent study by the Department of Health, Education, and Welfare that estimates that at least 20% of cancer deaths in this country in the near future may be due to past occupational exposures. They point out that such estimates are limited by the inadequacies of available data on cancer incidence and on worker exposure, adding that no firm quantification of the risks associated with carcinogens in the workplace can be made. They conclude that reducing occupational exposures to toxic substances offers important prevention opportunities. While levels of some carcinogens in the workplace have been lowered, levels of other such agents has been skyrocketing.

Vilma Hunt documents the early history of lead, phosphorus, and ionizing radiation regulation, each marked by political controversies. She briefly notes developments in federal authority to regulate and protect workers, such as the Coal Mine Health and Safety Act of 1969, the Occupational Health and Safety Act of 1970, and the Toxic Substances Control Act of 1976. Federal regulations of industry may provide some improvement in worker protection. But Hunt concludes that the right to know, like acknowledged civil rights, must be exercised if the relationship between work conditions and worker health are to be in positive balance in the future.

When the health risks involved are more speculative or unknown, the difficulties in setting effective national health policy become considerable. Moreover, when these risks are presented as things over which people have no control, there are real limits to what individual action can achieve.

The Environmental Defense Fund (EDF) warned potential nursing mothers in the early seventies that some of them might have toxic milk in their breasts. Stephanie Harris' review of the health risks and benefits of nursing or bottle feeding infants dramatically underscores the dilemmas facing individual health consumers. The psychological and early immunological benefits of breast feeding may sometimes now have to be compared with the potential health hazards of contaminated mother's milk and the less nourishing infant formula. To add to the problem, there is no inexpensive, accessible resource from which potential nursing mothers can acquire information about contaminants in their milk supply. Tests can cost $200, making this a decidedly upper middle class venture. The issue of breast or bottle encapsulates the contradictions and limits of individual responsibility for health today.

Stephanie Harris points out that no sector of the environment remains untouched by the global pollution caused by the family of chemicals called chlorinated hydrocarbons (or organochlorines). While promoting individual responsibility is an important part of sound health policy, it is equally important to ensure environmental and occupational protection against hazardous substances which may cause heart, respiratory, or other chronic irreversible illnesses.

J. Clarence Davies, Sam Gusman, and Frances Irwin review the concept of "unreasonable risk" as it will be applied to federal statutes regulating environmental hazards. They note that most recent environmental statutes implicitly or explicitly require the evaluation of potential health and environmental risks with market and non-market economic costs and potential health hazards. They indict conventional cost-benefit analysis for its one-value limits, which reduce all such analyses to monetary comparisons. Multi-value cost-benefit studies may be more appropriate, although considerably more cumbersome, to integrate in the decision-making process. In deciding what constitutes an unreasonable risk, several different kinds of information have to be assessed: information on health and environmental risks; information on market economic impacts, including the existence of alternatives and the likely costs of their development where they do not exist; and estimates of the non-economic costs, including effects on the quality of life and the environment. They note that, not surprisingly, no federal statute or case law yet stipulates how such determinations must be made, perhaps because a portfolio of approaches is required. There are few situations that can be imagined where universal decision algorithms or rules are to be desired, since so much of the relevant information will vary. In all this, the role of the federal regulator is that of an assessor of a decision package. There are no absolutely objective ways to make regulatory decisions.

An appendix to the Davies, Gusman, and Irwin chapter, by Gregory Wetstone, summarizes 14 key environmental statutes regulating hazardous substances. All of these laws are intended to grant the respective government agencies sufficient authority and direction to take effective action. A chart of these statutes indicates that, in providing this direction, many of these measures present the agencies with diverse criteria for making their decisions on whether the health or environmental risks associated with a particular substance or activity are reasonable. Thus, determinations of unreasonable risk will necessarily involve tentative assessments of complex factors.

Taking a different approach to the question of the role of economics in decision-making, Michael Zubkoff and Eugene Nelson draw on traditional economic theory to discuss the government's role in providing incentives for health promotion. They concentrate exclusively on lifestyle issues, and ask when government intervention can be justified. Their answers reflect traditional public finance criteria, which suggest that health activities that are entirely appropriate endeavors for the private sector may be improper for government. They note that the question of when intervention is justified is strongly related to what tools may be used for the intervention. They outline categories of intervention: incentives, education, subsidization, taxation, and regulation.

Insurance Issues. This section presents strategies and problems of preventive medicine and health care support as seen by the health insurance industry and trade unions, and examines issues relating to the national health insurance debate. Congressman George E. Brown proposes a five-point program for improving the health of the American people. He points out that our economic system provides little, if any, incentive to encourage the concepts of institutional and personal responsibility for health, self-help, or long-term prevention of illness and disease. Increasingly, every aspect of our personal lives is being assigned a quantitative economic value. Given this gradual evolution of the importance of economic criteria to public policy decision-making, it is little wonder that the current debate over national health insurance centers on such phrases as "percent of the GNP," "increase in the cost of living index," or "contribution to the inflation rate." Brown points out that there are serious dangers in placing such emphasis on economic criteria. These figures generally do not reflect non-market costs such as the costs of environmental pollution or occupational diseases. Nor do these figures reflect which of the costs should be adjusted to account for *prevention* of pollution or disease. There is presently no national accounting system to assess health costs and benefits. They are external to most economic analyses; hence, they tend to be understated, if considered at all, or relegated to the "other" category, as less serious than market economic factors. Brown contends that we will be able to develop sound health policies only when health factors are fully accounted for as part of the GNP. He notes that many of the difficulties of proposed federal regulations are that opponents can marshall overwhelming data, with models of their efforts, while no such material is available to advocates of environmental regulation. L.B. Lave and E.P. Seskin[35] have recently noted that while the costs of air pollution control to industry may be about $15 billion annually, the potential health savings can be conservatively estimated at about $23 billion. Further work by David S. Brookshire, Thomas D. Crocker, Ralph C. D'Arge, Saul Ben-David, Allen V. Knesse, and William D. Schulze has estimated the direct effect of air pollution on economic factors.[36] For a data set of 60 American cities, they found that air pollution appears to influence labor productivity and is related to time spent being ill. Although these analyses can be faulted on many counts, they constitute a beginning of the sort of accounting that Brown and others feel needs to be developed.

Clarence Pearson describes the history of the health insurance industry in health education ventures, many of which are still unevaluated despite their long existence. He reports that data from studies on in-patient hospital education have been especially encouraging. One hundred congestive heart failure patients were assigned to one of two groups. Those who received systematic education about their condition had one-third as many readmission days in the hospital as those who received no such education. In another study of patients receiving pre-operative education before abdominal surgery, those who received such education returned home an average of 2.7 days earlier than those who were given minimal information. This is consistent with other reports that give health education an economic, as well as a health, savings.

Duane Carlson's chapter about the experiences of Blue Cross and Blue Shield in promoting health and preventing disease also notes examples of cost-effective and health-effective programs. Several screening programs have been devised to identify high-risk individuals before their diseases have advanced and to provide them with prophylactic treatment. Thus, one screening found 20 cancer cases which were asymptomatic and had not spread. The average treatment cost was approximately $2000. This compares with $20,000 when the disease has spread, assuming the patient survives the first year. For this screening of some 10,000 patients, the costs were $8.50 per male and $12.50 per female. Five hundred of these people had previously undetected hypertension and are now under treatment. Carlson reports on another venture, where subscribers in either of two prepaid group practice programs with prevention and promotion projects spent significantly less time in the hospital than other subscribers.

While these reports are of admittedly small populations, they strongly indicate the potential for health promoting and disease preventing programs. However, it should be noted that most of these programs encounter people at the secondary or tertiary phase, when early detection offers help and economic savings. Devising true, primary prevention programs may prove more difficult because such programs involve preventing environmental exposure and influencing lifestyle decisions.

Matthew Greenwald discusses problems associated with changing current health insurance practices to include preventive health care coverage. He examines economic factors and other concerns which would have to be considered before insurance programs could fully realize their potential for promoting healthier lifestyles. Greenwald discusses some of the problems encountered in incorporating coverage of medical screening and health education into health insurance policies. He also notes the difficulties inherent in the use of the risk classification system to encourage healthful activities and to provide incentives for health (such as charging lower rates for health and life insurance to those who have positive health habits and giving premium reductions to those who improve their standing, as determined by certain indices of health). Although the health insurance mechanism can be used to provide incentives for health behavior, one must guard against unintended negative consequences, including the danger of "legislating lifestyles." Greenwald proposes the raising of health insurance deductibles and the raising of co-insurance levels as two possible mechanisms to provide a direct financial incentive for good health and more appropriate utilization of the health care system. He concludes that the basic solution to health care problems lies not only in increasing access to the health care system, but in encouraging people to develop healthier lifestyles that will reduce their need for access. He believes the health insurance business can contribute to health promotion through increased research and improved communication efforts.

Joanne Grozuczak of the United Mine Workers Health and Pension Fund (UMWHPF) works with a patient population that has a substantial environmental exposure problem. Mine workers also have an equally formidable economic problem—a support fund dependent upon the amount of coal mined per month. During the recent strike, the UMWHPF faced double jeopardy. Labor and health's linkage began in the thirties, but had a decidedly catastrophe-oriented focus.

Workers were to be protected from health disasters. In 1946, the UMWHPF became the first major employer-financed collectively-bargained health plan. Since then, nearly every major unionized industry has provided some form of health benefit. Despite this commitment to resources, as Grozuczak notes, there has been no marked improvement in workers' health since the forties. In fact, some analysts argue that miners are in worse health with respect to death due to accidents.[37] The Public Health Service estimates that 390,000 cases of occupational disease occur annually and that occupational disease causes more than 100,000 deaths each year. This does not represent a final tally of the threat posed by workplace hazards. Grozuczak argues for creation of more creative federal and labor strategies for health promotion and disease prevention. Restrictive tariffs on imports manufactured under unhealthy working conditions might reduce the present economic advantage for products made where occupational safety and health requirements do not exist. This could give American products a competitive advantage and indirectly spawn safer working conditions for foreign labor.

Health Promotion:　Action and Strategies. This section reviews seven selected areas and problems which appear to be particularly timely for health promotion efforts and programs. It begins with a review of efforts in the area of obesity control. One of the leaders in that effort, Albert J. Stunkard, observes that the practice of health promotion can benefit from studying the treatment of obesity. Obesity management is of interest to health promotion for reasons far beyond its contribution to prevention of ill health. Stunkard describes what might be called the classic single-factor approach to the control of obesity, noting that future approaches are not likely to be limited to such inefficient, one-by-one forms of intervention. Obesity is, in very large part, the result of the way we live. The most effective way to control obesity is to alter our lifestyles. As Stunkard emphasizes, lifestyle alteration requires changes in powerful social and economic forces. A number of recent programs indicate future cooperative efforts by industry, media, and government, as well as educational and voluntary agencies. The role these various agencies can play in health promotion concerning obesity is contained in the recommendations of the Fogarty International Conference on Obesity, held October 9, 1977. Stunkard points out that combining the capabilities of these various sectors to develop integrated programs of weight control could bring as yet unimagined benefits.

The chapter by Pekka Puska describing the North Karelia Project is a detailed description of a unique effort by an entire community to control cardiovascular disease. North Karelia, a county in the eastern part of Finland, has one of the highest mortality rates from coronary heart disease in the world. Men in their thirties routinely experienced angina and heart attacks. Faced with this exceptional problem, representatives of the local population signed a petition in 1971 asking for national assistance to reduce the high frequency and mortality of cardiovascular disease. After elaborate and careful planning, the North Karelia project was launched in 1972 to meet the urgent needs of the local population. This program represents one of the largest systematic planned programs in health promotion ever undertaken by a community, and stands as a model for future efforts. The main objective of the program was to decrease the mortality and morbidity of acute myocardial infarction and stroke in the population. Intermediate objectives included a reduction in smoking, changes in dietary habits, and control of hypertension. This project is an example of a systematic, well-controlled, large-scale planning effort undertaken by an entire community. It incorporated elements of primary prevention, treatment of acute phase, rehabilitation, evaluation, and research. Furthermore, as Puska points out, implementation of the program has been integrated into the service structure and social organization of the community, an important feature responsible for its success. Although the study is still ongoing, preliminary evidence indicates that there are significant changes in the lifestyle indicators, and that favorable changes in the mortality and morbidity rates are also indicated.

A long-overlooked area for developing incentives for health is in educational and medical services to teenagers. Emily H. Mudd and her collaborators in the Department of Obstetrics/Gynecology and the Department of Psychiatry at the University of Pennsylvania, Philadlelphia, describe an innovative program aimed at developing sound principles of self-management among young people concerning their own roles in the promotion and preservation of health. Their pilot program focused on the provision of initial and continuing guidance to teenagers on all aspects of sexual activity, particularly in the area of contraceptive use. Their pilot study of contraceptive use among never-pregnant, unmarried, high school girls showed that among those who requested contraceptive services, a high percentage (63%) stayed in the program for two years and managed contraceptive use effectively. Unintended pregnancies occurred in only 10% of the enrollment over three years. Contraceptive use involved conflicting social, emotional, parental, and peer pressures which affected utilization and continuation. The findings of Mudd *et al.* do not support the idea that teenagers become pregnant because they choose to do so. Most teenage pregnancies are probably truly unwanted. Their study indicates that developing incentives for health among adolescents is an overlooked area that merits further attention, and demonstrates the value of developing incentives for health among teenagers through appropriate educational and emotional support that teaching health care services can provide.

Richard Lauzon and Sandy Keir describe health promotion activities undertaken by the Canadian Ministry of Health and Welfare. These authors present an epidemiological approach to improving the physical activity participation rate of the relatively sedentary North American population. This model stresses the need to adopt a comprehensive perspective in the modification of maladaptive lifestyle behavior, and suggests a taxonomy of activities designed to influence health-related behavior. They illustrate the selected influence activities identified by the modified epidemiological model with a number of products, services, and activities initiated by the Fitness Division of the Fitness and Amateur Sports Branch, an agency of the Canadian Federal Health Department. Of particular interest and potential for wide use is the Canadian Home Fitness Test (CHFT), a two-stage, double-step test of cardiorespiratory fitness, developed as a self-administered testing tool. Another innovative product is the Fit-Kit, a comprehensive fitness testing and information package intended to convey some insight to users about their personal level of fitness, and to provide information about fitness and health in general. The Fit-Kit also suggests fitness enhancing activities as well as providing the means for individuals to evaluate their own progress.

Brent Arnold of Xerox discusses the current interest in physical fitness programs by corporations and reviews some of the initiatives being undertaken in the area. He points out that despite its current vogue, there is little quantitative research in the field of employee fitness as it relates to productivity, absenteeism, employee turnover, and morale. Studies are needed to demonstrate the effects of increased exercise on job performance.

Also from the corporate perspective, James Manuso discusses social, legal, and economic reasons for a growing cottage industry of corporate mental health policies and programs. Increasingly, employees, corporations, and unions are being educated concerning the potential benefits of preventive mental health measures. Manuso talks about the occupational stress sources peculiar to corporations and partially responsible for some stress-related disorders. The cost to the employing corporation of unchecked stress overloads is tremendous. Using the Equitable Life Assurance Society as an example, Manuso describes a variety of preventive policies for mental health and programs, including an in-house stress management training program which has been shown to be extremely cost-effective. He concludes that stress management programs can increase productivity and decrease medical costs, while decreasing the number of potential stress carriers who would otherwise diffuse stress throughout the delicate social network of the corporation.

From a theoretical perspective, John H. Proctor examines the need and potential for health information cooperatives tailored to meet local community needs. Such cooperatives, "Health-LINCs" (*L*ocal *I*nformation *N*etwork *C*ooperatives) would provide a means for linking people with other people in more active, informed ways and for linking consumers with health care providers to facilitate sharing of technical information. Participation and responsibility for self-help could be increased, as well. Proctor suggests that health information cooperatives could be a part of health promotion organizations (HPO) as proposed by Ng, Davis, and Manderscheid. These "Health-LINCs" could, in fact, become part of the existing and increasingly popular health maintenance organizations (HMO).

H. Frank Newman discusses the concept and evolutionary development of the HMO's, a form of prepaid group practice that is gaining increasing recognition by the government. Paul Ellwood, the originator of the term "health maintenance organization," defined an HMO as "an organization which delivers comprehensive care—including preventive services, ambulatory and in-patient physician services, hospital services, laboratory and X-ray services, and indemnity coverage for out-of-area emergency services—to voluntarily enrolled consumers on the basis of fixed price contracts." As Newman points out, HMO's have gained the interest of Congress and the administration primarily because of concern about the cost of health care and the challenge of bringing these costs under control. He cites studies done by the Research and Statistics Branch of the Social Security Administration indicating savings of 20-25 % in providing care to Medicare beneficiaries. Newman is quick to point out, however, that HMO's do not offer a panacea to all the health problems of health care delivery in the United States. Many people do not like the idea of getting care from a structured, organized system. Furthermore, HMO's are difficult to set up in rural and sparsely populated areas, although some versions of the plans show promise.

Newman traces the evolution of the Kaiser-Permanente health maintenance program, the nation's largest prepaid group practice, from its inception, and reviews its efforts in the areas of disease prevention, disease detection, health maintenance, and health promotion. He maintains that the systemized approach exemplified by the Kaiser-Permanente program provides an opportunity to develop a cost-effective system of comprehensive medical care involving disease prevention, early disease detection, health insurance, and health promotion. Additional data must be collected from other demonstration programs to assist in developing health care delivery and health promotion programs that are cost-effective and acceptable to American consumers.

REFERENCES

1. *Forward Plans for Health, (FY 1978-82).* U.S. Department of Health, Education, and Welfare (GPO 0017-000-00172-8), 1976.
2. *Healthy People, The Surgeon General's Report on Health Promotion and Disease Prevention.* U.S. Department of Health, Education, and Welfare, DHEW (PHS) Publication No. 79-55071, 1979.
3. Schneiderman, M., *National Conference on the Environment and Health Care Costs.* House of Representatives Caucus Room, Cannon House Office Building, August 15, 1979.
4. Gori, G.B. and Richter, B.J., "Macroeconomics of Disease Prevention in the United States," *Science 200,* pp. 1124-1130, June 1978.
5. Illich, I., *Medical Nemesis.* New York: Random House, 1976.
6. Navarro, V., "The Political and Economic Determinants of Health and Health Care in Rural America," *Inquiry.* **13,** *2:* 111-121, June 1976.
7. Engels, *Condition of the Working Class in England in 1848,* translated and edited by W. O. Henderson and W. O. Chaloner. Palo Alto: Stanford University Press, 1958.

8. Engel, G., *"Health and Disease,"* Perspectives in Biology and Medicine, pp. 459–485, Summer 1960.

9. Rosen, G., "The Bacteriological, Immunologic and Chemotherapeutic Period 1875–1950," *Bulletin of the New York Academy of Medicine.* **40,** *6:* 483–493, June 1964.

10. McKinlay, J.B. and McKinlay, S.M., "The Questionable Contribution of Medical Measures to the Decline of Mortality in the U.S. in the 20th Century," *Millibank Memorial Fund Quarterly; Health and Society.* **55,** *3:* 405–428, 1977.

11. *Ibid.,* p. 422.

12. *Ibid.,* p. 423.

13. *Illich, op. cit.*

14. *Ibid.;* LaLonde, M., *A New Perspective on the Health of Canadians: A Working Document.* Ottawa: Ministry of Health and Welfare, 1974; and Mc Keown, T., *The Modern Rise of Population.* London: Edward Arnold, 1976.

15. Rall, D.P., "The Role of Laboratory Animal Studies in Estimating Carcinogenic Risks for Man," paper presented to International Association for Research on Cancer Symposium, "Carcinogenic Risks–Strategies for Intervention," Lyon, France, 1977.

16. Davis, D.L., "Multiple Risk Assessment as Preventive Public Health Strategy," in J. Staffa (Ed.), *FDA Symposium on Risk/Benefit Decisions and Public Health,* 1979.

17. *First Annual Report to Congress by the Task Force on Environmental Cancer and Heart and Lung Disease,* Douglas M. Costle, Chairman. Washington, D.C.: U.S. Government Printing Office, 1978.

18. National Cancer Institute, National Institute of Environmental Health Sciences, National Institute for Occupational Safety and Health, "Estimates of the Fraction of Cancer in the United States Related to Occupational Factors," 1978, draft paper.

19. Waldbott, G.L., *The Health Effects of Environmental Pollution.* St. Louis: C.V. Mosky, 1978, p. 59.

20. *Ibid.,* p. 300.

21. "A Survey by the Association of Teachers of Preventive Medicine Submitted to the National Task Force on Environmental Cancer and Heart and Lung Disease." Unpublished, 1978.

22. Tanaka, S. and Lieben, J., "Manganese Poisoning and Exposure in Pennsylvania," *Arch. Environmental Health.* **19:** 674–84, 1969; and Matsui, K. *et al.,* "Studies on the Metal Fume Fever and Pneumoconiosis due to Welding Work in the Holds," *Japanese Journal of Industrial Health.* **7:** 3–7, 1969.

23. Matsui. *et al., op. cit.*

24. Needleman, H.L., Gunnoe, C., Leviton, A., Reed, R., Peresie, H., Maher, C., and Barrett, P., "Deficits in Psychologic and Classroom Performance of Children with Elevated Dentine Lead Levels," *New England Journal of Medicine.* **300,** *13:* 689–695, May 29, 1979.

25. Fabrega, H., Jr., *Perspect. Biol. Med.,* Summer 1972.

26. Heller, S.I., M.D., and Ng, L.K.Y., M.D., personal reports.

27. Fabrega, *op. cit.*

28. Lalonde, M., *A New Perspective on the Health of Canadians: A Working Document.*

29. Fabrega, *op. cit.*

30. Lalonde, *op. cit.,* p 20.

31. *Ibid.*

32. *Ibid.*

33. *Ibid.*

34. *Ibid.,* p. 63.

35. Lave, L.B. and Seskin, E.P., *Air Pollution and Human Health.* Baltimore: Johns Hopkins University Press, 1977.
36. Brookshire, D.S., Thomas, D.C., d'Arge, R.D., Ben-David, S., Kneese, A.V., and Schulze, W.D., *Methods of Development for Assessing Air Pollution Control Benefits,* Office of Research and Development, Environmental Protection Agency, EPA/60 0/5-79-001 (five volumes).
37. Seltzer, C., "Health Care by the Ton: Crisis in the Mine-workers' Health and Welfare Programs," *Health-PAC Bulletin No. 79,* pp. 1–8, 25–33, November/December, 1977.

Health Enhancement, Stress and Wellness

2

Stress and the Promotion of Health

Hans Selye, C.C., M.D., Ph.D., D.Sc.

President, International Institute of Stress

On all levels of life, from the unicellular organism to man and even entire societies, health is largely determined by stable balance — what Walter Cannon called homeostasis. When that balance is disrupted, "dis-ease" sets in. The idea of health, thus expressed, is simple enough; yet I feel that a knowledge of the biological stress syndrome can elaborate on, and develop, the concept of homeostasis to the point where it will offer insights relevant to both public and private policy in health promotion and disease prevention. Specifically, it can clarify the newly emerging view of health as a problem of the whole person's approach to life, by making one aware of the intimate links that have been demonstrated to exist between man's mind — which is in large measure under the control of the individual — and his body.

Stress, Health, and Disease

Interest in biologic stress as it influences the lives of individuals and even entire societies has grown enormously during the past few decades. There has been a phenomenal increase in the number of laboratories, technical and lay articles, books, lectures, and journals dealing with the far-reaching implications of stress in virtually all fields of human endeavor, including medicine, physiology, psychology, psychiatry, sociology, and philosophy. Even the lay press, television, and radio are constantly discussing stress, but frequently there is no real awareness of the objective scientific proofs upon which the idea of stress rests.

First we must clearly realize that *stress is a condition, a state*, and as such it is imponderable, though *it manifests itself by measurable changes* in the organs of the body. Using these alterations as indicators of stress, we should be able to come closer to an understanding of stress itself.

The manifestations of stress are extremely complex. Our understanding of them was made possible through countless animal experiments performed all over the world, starting perhaps with Walter Cannon's classic investigations in cats and dogs.[1]

Cannon proved that higher animal species, including man, defend themselves against various types of aggression, insult, or injury by a single fundamental response, which he called the "fight or flight" response. He showed that challenges to the animal's normal resting equilibrium were met by this stereotypical reaction, which varied in intensity with the force of the challenge. The reaction, he theorized, was built into the animal's defense system as a safety measure to ensure its survival.

First Mediator. We still do not know how a nonspecific stimulus is produced, except that something must convey the message, from the directly affected region to the centers of adaptation, that a challenge or "stressor" exists. Nothing is known about this first effect — it could be a nervous impulse, a chemical substance, or even the depletion of an indispensable metabolic factor — so we simply call it the "first mediator." We cannot even be certain that it is an excess or deficiency of a particular substance. Apparently, the stress response is often initiated by emotional arousal, for man is endowed with a highly developed central nervous system; but stress reactions also occur in plants and in lower animals that have no nervous systems, and patients under deep anesthesia show typical stress responses to such stressors as trauma, hemorrhage, and so on. Thus, it can be seen that conscious psychic disturbances are not indispensable for typical somatic stress reactions to occur. It is tempting to speculate at this point that cell consciousness is common to all life forms and that cells respond to stressors, always with the purpose of re-establishing the homeostatic balance or equilibrium.[2]

Hormonal Mechanisms. Although the "first mediator" has still to be identified, we do know that, at least in man and other mammals, eventually the stressor acts upon the hypothalamus, a complex bundle of nerve cells and fibers that serves as a bridge between the brain and the endocrine system, and particularly upon the ME (median eminence). The message is relayed by means of CRF (corticothrophin releasing factor) to the first endocrine gland in this chain, the pituitary; the result is a discharge of ACTH (adrenocorticotrophic hormone) from the pituitary into the general circulation. Upon reaching the adrenal cortex, ACTH triggers the secretion of corticoids, mainly glucocorticoids, such as cortisol or corticosterone. These "stress hormones" supply a readily available source of energy for the adaptive reactions necessary to meet the demands made by the stressor agent. The corticoids also facilitate various other enzyme responses, and they suppress immune reactions and inflammation, thereby helping the body to coexist with potential pathogens. This complex chain of events is cybernetically controlled by several biofeedback mechanisms. (See Figure 2-1.)

At the same time as these events are taking place, another important pathway is utilized to mediate the stress response. Other stress hormones, such as catecholamines, are liberated to activate mechanisms of general utility for meeting the various demands for adaptation. Epinephrine (often called adrenaline), in

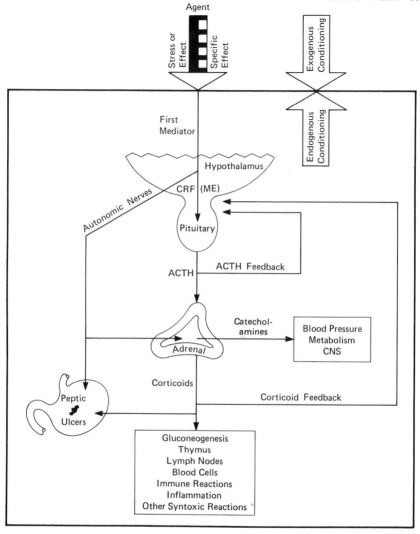

Figure 2-1. Principal pathways mediating the response to a stressor agent and the conditioning factors which modify its effect. (As soon as any agent acts upon the body—the thick outer frame of the diagram—the resulting effect will depend upon three factors, indicated by the broad vertical arrows pointing to the upper horizontal border of the frame. All agents possess both nonspecific stressor effects—the solid part of the arrow—and specific properties—the interrupted part of the arrow. The latter are variable and characteristic of each individual agent; they will not be discussed here other than to state that they are inseparably attached to the stressor effect and invariably modify it. The other two heavy vertical arrows, pointing toward the upper border of the frame, represent exogenous and endogenous conditioning factors which largely determine the reactivity of the body. It is clear that since all stressors have some specific effects, they cannot elicit exactly the same response in all organs. Furthermore, even the same agent will act differently in different individuals, depending upon the internal and external conditioning factors which determine their reactivity.) *Reprinted by courtesy of Butterworths, Reading, Massachusetts, from H. Selye, Stress in Health and Disease, 1976.*

particular, is secreted to provide energy, to accelerate the pulse rate, to elevate blood pressure and the rate of blood circulation in the muscles, and to stimulate the central nervous system (CNS). The blood coagulation mechanism is also triggered as a protection against excessive bleeding if injuries are sustained in the encounter with the stressor. All these coping measures help the organism in its "fight or flight" response.

Innumerable other hormonal and chemical changes check and balance the body's functioning and stability, constituting a virtual arsenal of weapons by which the organism defends itself for survival.[3]

Nervous Mechanisms. The hypothalamus functions through the two divisions of the autonomic nervous system: the sympathetic and the parasympathetic nerves. In addition to regulating growth, sex, and reproduction, it is responsible for stimulating the emotions of fear, rage, and pleasure, to name a few. The sympathetic system passes through the spinal cord to specific organs through large ganglia, or nerve clusters. The functions of this system manifest themselves in muscular movements of the stomach, intestine, and bladder. Face muscles contract or contort under the influence of the emotions. The pupils dilate, the nostrils flare, and the throat passage widens. Breathing becomes fast, raising the pulse rate and carrying extra oxygen to vital areas. Digestion by the stomach and intestine is temporarily suspended. The muscles controlling the bowels and bladder become loose. These are some of the physiologic features of the "fight or flight" reaction.

Now the body is mobilized for action. There is evidently increased strength and vigor while digestion has stopped along with other functions that are not needed for fight or flight. Now, the accelerated clotting time will heal wounds rapidly and the proliferation of white blood cells will counteract infection. Perspiration cools the entire organism through evaporation of sweat, and bodily wastes are eliminated as well.

Though much more detailed scientific investigation would be needed before we could arrive at a comprehensive and systematic analysis of the separate adaptive reactions indispensable for the maintenance of life under special conditions, all these phenomena are just a few examples of the oft-noted fact that mind and body are closely integrated.

The General Adaptation Syndrome. The external signs of stress are adrenal enlargement, thymicolymphatic involution, and gastrointestinal ulcers; but the stress reaction evolves over time, in three stages: the alarm reaction, the stage of resistance, and the stage of exhaustion. The *alarm reaction,* which is a generalized call to arms of the body's defense forces, is characterized by the signs just mentioned. In the *stage of resistance,* the organism becomes adapted to the challenge and even begins to resist it, and the chemical changes are the exact opposite of those of the alarm reaction.

But just as a machine gradually wears out even if it has enough fuel, so does a living organism sooner or later become the victim of constant wear and tear. Subjected to still longer exposure to the stressor, it enters the third and final *stage of exhaustion.* Symptoms appear which are strikingly similar to those of the alarm reaction, only this time they are irreversible, and the organism dies. Apparently, it has used up its supply of "adaptation energy."

This triphasic response, which I call the *general adaptation syndrome* (G.A.S.), gave us the first indication that the body's adaptability is finite. It is tempting to view the G.A.S. as a kind of accelerated aging. It appears as though, because of more intense stress, the three major periods of life — infancy (in which adaptation has not yet been acquired), adulthood (in which adaptation has developed to the usual stresses of life), and senility (in which the acquired adaptation is lost again) — are here telescoped into a short space of time.[4]

Conditioning Factors and Diseases of Adaptation.   Both the intensity and the consequences of the stress response are largely influenced by heredity, age, previous exposure to stress, nervous stimuli, the nutritional state of the organism, and many other factors. All these conditioners alter the production of adaptive hormones and, consequently, the stressor effect modifies the entire state of the body. Perhaps the most important consideration here is the way each individual views or evaluates a given situation in the light of his needs, aspirations, and past experiences. Under the influence of such internal or external (endogenous or exogenous) conditioning factors, a normally well-tolerated degree of stress can become pathogenic and cause *diseases of adaptation,* selectively affecting those parts of the body that are particularly sensitized both by the conditioning factors and by the specific effect of the stressors. By "diseases of adaptation," we mean maladies that are caused principally by errors in the general adaptation process. For example, under certain circumstances, animals in a state of severe stress develop such diseases as hardening of the arteries, kidney disorders, severe bleeding peptic ulcers, physiologic changes reminiscent of arthritis, and other maladies closely resembling heart accidents, mental exhaustion, and so on.

These same phenomena can be observed every day, all around us. For years, most of us resist the stresses caused by occupations, frustrations, physical fatigue, tension, overwork, cigarette smoking, excessive alcohol consumption, chronic infections, and numerous other agents that demand constant adaptation. Then, finally, there comes a day when a normally well-balanced person begins to show signs of increased blood pressure, suffers a heart attack, or notices the signs of a gastrointestinal peptic ulcer.[5]

However, no disease is purely a disease of adaptation, any more than a disease of the heart or an infectious disease is a "pure" disease in which adaptive phenomena play no part. The term "disease of adaptation" should be used only when the maladaptation factor appears to be more important than any eliciting pathogen itself.

Among the derailments of the G.A.S. that may cause disease, perhaps the most important are absolute excess, deficiency, or disequilibrium in the amount of adaptive hormones (e.g., corticoids, ACTH, and growth hormone) produced during stress. But while it is true that the hypothalamus-pituitary-adrenal mechanism, which produces these hormones, plays a prominent role in the G.A.S., other organs participate in the latter (for example, the nervous system, liver, and kidney), and these may also respond abnormally to become the cause of disease during adaptation.

Health in the Twentieth Century

Today's medical practice, at least as we know it in the West, has only just started to explore the close interrelation of body and mind. Science has not been able to fully clarify the nature of man, although it has been well-established that "man's ability to adapt in order to remain free of illness depends not only on his own inherent capacities and past experience, but also on his motivation and the support and refreshment that his environment can afford him."[6] Yet the goal of medicine should be to understand the patient as a person, to establish the circumstances that precipitated his illness, the underlying conflicts, hostilities, and griefs – in short, the bruised nature of his emotional state. The modern physician ought to know as much about emotions and thoughts as about disease symptoms and drugs. This approach would appear to hold more promise of cure than anything that medicine has given to man to date.[7]

Clearly, the field of stress has much to offer in this regard. If I may venture a prediction, in my opinion, research on stress will be most fruitful if it is guided by the principle that to combat the stress factor in our lives, we must learn to imitate and, if necessary, to correct and complement the body's own autopharmacologic efforts.

This view of health and disease, then, is that they are not merely individual interactions between pathogens and human beings, and that they involve, rather, the entire spectrum of other relationships, including those with one's spouse, employer, children, neighbors, and spiritual or medical advisers. Too much consideration has been directed toward specific pathogens and toward specific disease models, and not enough toward the patient and how he developed his particular disease. Only when we shift our focus from diseased parts to the whole being, can we learn more about what activates the adaptation syndrome at all levels within the organism, and understand why stress affects different people in different ways.

Nowadays, the skills and knowledge demanded by any job, as indeed by the goals of society itself, are developing, or at least changing, at such an unprecedented rate that our first objective must be to learn how to cope with the stress of adaptation to change as such, both in our work and in our social goals. Only thus can we hope to succeed in overcoming the distressing loss of stability, and perhaps to even enjoy the challenge of adjustment to ever-changing tasks, aspirations, and possibilities.

There can be no doubt that stress diseases are on the increase. Cardiac maladies, gastrointestinal disturbances, and mental disorders, all stress-induced, are striking people down in their 30's, 40's, and early 50's. Heart diseases, mostly due to stressful events and lifestyles, have reached epidemic proportions in the United States, and these disorders seem to be on the rise with the American gross national product.[8]

Of course, the need to adjust to constant change arises from the fact that the more we know and the larger the number of people who acquire knowledge, the faster the pace of development, or at least of exploratory change, in all fields. This situation is primarily created by recent progress in mathematics, physics, chemistry, and engineering (with its resulting industrial implications: computers, automation, and extraordinary acceleration in the rate at which people and information travel and alter the world).

Man's highly developed brain has produced sophisticated technology, and has generated an unprecedented speed and spread of information. He has now to communicate with the teeming multitude around him, and his interrelations are fraught with pleasures, mood changes, threats, and an incredible number of situations and events that cause excessive stress. His personal contacts now have more and more pleasant and unpleasant connotations, because he feels the growing need to control events in his life and his environment. But such control is sometimes beyond the individual's power. He therefore tries to anticipate and prepare, plan and act accordingly, and, usually, anticipation of events proves to be more stressful than the actual events themselves. Some have even called the twentieth century the Age of Anxiety, of Uncertainty, or of Future Shock.[9]

Today's technologic progress or process has advertently or inadvertently reduced the quality of man's life, his food, his environment, and even his behavior, all of which determine health and well-being. Technologic societies are totally committed to economic or industrial growth. Steady-state policies rarely exist. The demands created by growth are increasingly far-reaching. They prey on the finite resources of this planet and steer us away from our basic instincts of survival and natural well-being. Somehow, many of us have surrendered our innate responsibilities to others: doctors, hospitals, institutions, the state.

This is not to say that change is unnecessary; no one would want to live a life of "no hits, no runs, no errors." Change could, and should, be a dynamic force in human growth and development. Its beneficial effects can be fully exploited with heightened self-awareness of individual strengths and weaknesses, capabilities, and limitations—all indicators of one's stress level. One should strike for the highest attainable aims but never put up resistance in vain.

It only takes a little reflection to realize that we cannot escape stress caused by awesome technologic changes. The big push from rural to urban areas has altered life dramatically. Dwelling in large apartment houses is nowadays so commonplace that it has become casual, yet when you come to think of it, such lifestyles did not exist more than a century ago. All this is endurable and sometimes even enjoyable, but only within the limits of human adaptability. If we compare this situation with the experiments performed on crowding among rats, we cannot but feel that it will somehow generate behavioral aberrations. Economic factors are dominating our lives. Just getting to work at the office often requires a high level of stress resistance. Crowding and an accelerated pace of life must induce almost unremitting arousal within the body.

There seem to be no proper escape routes for the individual. Many turn to drugs, alcohol, tobacco, coffee, or snacking foods, but these only mask the symptoms of distress, temporarily displacing distress by euphoria or an artificial feeling of well-being. Few realize that these escapes are stressors in themselves, adding to the overall stress of our lives. Some choose suicide, the incidence of which usually rises in times of emotional strain or economic crisis.

It should be clear, then, that we need to tune ourselves down, to unwind. If we do not learn the skills to relax and allow our bodies time and a chance to cure themselves, we will always be living well above our level of stress resistance, depleting our limited fund of adaptation energy. We must learn how to eliminate chronic anxiety, and take things as they come, without perceiving them as exaggerated threats to our well-being.

The integrating concept of body, mind, and spirit is assuming phenomenal popularity and importance. The holistic approach aims at naturally enhancing our total self-awareness and well-being. By learning to gauge our innate energy and potential weaknesses and strengths, each of us can learn how to improve our health and behavior. It requires a great deal of self-discipline and development of will power.

Above all, we must not lose sight of the vital, innate awareness that each of us is responsible for his or her own health and well-being. We need unequivocally to adopt this guiding principle, or we will continue to be plagued by stress-induced diseases.

Man has always been preoccupied with his health and has wanted to improve it, both as regards the mind and the body. Throughout history, innumerable great thinkers have approached the problem from the point of view of theology, psychology, sociology, and, of course, particularly medicine, but whatever the approach or technique favored, the point of view was always specialized. Only now are we really beginning to look upon health as a holistic problem. After all, we are thinking of the health of the man as such, and we will never arrive at a satisfactory solution if all of us take different reductionist points of view. Individually, we are interested in improving health by research limited to molecular biology, electron microscopy, pharmacology, behavioral philosophy (including religious codes), sociology, politics, economics, or any of the other specialized disciplines, but one must not look upon his or her particular field of expertise as the only, all-encompassing solution to man's troubles and the only road to happiness. There is no great point in elucidating or improving one part of the human machine, blinding ourselves to the fact that another vital part is meanwhile deteriorating and destroying the whole.

Primarily, we should convince the world that the point is not to improve our troubles with the "cost of living index" with tricks through which we can get more money for less work and make available more of the "comforts" of civilized society such as luxurious automobiles and television sets. Just as wars will not be avoided by more sophisticated weaponry, so disease can never be completely eradicated merely by improvements in pharmacology, immunotherapy, or any other purely medical means. The great decision-makers of our times must give more attention to the quality of life.[11] No scientific discoveries, such as nuclear fission, space travel, or psychopharmacologic drugs, are in themselves good or evil for man; the great conflagrations and dangers of the future life are within the motivation of the decision-makers to use them one way or another.

REFERENCES

1. Cannon, W.B. *The Wisdom of the Body.* New York: W.W. Norton & Co., 1939.
2. Selye, H., *Stress in Health and Disease.* Reading, Massachusetts: Butterworths, 1976.
3. *Ibid.*
4. Selye, H., *Stress Without Distress.* Philadelphia-New York: J. B. Lippincott, 1974.
5. Blythe, P., *Stress Disease: The Growing Plague.* New York: St. Martin's Press, 1973; Wolf, S. and Goodell, H., *Harold G. Wolff's Stress and Disease, Second Edition.* Springfield, Illinois: Charles C Thomas, 1968.
6. Wolf, S., and Goodell, H., *Behavioral Science in Clinical Medicine.* Springfield, Illinois: Charles C Thomas, 1976.
7. *Ibid.*
8. Knowles, J. H. (Ed.), *Doing Better and Feeling Worse: Health in the United States.* New York: W. W. Norton & Co., 1977.
9. Albrecht, K., *Stress and the Manager.* Englewood Cliffs, New Jersey: Prentice-Hall, 1979; Sarason, I. G., and Spielberger, C. D. (Eds.), *Stress and Anxiety, Volume 3.* Washington–London: Hemisphere, 1976.
10. Selye, *Stress Without Distress, op. cit.*
11. Knowles, *op, cit.*

3

Toward a Conceptual Formulation of Health and Well-Being*†

Lorenz K.Y. Ng, M.D.

Division of Research, National Institute on Drug Abuse, Rockville, Maryland
and World Man Fund

Devra L. Davis, Ph.D.

World Man Fund and Environmental Law Institute

Ronald W. Manderscheid, Ph.D.

National Health Study Center, National Institute of Mental Health

Joel Elkes, M.D.

Department of Psychiatry, McMaster University Medical Center, Canada

Definition of Health as Absence of Illness

Traditionally, health has been defined by what it is *not*. Just as peace has been defined as the absence of war, and sanity as the absence of insanity, health has been defined as the absence of illness. When we say that a person's health is good, we mean that he or she is not suffering from any serious disease. As disease becomes less severe, we say that health "has improved." Lester Breslow[1] has pointed out that this focus on pathology in the measurement of health probably arose because, for most of human existence, the health problem facing society in general, and medicine in particular, has been in overcoming disease. Morbidity and mortality caused by microorganisms, toxic agents, injury, and nutritional deficiency have plagued – and still plague – much of humanity.

---

*Presented at the Annual Meeting of the American Association for the Advancement of Science. Symposium on Health Enhancement: Prevention and Promotion, Houston, Texas, January 4, 1979.

†The ideas and opinions expressed herein are solely the authors' and do not represent the official viewpoint of the agencies listed above.

Under such conditions, it was only natural to concentrate on defining and measuring the specific entities against which medical science had something to offer, or at least those areas in which science could provide some hope of achievement.

Indeed, medicine's health mission in combating disease has had an impressive and successful history. So successful, in fact, that one might come to accept from modern medical practice that health is simply the absence of all known diseases. For example, Harrison's textbook, *Principles of Internal Medicine,* is a veritable compendium of diseases and specific ways of diagnosing and treating such diseases. So well-accepted and unquestioned is the concept of health as the absence of disease, that the term "health" does not occur in Harrison's index.

The Biomedical Model of Disease

Western allopathic medicine has been dominated by a philosophy which can be traced to the seventeenth century French philosopher Descartes, who split the human being into mind and body. This mind-body dualism permitted the study of the body without bothering with the mind (which was believed to have more to do with the soul and hence properly remained within the domain of the church). This separation led to enormous advances in science and medicine by enabling scientists and doctors to study the body without worrying about the soul, and was largely responsible for the anatomical and structural base on which scientific Western medicine eventually was to be built. Traditional Western medicine came to view the body as a machine, and disease as the consequence of a mechanical breakdown or as a condition due to a defective part. The biomedical model, therefore, has come to be accepted as the model for understanding the disease process, employing molecular biology as its basic scientific discipline. Identification of the causal mechanisms of disease has been the pre-eminent goal of this model and has led to the elucidation and treatment of many heretofore unknown and untreatable diseases.

Largely due to its success, the biomedical model has had an enormous impact not only on medical research but also on the health care delivery system. An entire industry has arisen, one that is oriented toward disease: its identification, treatment, and amelioration. Based on this orientation, a language has evolved in which individuals with identifiable diseases are called "patients" and are treated by a special group of individuals called "doctors," whose task is to treat and cure the particular identifiable disease or at least to restore the patient's condition to an accepted norm. A system of insurance has been devised largely for sick care. For the most part, our health care providers treat individuals once they become sick, but do not concern themselves with the factors that lead to illness. Economic incentives are largely sickness-oriented, in that individuals receive financial reimbursements from their insurance plans only when they are ill (these plans are euphemistically called "health insurance," whereas in fact they are "sickness insurance"). Generally, physicians are paid only for treating illnesses, and there is little incentive to focus on methods for preventing illness or for promoting health.

Our medical research enterprise is directed toward providing interventions to attack the causes of disease. Fabrega[2] discusses some of the problems attendant to this person-centered, temporally-bounded, and discontinuous view of disease:

Many of the present problems of health care and its delivery may be traced, at least in part, to problems stemming from the dominating influence of an organismic conception of disease. As implied above, an episodic view of disease underscores the need for only episodic treatment and militates against the comprehensive and continuous evaluation that some patients require. When the disease "appears" as defined by a set of symptoms, a person may then seek help and have his discomfort validated and pay for it on the basis of a completed service.

In this view, the roles are well-defined for the health care providers, the patients, and the health care system: health care providers treat diseases; patients present themselves for passive cures; the health care system rewards illness by reimbursing providers for services rendered in diagnosing and treating a consensually validated set of conditions identified as a "disease state." This doctor-patient transaction is further governed by an ethic that has been characterized as the "technologic imperative" — namely, that if something can be done, it will be done, no matter what the cost.

Limits of the Biomedical Model: Changing Concepts of Health

The biomedical model of disease and its treatment has been successful beyond all expectations, but at a cost. It is an irony of history that at the very time that we are witnessing major strides in molecular biology and genetic research, we are simultaneously experiencing a crisis of confidence in the ability of medical science to improve the health status of our post-industrialized society. Aaron Wildavsky[3] has expressed this sentiment cogently:

According to the Great Equation, medical care equals health. But the Great Equation is wrong. More available medical care does not equal better health. The best estimates are that the medical system (doctors, drugs, hospitals) affects about 10% of the usual indices for measuring health: whether you live at all (infant mortality), how well you live (days lost due to sickness), how long you live (adult mortality). The remaining 90% are determined by factors over which doctors have little or no control, from individual lifestyle (smoking, exercise, worry) to social conditions (income, eating habits, physiological inheritance), to the physical environment (air and water quality). Most of the bad things that happen to people are at present beyond the reach of medicine.

Increasingly, there is recognition that the critical factors contributing to our morbidity and mortality relate as much, if not more, to behavioral, social, and environmental factors, as they do to the quality of our medical care system. Western medicine, which has conceptualized health as the absence of physical or physiological disease, has relegated behavioral, social, and environmental factors to a minor role. Such a view is no longer tenable, considering the enormous technological changes that human society has undergone in the past century. As Rene Dubos[4] said:

It is no longer permissible to take comfort in the belief that various types of vascular disease, cancers, chronic ailments of the respiratory tract, have become more prevalent simply because people live longer in affluent societies. The increase in chronic and degenerative diseases is due, in part at least, and probably in a very large part, to the environmental and behavioral changes that have resulted from industrialization and urbanization.

The recognition of the import and influence of environmental and lifestyle factors on health status if further supported by the Canadian experience of the past decade. Studies by the Long-Range Health Planning Branch of the Canadian Ministry of Health and Welfare, summarized in the Lalonde document entitled, "A New Perspective on the Health of Canadians,"[5] suggest that little improvement has occurred in the overall health of that nation, despite rapid improvement in the quality of prepaid health insurance over the past 15 years, which culminated in the introduction of National Universal Medicare in 1967. Although this program made health services available to all Canadians, it has had little impact on morbidity and mortality rates. An analysis of the principal causes of morbidity and mortality reveals that environmental and lifestyle factors contributed so greatly as to constitute the keys to effective control.

Prevention: A Rediscovery

In America, the leading causes of premature disability and death are no longer infectious diseases, but are associated with where and how we live. Cardiovascular incidence, heart disease, respiratory illness, and cancer kill nearly two million people annually and leave many more disabled and in pain. The increasing prevalence of chronic degenerative diseases, coupled with rising health care costs, have engendered a renewed public interest in disease prevention, the catchword of the day. On the one hand, prevention is being criticized as suffering from overpromotion in the face of underachievement. On the other hand, it is also being proposed as a panacea for our mounting health care problems. The issues are multifactorial and complex. Presumed benefits arising from a successful disease prevention program may be accompanied by a host of major problematic implications. For example, if we can prevent the transmission of genetic diseases (a definitely worthwhile goal), we may also substantially alter the present genetic makeup of society.[6] If we succeed in preventing some of our chronic diseases, we are likely to profoundly alter the demographic characteristics of our population. For example, if we prolong life, we may cause major redistribution and dislocation in the economy.[7] On this latter point, it has been pointed out that even the complete eradication of heart disease, cancer, and stroke — currently the major mortal diseases — would, according to some calculations, extend the average life expectancy at birth only by approximately six or seven years, and at age 65, by no more than one-and-a-half to two years.[8] Furthermore, quite apart from questions regarding the effectiveness of prevention strategies, issues of social priorities will have to be addressed. In the midst of already scarce resources, how shall we select prevention programs versus increasing and improving medical care services to those in need, such as those in the rural areas and some urban inner cities of our country?

Even beyond the elderly, the prospect of having increasing numbers of individuals who may be prematurely chronically ill and impaired, but nevertheless will have many years of life before them, raises questions of living and the quality of life which our conceptualization of health must begin to take into account. Whatever the evidence for or against preventive strategies may turn out to be, prevention represents only one side of the total health equation. The prevention of disease must be linked also to the promotion of positive health strategies. Telling people what *not* to do to avoid becoming sick is not enough. Our research must also help us determine what we *can* do, in a positive way, to remain or to become healthy.

The concept of positive health brings us closer to the etymological derivations of the word, "health," which literally means "wholeness." It should be noted that both the Greek and the English words for health are totally unrelated to all the words for disease, illness, or sickness. Rather, "health" connotes the sense of wholeness or completeness, or the sense of "working or functioning well."[8] This generic definition is embodied in the conceptualization given by the World Health Organization, which defined health as "a state of complete physical, mental, and social well-being, and not merely the absence of disease or infirmity."[9] Therefore, the challenge for health enhancement is not just prevention of disease. It must incorporate the twin concepts of disease prevention and health promotion, involving positive strategies oriented toward wellness and well-being.

The development of a biopsychosocial model of wellness and well-being poses a challenge for all of society. While the focus of such a model is the wellness and well-being of the individual, we must recognize that the individual functions as a social human being in a social environment with social roles. This model must take into account the organismic, psychological, and social dimensions of the individual human being. Advances in biobehavioral science over the past several decades are making this task possible, as manifested by the progress being made in the area of psychosomatic medicine, and, more recently, in the area of behavioral medicine. Also over the past decade, social science researchers have made considerable advances in the development of social indicators to measure changes in various societal characteristics. Techniques of large-scale sampling with reduced bias are now well developed, both theoretically and practically. Social scientists have a capacity to obtain data from the national population or any important segment of it. This state of the art was summarized in an important document issued by the Department of Health, Education, and Welfare in 1969, entitled, "Toward a Social Report." This document was developed as an attempt on the part of social scientists to look at several important areas and digest what is known about progress toward generally accepted goals. The areas treated were health, social mobility, the condition of the physical environment, income and poverty, public order and safety, and learning, science, and art. The report pointed to the need to develop measures which reflect the quality of life in addition to its quantity: "We have measures of deaths and illness, but no measures of physical vigor or mental health. We have measures of the level and distribution of income, but no measures of the satisfaction that income brings . . . We have some clues about the test performance of children, but no information about their creativity or attitude toward intellectual endeavor." The groundwork has been laid for the conceptual formulation of a truly integrative biopsychosocial model of health that is oriented toward wellness and well-being. As Angus Campbell[10] has said: "It is time for a major investment of effort into the development, refinement, and standardization of the kinds of scales and other measures needed to carry forward a program of documentation and analysis of the dimensions of human experience." Obviously, one of these dimensions is wellness. Efforts to develop indicators in this area could provide a framework for systematic studies of the relationship between the quantity and the quality of life.

Toward a Wellness Concept of Health

In contradistinction to an illness model of health, a wellness model does not view health defensively, as the absence of illness, but affirmatively, as a continual process of learning, growth, and development throughout the life cycle. It has been suggested that "wellness" expresses the quantity of the state of being well, whereas "well-being" refers to its quality. Both are dimensions of positive health. No single theory provides an adequate background for an understanding of the wellness process. From a heuristic standpoint, one may reasonably start with the hypothesis that wellness is a process that can be taught, learned, and acquired by the human organism throughout development. Like illness, human wellness does not become a complete entity all at once. Like the development of an illness, the development of wellness may be conceived as a cumulative process, over time, that can be influenced by environmental, physical, behavioral, psychological, and social factors. Bruhn, et al.[11] have suggested that Erikson's typology of eight developmental stages of man offers a beginning in the search for an understanding of the wellness process. They have proposed an index for assessing wellness based upon the individual's completion of the minimal wellness tasks appropriate to each developmental stage. These authors correctly point out that children grow up in our society exposed to our concept of health as the absence of illness. There is no parallel concept available to a child to help him or her learn about wellness, as there are concepts for developing such other positive values as honesty, industry, or kindness to animals. For this reason, the authors argue, it is important to identify both the tasks that are appropriate for learning about wellness at various points along the developmental continuum and those tasks that will enhance an individual's motivation to work toward wellness.

Bruhn *et al.'s* proposal is a step in the right direction. It provides a framework for developing a taxonomy of identifiable markers congruent with the wellness process. Along with these biobehavioral markers, we need also to delineate the components and correlates of mental and social well-being. Subjective well-being has become a topic for serious empirical study only within the past decade or two. During this period, a number of seminal studies have suggested the importance of a multidimensional approach to the measurement of positive mental health.[12-15] These studies have shown that the feeling state of well-being is not a unidimensional construct, but rather is the reflection of a complex interaction of psychological processes. Bradburn[12] was able to demonstrate an orthogonal relationship between what he called negative affect and positive affect, as well as to document a correlation between positive affect and indicators of social involvement and new or varied experiences. In a more recent study, Beiser[13] has identified a third affective state that he has called "long-term satisfaction" and suggests that these three affects — negative affect, positive affect, and long-term satisfaction — contribute to feelings of general well-being. Beiser and his colleagues have suggested that well-being is the resultant effect of a complex intra-psychic process in which a person's general level of satisfaction with life interacts with more short-lived and fluctuating affective states. Evidence from available studies strongly suggests that, contrary to much popular and clinical belief, the absence of factors promoting negative affect does not automatically insure the emergence of positive feeling states, and vice-versa.

One might ask, and reasonably so, what possible values do such descriptives have? The answer to this question becomes apparent when one views the evolution of the disease model in a historical perspective. Starting out with a taxonomy based on observable states, the biomedical model of disease progressed from the identification of symptoms, to clusters of symptoms, to syndromes, and, finally, to diseases with specific pathogenesis and pathology. This is the basic sequence upon which the elucidation of disease has progressed. A comparable model of health focused on wellness and well-being could similarly provide guidelines for research and innovative policy initiatives.

In fact, preliminary evidence suggests that positive affect may be accompanied by concomitant changes in the body. Let us remind ourselves once again of the famous case example of Norman Cousins and his successful employment of "laughter therapy" for a condition his doctor had diagnosed as very rare and universally fatal. Cousins asked himself: "If negative emotions produce negative chemical changes in the body, wouldn't the positive emotions produce positive chemical changes? Is it possible that love, hope, faith, laughter, confidence, and the will to live have therapeutic value? Do chemical changes occur only on the downside?"[16] Cousins' personal experiment brought positive results beyond the capabilities of orthodox medicine.

Toward a Wellness Model of Health

Bruhn et al.[11] have proposed a formulation which views wellness and illness as being at extreme ends of a "Health Continuum," as shown in Figure 3-1. We would, however, prefer to conceptualize the relationship between "wellness" and "illness" as two independent dimensions that can be combined to generate a four-fold typology as shown in Figure 3-2. Type 1, the well who are not ill, is an ideal state of health. Type 2, the ill who are well, is characterized by individuals (such as the late Senator Hubert Humphrey) who can overcome the adversity of illness and maintain a positive outlook on life and on themselves. Type 3, those who are neither well nor ill, represents the vast majority of the American population – people who, while not ill, do not have a positive orientation toward health. Type 4, the ill who are not well, characterizes most individuals afflicted with chronic illness: their lives deteriorate, and they withdraw from active social involvement. The figure emphasizes that efforts toward health are not restricted solely to those who are not ill. Less clearly shown, however, is the notion that it is possible to move from type to type over time. Initial efforts at prevention and promotion need to be directed toward moving people from Type 2 to Type 1. It should be noted that Types 1 through 4 correspond roughly to Sidney Garfield's four categories: well, worried well, asymptomatic sick, and sick.[17] Our present so-called "health care system" is, in reality, a medical care system which deals principally with the horizontal ILL/NOT ILL dimension. A truly comprehensive "health care system" must include also the WELL/NOT WELL dimension. The

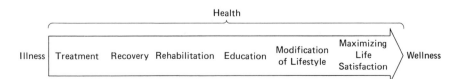

Figure 3-1. The health continuum.

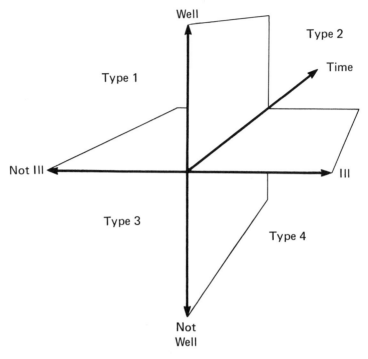

Figure 3-2.

whole must be viewed in a hierarchical perspective encompassing the biological, psychological, and social domains.

The conceptualization proposed for health and illness provides a useful framework not only for research but also for health care planning. Good health is viewed not as a commodity that can be purchased or as a state that can be legislated into existence. The presence of disease or ill health does not exclude the potential to experience wellness and well-being. An unfortunate individual may be born with a genetic birth defect, or be confronted with an acquired illness at a certain point in life, but such an individual still possesses the potential to attain wellness. As Bruhn et al.[11] have stated: "Everyone has a different potential for wellness, given their genetic inheritance and life circumstances . . . The movement toward wellness of a chronically ill person might include: (a) developing his full potential as a person, given his physical limitations; (b) improving his behavior relative to his fragile health condition so as to minimize future risks; and (c) expanding his self-sufficiency to accomplish what he believes to be important in his life. The maximum potential for wellness must be left to each individual to define or determine. However, there are minimal wellness thresholds; these should be viewed as rights or potentials for everyone." The late Sen-

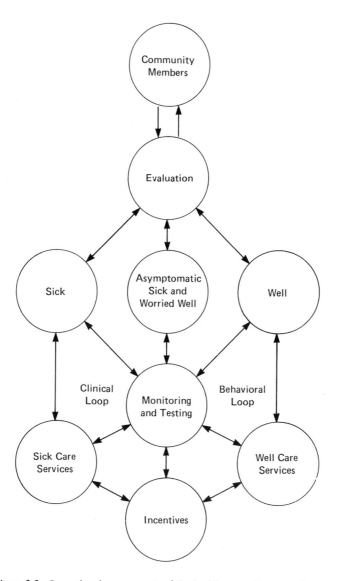

Figure 3-3. Operational components of the health promotion organization.

teaching people to take greater responsibility for their own health, and 2) create incentives for health promotion and disease prevention by stimulating a closer working relationship among government, business, labor, and the medical care system.

The HPO would provide initial screening and diagnostic services for all participants. From these results, a health status report would be constructed. This report would be amended periodically to reflect an individual's progress in achieving personalized health goals. On the basis of the health report, individuals would be requested to participate in various programs designed to enhance health status by changing attitudes and behaviors that are health-aversive. For example, the health enhancement program would include stress-reduction and relaxation training, courses in nutrition and diet, biofeedback training, exercise regimens, and courses in medical self-care. It should be emphasized that each person's program would be individually tailored to his or her health status report.

Obviously, an appropriate incentive system would be essential for the HPO to insure that new members would be recruited and that participants would be motivated to follow their individualized programs. Thus, it would be essential for the HPO to stimulate linkages among the major societal institutions. For example, government could provide tax reduction incentives for participation, the insurance industry could design special health insurance programs for members, and business could incorporate HPO activities into the fringe benefit package provided for employees.

The incentive system described above is oriented toward the individual. However, health is not only a personal concern. It would also be essential for the HPO to stimulate inter-institutional incentives to encourage the development of "passive" strategies that would promote health. For example, government could provide tax incentives to industry for pollution abatement, for enhancing the health quality of the workplace, for improving the diet of Americans, etc. To be successful, the HPO must be oriented toward institutions as well as toward individual people. Alone, either approach can be only minimally successful.

The HPO is envisioned as a community endeavor that would function as the "wellness" component of pre-existing medical sick-care facilities. Through adjunctive status and through extensive use of paraprofessionals and community volunteers, operating costs could be kept to a minimum. Although not all of the goals of the HPO could be attained initially, the model seems to provide a viable mechanism for enhancing health.

Small-scale demonstration projects will be required to document the utility of the present model and to suggest improvements in the design.

Conclusion

Although the present report demonstrates that a conceptual model of health and well-being is still in the nascent stage, adequate knowledge is already available to conduct demonstrations of HPO-type organizations in conjunction with a rigorous and diverse program of research. From these twin endeavors, meaningful directions and policy initiations can emerge in the near-term future. Granted the magnitude and import of the issue, prompt action is necessary. Indeed, in an era of cost containment and reduction, it seems odd that more effort has not been directed toward the twin goals of prevention and promotion, the most-cost-effective policies in the long term.

REFERENCES

1. Breslow, L., *J. Epidemiology* 1:347–359, 1972.
2. Fabrega, H., Jr., *Perspect. Biol. Med.*, Summer 1972.
3. Wildavsky, A., *Daedalus* 106:105–124, 1977.
4. Dubos, R., *Medicine, Man, and Environment.* New York: Praeger, 1968.
5. LaLonde, M., *A New Perspective on the Health of Canadians: A Working Document.* Ottawa: Ministry of Health and Welfare, 1976.
6. *Report by the National Commission for the Protection of Human Subjects of Biomedical and Behavioral Research,* 1978.
7. Gori, G. B. and Richter, B. J., *Science* 200:1124–1130, 1978.
8. Kass, L.R., *The Public Interest,* Summer 1975.
9. *Constitution of the World Health Organization in The First Ten Years of the WHO.* Geneva: Palais des Nations, 1958, p. 459.
10. Campbell, A., in *The Human Meaning of Social Change,* A. Campbell and P.E. Converse (Eds.). New York: Russell Sage Foundation, 1972.
11. Bruhn, J.G., Cordova, F.D., Williams, J.A., and Fuertes, R.G., *J. Community Health* 2:209–221, 1977.
12. Bradburn, N.M., *The Structure of Psychological Well-Being.* Chicago: Aldine, 1969.
13. Beiser, M., *J. Health and Social Behavior* 15:320–327, 1974.
14. Brenner, B., *Social Indicators Research* 2:315–331, 1975.
15. Jahoda, M., *Current Concepts of Positive Mental Health.* New York: Basic Books, 1958.
16. Cousins, N., *New England J. Medicine* 295:1458–1463, 1976.
17. Garfield, S.R. *et al., New England J. Medicine* 294:426–431, 1976.
18. Vice President Walter F. Mondale's Eulogy for Senator Hubert Humphrey, delivered at the United States Capitol Memorial Service on Sunday, January 15, 1978.
19. Sullivan, D.F., *National Center for Health Statistics, Vital and Health Statistics, Series 2, No. 42,* Washington: Public Health Service, July 1971.
20. Elinson, J., in *Health, Medicine, Society,* M. Sokolowska, J. Holowka, and A. Ostrowska (Eds.). Warsaw: PWN-Polish Scientific Publishers, 1975.
21. Belloc, N.B. and Breslow, L. *Preventive Medicine* 1:409–421, 1972.
22. Belloc, N.B., *Preventive Medicine* 2:67–81, 1973.
23. Tomatis, L., "The Value of Long-term Testing for the Implementation of Primary Prevention," H. Hiatt, J.D. Watson, and J. Winston (Eds.), *Origin of Human Cancer, Book C: Human Risk Assessment.* Cold Spring Harbor Laboratory, pp. 1339–1358, 1977.
24. Davis, D.L. and Rall, D.P., "Estimating Risks as the Basis for Preventive Policies," in L.K.Y. Ng and D.L. Davis (Eds.) *Strategies for Public Health: Promoting Health and Preventing Disease.* New York: Van Nostrand Reinhold, forthcoming.

25. Davis, D.L., "Multiple Risk Assessment as a Preventive Strategy for Public Health," in J. Staffa (Ed.), *FDA Symposium on Risk/Benefit Diseases and the Public Health.* forthcoming.

26. Schneiderman, M., "The Links between Environment and Health," paper presented to the National Conference on the Environment and Health Care Costs. U.S. House of Representatives, August 15, 1978.

27. Public Health Service, *Forward Plan for Health, FY 1978-82.* DHEW Publication No. (OS) 76-50046. Washington, D.C.: U.S. Government Printing Office, 1976.

28. Ng, L.K.Y., Davis, D.L., and Manderscheid, R.W., *Public Health Reports* 93:446-455, 1978.

4

Holistic Medicine: Health Care of the Future?

Paul J. Rosch, M.D., F.A.C.P.

American Institute Of Stress

> *I absolutely flatly deny that I am a soul,*
> *or a body, or a mind, or an intelligence,*
> *or a brain, or a nervous system,*
> *or a bunch of glands,*
> *or any of the rest of these bits of me.*
> *The whole is greater than the part.*
> *And therefore, I, who am man alive,*
> *am greater than my soul,*
> *or spirit, or body, or mind,*
> *or consciousness, or anything else*
> *that is merely a part of me.*
> *I am a man and alive.*

> D.H. Lawrence, *Women in Love*

The concept of holistic medicine, as well as the closely related subject of the role of stress as a cause of illness, has captured the attention of both the medical profession and the public at large in an unprecedented fashion. Recently, a lead article by Norman Cousins, entitled "The Holistic Health Explosion," in the *Saturday Review of Literature* outlined the reasons for the great health revolution now sweeping this country. At the same time, editorials on the subject appeared in the *Journal of the American Medical Association* and *The New England Journal of Medicine;* the *Wall Street Journal* was running a four-part series on the role of stress in hypertension, heart disease, ulcers, arthritis, cancer, and a variety of other disorders; and 100,000 physicians were participating in a three-year nationwide educational program to learn how to recognize and manage "stress disorders."

This does not appear to be just another passing fad. Courses and seminars on holistic medicine are being held at Stanford University and the University of Pennsylvania Medical Schools, and a host of other courses are being sponsored by other, equally prestigious institutions, many of which are accredited for physicians' Continuing Medical Education. The government is exploring holistic medicine as a means of reducing health costs, and, two years ago, a conference—"Holistic Health: A Public Policy"—was held under the aegis of the Department of Health, Education, and Welfare, which has also provided seed money for the Institute for the Study of Humanistic Medicine in San Francisco.

Granger Westberg, a hospital chaplain, with the aid of physicians he worked with on the (A.M.A.) Committee on Medicine and Religion, started a clinic based on holistic principles in Springfield, Ohio. It was so successful that three more were organized in Illinois. Several thousand doctors attended an Association for Holistic Health Conference in San Diego in July 1977, and since then we have seen the formation of the American Holistic Medical Association in La Crosse, Wisconsin, the East/West Center for Holistic Health in New York City, the Holistic Health Center in St. Petersburg, Florida, the Omega Institute for Holistic Studies in New Lebanon, New York, the Holistic Life University in San Francisco, the Association for Holistic Health in Del Mar, California, and the Holistic Health Organizing Committee in Berkeley, California, to name only a few. Thus, the movement is not limited to a handful of zealots in California, as is often assumed, but is truly nationwide. The second conference, on "New Horizons in Holistic Health," was held in Chicago in May 1979, and, in September 1979, the First International Conference on Holistic Health was sponsored in part by San Diego State University. One can subscribe to any number of holistic health periodicals, such as *Holistic Health Review, Journal of Holistic Health,* and a variety of others published by the above organizations and numerous academies, societies, and associations devoted to the same principles, but not bearing the term "holistic."

What is the reason for all this interest? Americans have always been characterized as a people preoccupied with their health, and America is certainly the land of the cult, so the soil would appear to be fertile for the planting of this particular seed. But there is obviously much more to it than that. The reasons are varied, but not difficult to understand when one is able to separate the wheat from the chaff. That can best be accomplished by trying to understand what the ideals of holistic medicine are, since numerous practices, doctrines, sects, and procedures are based on these ideals.

Origin of the Words Holism and Holistic

Although frequently attributed to a variety of contemporary individuals, "holism" and "holistic" are words which were "invented" by Jan Smuts and appeared in 1926 in his book, *Holism and Evolution.* Smuts is best known as a general and field marshal in the British Army, and later as Prime Minister of South Africa. However, he was also a highly skilled barrister and a trained philosopher, and he contributed the essential framework for the League of Nations. *Holism and Evolution* describes an evolutionary concept wherein "holism underlies the synthetic tendency in the universe." Smuts theorized that an entity grows and evolves, and at some point in its maturation becomes complete, at which time the whole is greater than the sum of its parts. It then progresses to new levels of existence, new "wholes," brought about by the creative force within, which Smuts termed "holism." Evolution, therefore, is "nothing but the gradual development and stratification of a progressive series of wholes, stretching from the inorganic beginnings to the highest levels of spiritual creation. Wholeness, healing, holiness—all expressions and ideas springing from the same root in language, as in experience—lie on the rugged upward path of the universe."[1]

You will not find "holistic" in most dictionaries, although it is in the supplementary volume of the new *Oxford English Dictionary* and is defined in Dorland's latest *Medical Dictionary* as "considering man as a functioning whole, or relating to the conception of man as a functioning whole, being derived from the Greek *holos* meaning whole." It is difficult to find the term "wholism" anywhere except in psychiatric or behavioral sciences dictionaries, where it is used interchangeably with "holism." Actually, the word springs from the Indo-European root word *kailo,* which meant whole, intact, or uninjured. This quite likely accounts for some of the appeal of the term "holism," since, when new words develop, the connotation of old ones tend to linger in the subconscious. Thus, we have the distinct scent of something transcendental because of "holy." Other words, such as health, whole, hallow, hale, and (certainly) heal, increase in attractiveness without our being consciously aware of it.

The Holistic Approach

The major difference between practitioners of holistic medicine and orthodox physicians would appear to be their orientation: the holistic practitioner is oriented toward the patient, rather than toward the disease or illness. This shift in emphasis carries with it several implications. The most important is that holistic medicine posits its focus on "wellness," which it visualizes not merely as the absence of illness, but as a very positive state that embraces not only physical, but also mental, emotional, and spiritual well-being.[2] It emphasizes the inseparability of mind and body in any attempt to evaluate or treat the patient, and places great importance on the body's own innate and natural potential for maintaining health (*vis medicatrix naturae*). As a consequence, it tends toward the utilization of naturopathic modalities of therapy, rather than reliance upon drugs or other artificial aids. Most important, it recognizes and affirms that the individual's health is his or her own responsibility, with the obvious corollary that the patient must be an active participant in any therapeutic endeavor. Prevention of illness and enhancement of health, rather than treatment of disease, are the goals.

In keeping with the original intent of the word, the holistic approach in psychiatric jargon represents Gestalt totality, the thesis that the whole is something different from the simple summation or accumulation of its parts. "From a holistic point of view, the human being is more than a mere aggregation of physiological, psychological, and social functions; the person as a whole has attributes that cannot be explained by the attributes of its constituent parts."[3] Thus, increasing knowledge of the structure or function of cells, tissues, or organs of the body does not increase our understanding of the totality, except by appreciating these parts as expressions of the functioning of the organism as a whole.

Holiology—to coin another new word—is therefore the study of the person in totality: the physical, mental, spiritual, behavioral, emotional, nutritional, ecological, and any other factors that might influence any aspect of well-being. Physiology, psychology, sociology, and psychobiology all represent disciplines dealing with specific aspects of the human function, and we have a number of sciences relating *to* the person, but no science *of* the person functioning in his or her totality. Holistic medicine aims at filling this need.

Euexia, A Definition of Health: The Distinction between Normal and Average

Holistic medicine is primarily distinguished by its concept of health. As physicians, we tend to assume that people who are not sick are by definition healthy. Sickness usually means that the patient is complaining of something, or that the physician has discovered some abnormality through examination or other testing. In fact, even if the patient does have some complaint, if the doctor cannot find something abnormal after extensive testing, the patient is still presumed to be healthy by virtue of the fact that there is no demonstrable evidence of abnormality. The logic of this negative reasoning is a function of the nature of traditional medical education; there is no positive definition of health that is taught in our usual medical training. Health is considered to be merely the absence of illness.

Our American health system is, in reality, a sickness system. One does not purchase health insurance — one purchases sickness insurance. Our health centers are sickness centers. If one wished to invest $50, $500, or $5000 in an effort to insure, promote, or enhance one's *health,* one would have a difficult time determining how to proceed in accomplishing this goal.

The holistic definition of health may be found in the Constitution of the World Health Organization: "Health is a state of complete physical, mental, and social well-being, and not merely the absence of disease or infirmities."[3] This is a positive definition, and one which provides the individual with something to strive toward in an active fashion. This is inherently different from the effort to promote health by simply *avoiding* sickness. In this context, one may view the lack of health at five levels:

1. Dissatisfaction
2. Discomfort

3. Disability
4. Overt disease
5. Death or dying.[4]

While we would normally tend to view these as progressive and more severe *stages* of illness, they might be accorded equal weight on a holistic scale which measures total health. Thus, it is possible to be "healthy" even when one is "sick," and the late Hubert H. Humphrey is often cited as an example of just that.

Another distinction that follows from the above is the difference between *normal* and *average*. Most of our recognition of disease is based upon an observation of an abnormal finding. There is little question that such a deviation suggests illness, but it is an error to assume automatically that a normal finding implies health. Normal values are generally determined from surveys of Americans presumed to be healthy. Many of them, however, are afflicted with hypertension, ulcers, arthritis, or obesity, or have habits that are anything but healthy.

What is required is a concept of *optimal health;* that is, the best achievable state of total wellness for a given individual. This is analogous to the *euexia* espoused by Hippocrates and Aristotle, and describes not only a state of excellent health, but also a proper way of life. Such a concept recognizes that the quality of life must ultimately depend upon the level of total health, in the holistic sense.

The Decline of the Healer and How it Came About

Holistic medicine is, to a large extent, filling a void that has been created by our own medical technocracy. The practice of medicine has become less and less an art, and more and more just another science, profession, or business. The doctor-patient relationship, so essential to the healing process, has been steadily disintegrating due to factors related to time, cost, expertise, and experience, as well as advances in technology. The depersonalization of the patient is not limited to physicians. Nurses now refer to "the case in Room 301" or "the perforated ulcer," but rarely refer by name to the individual entrusted to their care.

The nurse-patient estrangement represents a marked shift in the degree of individual care rendered by nurses only 20 years ago. Then, the charge nurse on the floor knew every patient by name, and was generally aware of certain personal problems that might have escaped the physician's attention. The nurse had an opportunity to speak with and observe the patient daily, and also to converse with relatives and other visitors. Part of the trend toward patient anonymity may be because a large portion of those services formerly performed by nurses, which enabled them to gain extra insight through direct patient contact, are today being performed by aides, orderlies, or other hospital personnel with whom the physician does not come into contact. Nurses' notes are now devoted to the problem-oriented record, not the patient-oriented record, and throughout the entire range of medical care, we find the sensitive, caring, human touch replaced by a form of smug psuedo-scientific technology.

A premium is placed on advances made in the laboratory or in the operating room, but the only reward for the physician exercising his or her skills at the bedside or in the consultation room is the physician's own satisfaction or the gratitude of the patient. Thus, we witness the phenomenon of more and more medical celebrities, but fewer and fewer old-fashioned heroes.

The Decline and Fall of the Art of Medicine

Most of the current patterns in medical care can be traced to the development of the present model of illness, which has its roots in Cartesian philosophy. In this mechanistic paradigm, the body was viewed as a type of machine, and illness represented some malfunction of its operation. The purpose of medicine was to repair that malfunction. Matters relating to the mind or soul were relegated to the separate province of the Church. We still see this attitude in patients who drop into the doctor's office, much as one would bring a car to a mechanic, asking or demanding repairs, although usually, in the latter instance, the individual expresses some interest as to why things went wrong with the vehicle, while in the former case, the patient often expresses no such concern.

The interrelationship between societal norms and concepts of health and the healing art has existed virtually since men organized themselves into societies. Illness, as well as health, therefore becomes definable in terms of social and cultural value systems. In classical Greece, health was a virtue, and ill people (the non-virtuous) were often despised. In Mesopotamia, illness was viewed as a punishment from the gods, and those afflicted were treated like criminals. In the Ndembu tribe of northern Rhodesia, it was believed that all serious or chronic illness was due to a breach in social custom, such as failure to respect ancestors or parents by the performance of certain ceremonial rites and tributes, and the offender was treated as a pariah until the wrong could be rectified.[5]

In nineteenth century England and Europe, however, tuberculars were treated as the objects of compassion in novels and opera (*La Boheme* or *The Lady of the Camellias,* or *La Traviata,* "The Unfortunate One"), a far cry from the biblical leper who was ostracized. The subject of societal attitudes toward cancer has been deftly explored in Susan Sontag's recent book, *Illness as Metaphor.*[6] In our present society, we are more apt to view the sick person as a dropout from the production line, and, in current parlance, as a consumer rather than a provider, with no particular onus of punishment attached. In fact, having a coronary is, in some ways, a badge of courage bearing testimony to the individual's intense, driving lifestyle, very much comparable to the traditional German dueling scar.

Beyond the appealing popularity of the holistic concept, there are many reasons why the public is turned off by modern medicine. Some of these reasons are related to the depersonalization of the patient, and other stem from factors related to the commercial aspects of the practice of medicine, as depicted in the media and as dictated by the policies of fiscal intermediaries concerned with cost containment.

In the past decade, physicians have been increasingly relegated to the roles of cogs in the overall machinery of the "health business." The official language of government characterizes the medical profession as one among many other vendors or providers of "health" services, lumped together in a mixed bag that includes the pharmaceutical industry, insurance companies, and hospitals. It is small wonder that the doctor's image in the public eye is that of just another businessman. Furthermore, the reimbursement policies for all types of health insurance reward the physician for doing something – for *cutting,* or for *looking* through some body orifice – but almost never for *thinking, caring,* or *feeling.* A doctor can spend two hours with a patient, utilizing skills and talents to arrive at an understanding and, it is hoped, a solution to the patient's problem that will prevent similar distress in the future. But the material reimbursement to either the physician or the patient for such a service is nil or minimal. On the other hand, if five or ten minutes are spent removing a skin blemish, or performing a proctoscopic examination, one will be remunerated handsomely. It is not surprising, therefore, that medicine is considered to be increasingly less of an art and increasingly more of a science (or a business, as young physicians, establishing their practices, recognize the financial criteria that govern their economic futures).

The distinct tendency toward specialization and subspecialization has undoubtedly led to greater knowledge and better treatment of various portions of the body, and is responsible for many advances in the state of the art of modern medicine. However, this type of zeroing in does not favor a holistic approach, and, in practice, often gives rise to an assembly-line type of production, wherein patients are treated in large clinics and shuttled from one specialist to another, with very little of that unique personal bond that represents the magic and the art of healing.

It is not entirely medicine's fault that this unhappy state of affairs exists. Television, radio, and the print media have created a population that is symptom-oriented. "Can't sleep? Try Sominex!" "Nervous, tense? Try Compoze!" "Acid indigestion, heartburn? Try Tums, Rolaids!" "Headache? Take Excedrin, Anacin!" "Headache and indigestion? Use Alka Seltzer, Bufferin!" And so on! Physicians may be a little more sophisticated in prescribing Dalmane, Valium, or Tagamet, but too often they are compelled by the demands of time and patient case loads into treating the tangible or visible effects of disease without proper attention to the causes. Far too frequently, physicians fail to realize that their ability to make a diagnosis based upon laboratory or X-ray procedures does not absolve them of the responsibility of investigating further into *how* the dysfunction came about, how it might have been prevented, or how its recurrence might be avoided. In its extreme, this preoccupation with the immediate relief of symptoms is as illogical as treating a diabetic infection with antibiotics without controlling the diabetes, or treating the pain of a fractured leg with morphine and not setting the fracture.

Another reason for public disenchantment with conventional medical practices has been the rapid rise in the educational level of the average American, and the ready availability, through various media, of information relating to new health discoveries as they arise. The increase in medical knowledge on all frontiers is occurring at such a rapid rate that it is impossible for physicians to be aware of every new advance or discovery, much less have the personal capacity to evaluate it. Often, the public knows of a new discovery as soon as (or even before) the physician does.

The advent of consumerism as a powerful force on the local and national scene is another factor that causes considerable problems. Americans are obsessed with health. They demand immediate healing much as they demand any other commodity. Why diet if you can obtain reducing pills? Why relax the pace of your life when you can take Valium? The tremendous success of antibiotics in treating infections has spoiled the average citizen, who assumes that all ills must yield to a pill of some sort.

On the other hand, the patient is really a passive participant in conventional medicine, a consumer without a specific role. Emphasis is placed upon what the *physician* must do. Even when we talk about patient compliance, it is in the sense of whether he or she is faithfully executing a physician's instructions, rather than taking an active part in the healing process. The consumer has little to do with the cost of care, which appears to be the major cause of concern today. Physicians, who are often forced into practicing a defensive type of medicine because of the threat of costly litigation, determine the type and number of tests and the nature of treatment. All too frequently, many of these tests and treatments are unnecessary or superfluous. The pharmacy, laboratory, or hospital determines the costs, and the patient rarely questions — much less controls — any of this, in marked contradiction to services in other areas, which may explain some of the inordinate costs. This is especially evident in those instances where the individual does take an active role in therapy, such as in Weight Watchers, Alcoholics Anonymous, or Smoke Enders, and where, although experts are relatively minimal, the results are not, particularly on a cost-effective basis.[7]

The increasing recognition of the harmful potential of many conventional medical practices and prescriptions has created serious problems. The experience with thalidomide, the advancing spectre of radiation-induced defects, controversies about widely utilized prescription items such as reserpine, estrogens, or even ubiquitous substances such as artificial sweeteners, have all contributed to a justified wariness, if not fear, in the mind of the public. The unknown long-term effects of medication and diagnostic radiologic procedures have encouraged a search for alternative (especially non-toxic) natural forms of treatment, sometimes based on anecdotal experience alone. This has been strengthened by the observation that previously unrecognized or discredited procedures, such as biofeedback, behavioral modification, acupuncture, transcutaneous stimulation, hypnosis, and vitamin and other types of nutritional therapy, are becoming widely accepted and utilized by orthodox physicians.

Because of all of these factors, patients are not as disposed to accept all medical decisions with the customary blind faith exhibited in the past. Rejection of naturopathic types of therapy, based simply upon the argument of lack of proof or rationale, no longer seems as compelling as it used to seem, especially if the treatment suggested has no harmful effects.

Holistic Hoax?

The problem today is that, since the concept of holistic medicine is so appealing, and since certain aspects of conventional medicine are evidencing a decline in attractiveness, everyone wants to get onto the bandwagon. Consequently, there is a great proliferation of organizations and cults that purport to serve rather lofty aims, but, in effect, are dedicated to other goals or are outright frauds. If one reads the brochures from various organizations, it is apparent that the practitioners of holistic medicine include numerologists, pyramid therapists, iridologists, and proponents of apricot kernel therapy, Rolfing, touch encounters, negative ionization, psychocalisthenics, self-massage, and a host of other seemingly baseless, but apparently harmless, techniques. To be sure, many of the proponents of these methodologies are sincere. They are convinced that their particular approach will find the same path of acceptance as biofeedback or meditation, and they may be emphatically negative about any other approach, even if it invokes the aura of holism.

Almost any one of these therapies will meet with some success, regardless of its merit, depending upon the enthusiasm of the sponsor and the faith of the subject. This will be augmented if the technique also provides an explanation as to *why* the patient is sick as well as *what* he or she must do to become well.[8] This is apparent from the experience of many older cultures,[9] and recent studies suggest that "it may well be that any practitioner, regardless of his discipline, who is responsive to the emotional needs of the patient, can achieve equal results . . . ."[10] Therapeutic trust has been for years the magic of medicine, and newer knowledge of endorphin secretion and the nature of the placebo effect suggests a physiologic rationale for this.

The subject is so vaguely defined in the public mind, and the boundaries of holistic medicine are so loosely and poorly drawn (by patients, as well as physicians), that it often becomes difficult to discriminate between valid, legitimate, promising modes of therapy, and worthless, or even fraudulent programs masquerading under the same wholesome and attractive title. Thus, holistic medicine today is comparable to a three-ring circus. Perhaps the main acts in the center ring embody the qualities of purity, body, and flavor, but there is a great danger that some of the side shows will supersede the main act in this variegated carnival.

The Crossroads

What should be the response and attitude of the responsible physician and the enlightened patient to all of this? It seems obvious that a physician must maintain an open mind about newer developments in diagnosis and treatment of disease, even if these developments do not appear to be consonant with the physician's own experience or training. Purely scientific research depends upon a type of objectivity which almost precludes all the qualities that are integral to discovery: insight, imagination, inventiveness, and freedom from false necessities of thought. Science alone does not have all the answers to problems relating to the healing process.

Yet one cannot unreservedly endorse treatment suggestions simply because they are natural or harmless, especially if they waste valuable time by foregoing therapeutic methods that might be helpful for lifesaving. Our present state of knowledge about nutritional requirements and the need for vitamin and mineral supplementation is woefully inadequate. While it would be illogical to subscribe to the doctrine that all illnesses are manifestations of nutritional deficiencies, it would be equally illogical to refuse to acknowledge that there may be increased requirements for such substances in individuals under stress, or those with lifestyle habits that would result in chronic imbalances or deficiencies.

Therefore, while it is wise to question and to be discriminative, and to adhere to scientific principles in our evaluation of various modalities of therapy as they arise, it may be imprudent to automatically reject the novel and the innovative just because they have no proven basis or because we cannot justify their apparent effects. Science always demands proof, and that is not always the same as evidence. Thus, we need to strike some kind of balance that permits us to retain a healthy skepticism until all the facts are in. At the same time, we must recognize that our mere inability to explain certain results or observations does not necessarily negate their validity. Some psi phenomena and the feats of various yogis serve as accurate examples of this. We should follow Pasteur's dictum: "Keep your enthusiasm, but let strict verification be its constant companion."[11]

The Future of Holistic Medicine

The drive toward modes of health improvement via natural techniques that aim to improve the individual as a whole has generated an increased interest in nutrition, particularly in vitamin and previously obscure mineral therapy; in physical fitness, particularly in exercise and jogging (with its spiritual as well as physical and biochemical benefits); in meditation; in faith healing; etc. This impetus has been accelerated by a growing recognition of the powers of the mind in the regulation of health. A steadily expanding appreciation of the potential benefits of "eustress," as exemplified by the health and longevity records of symphony conductors, successful professionals and artists, and communities of individuals such as Mormons, Christian Scientists, nuns, and Seventh Day Adventists, reinforces the link between emotional and physical well-being.

Western medicine has only recently come to appreciate that good health is not merely the absence of disease, but a state of positive well-being in which the body and the mind are inseparable. We are long overdue in focusing our attention on health enhancement as well as on the prevention and treatment of illness. The Chinese have been doing this for milennia, and traditionally reimburse the physician for helping the patient to *stay* well, which, on reflection, seems to be a more sensible basis for a doctor-patient relationship.

There is nothing new about any of this. Juvenal's *mens sana in corpore sano* (a sound mind in a sound body) said it most explicitly, and it is as old as the history of medicine itself. In one of Plato's dialogues, it is noted: "Hippocrates, the Ascelepiad, says that, 'The nature of the body can only be understood as a whole, for this is the great error of our day in the treatment of the human body, that physicians separate the soul from the body.' " The Greek stem word (δλος) is found throughout the New Testament,[12] and the Apostle Paul wrote, "May the God of Peace Himself sanctify you wholly, and may He preserve you whole and entire in spirit, and in soul, and in body, without blemish . . . . " (1st Thessalonians, Chapter 25, Verse 23).

The era of the awe-inspiring, aloof, authoritarian physician, the demigod before whom the supplicant patient worshipped, is disappearing. Although this type of attitude can be very useful and beneficial, and is essential to the healing art of the shaman, it is not likely to flourish in the current climate of consumerism and increased public education. And, in any event, a firm relationship, built upon mutual respect, trust, and understanding, if entered into enthusiastically by both parties, may achieve far greater results.

In its essence, holistic medicine states that there are no illnesses, only patients and, to paraphrase Maimonides, physicians must treat not the disease, but the patient who is suffering from it.[13] Few medications can substitute for the warmth, compassion, and empathy of a physician, and so it is necessary for the physician to bring something else to the patient other than diagnostic acumen and knowledge of drugs and procedures. This implies that physicians must be sensitive, cultured, and — yes — even healthy individuals themselves, with an emphasis on "skills rather than pills."[14] Although the original quote is Caleb Parry's, Sir William Osler noted: "It is sometimes more important to know what kind of patient has the disease than what kind of disease the patient has."[15]

Allopathic and holistic medicine are neither mutually exclusive nor incompatible, and the wise physician and patient will choose from the best that both have to offer. As Abraham Lincoln once wrote to his law partner: "Let not a worship of the past nor a confusion of the present keep us from an attempt to wisely plan for the future."[16] There are many discoveries open to the educated, inquisitive, but uncluttered mind, and as we mature in our knowledge, appreciation, and wonder of the healing art, we should feel "only the check-rein, not the curb, the blinder or the hobble."[17]

Holistic medicine is ill-defined and much maligned, but its roots are solid and cannot be ignored or dismissed. The pendulum may be swinging too far or too quickly in a direction away from conventional medicine, but the limits of the arc it prescribes may provide a vantage point that will ultimately restore the balance and equilibrium so essential to the healing art and to health.

REFERENCES

1. Smuts, Jan, *Holism and Evolution*. London: MacMillan,: p. 54, 1926.
2. Angyal, A., *Foundations for a Science of Personality*. Cambridge, Mass.: Harward University Press, 156, 1941.
3. *The First Ten Years of the World Health Organization*. Geneva: World Health Organization, 1958.
4. White, K. L. "Primary Medical Care for Families: Organization and Evaluation," *The New England Journal of Medicine"* 277: 847, 1967.
5. Turner, V. W., "A Ndembu Doctor in Practice," in A Kiev (Ed.), *Magic, Faith and Healing.* Glencoe, N.Y.: Free Press, p. 231, 1964.
6. Sontag, Susan, *Illness as Metaphor.* New York: Farrar, Straus and Giroux, 1978.
7. Rappaport, R. N., *Community as Doctor: New Perspectives on a Therapeutic Community.* Scranton, Pa.: Harpen, Row, p. 10, 1960; and Rabkin, J. G. and Struening, E.L., "Life Events, Stress and Illness," *Science* 194- 1013-1020, 1976.
8. Mason, R. C., Clark, G., Reeves, R. G. *et al.,* "Acceptance and Healing," *Journal of Religion and Health* 8: 123, 1969.
9. Alland, A., *Adaptation in Cultural Evolution: An Approach to Medical Anthropology.* New York: Columbia University Press, p. 115, 1970.
10. Kane, R., Oldsen, D., Leymaster, C. *et al.,* "Manipulating the Patient: A Comparison of the Effectiveness of Physician and Chiropractic Care," *Lancet* 1: 1333, 1974.
11. Quoted in Dock, W., 'Treatment of Myocardial Infarction," *Lancet* 1: 1106, 1974.
12. Thayer, J. H., *Greek-English Lexicon for the New Testament.* Grand Rapids, Michigan: Zondervan, p. 443, 1976; and Darton, M. (Ed.), *Modern Concordance to the New Testament.* New York: Doubleday & Co., pp. 661-662, 1949.
13. Muntner, S. (Ed.), *The Medical Writings of Moses Maimonides,* Treatise on Asthma. Philadelphia: J.P. Lippencatt, 1963.
14. Elkes, Joel, "Health Enhancement and Behavioral Medicine II," from BMA Symposia on Stress and Behavioral Medicine, Audio Cassette Program, New York, 1978.
15. Cited in Osler, William, *Aequanimitas with Other Addresses.* New York: McGraw Hill, p. 54, 1932.
16. Quoted in Daines, William P., "Message from the President," Twenty-Second Annual Meeting of the American Society of Internal Medicine, San Francisco, May 4-7, 1978.
17. Bean, W. B., "Right and Wrong," *Archives of Internal Medicine.* 117: 613, May 1966.

5

On Awareness and the Good Day

Professor Joel Elkes, M.D.

Department of Psychiatry, McMaster University Medical Center, Canada

The convergent cones of past and future steadily press on the moving point that is the "now" of today. In this continuous transformation, each day becomes a piece of personal history, forming a unit of life. Of late, however, this now of today has become a neglected entity because a future-oriented culture, preoccupied with plans and maps of things to come, is apt to overlook the present. There is still a preoccupation with the concept of noxious *cause,* a carry-over from the traditions of Pasteur and Rudolf Virchow. The "invader" and the environment are held responsible, and the person is seen as the passive victim of outer circumstances. No one will deny the role of the environment, particularly the early, social, and physical environments, in the genesis of psychological and biological competence. Yet, we must ask whether the successes of modern theoretical biology and medical practice have emphasized outer cause at the expense of personal competence and responsibility, while ignoring the mode of life as a pathogen, despite compelling evidence.[1]

Remembering takes the place of awareness. Organismic sensing gives way to a causal chain which stops just short of present enactment. Symbolic learning (insight) is apt to assume an intellectual and affective autonomy, rather than being tested through day-by-day performance. A shift of the locus of control[2] to the "without" creates psychological dependence. The mere disappearance or attenuation of the unpleasant ("I do not feel depressed today" or "My headache is gone") is sought as an end-point rather than a mid-point in a person's goal-seeking behavior. It would seem that psychiatry, as medicine, has become preoccupied with *relief.* Enhancement of well-being is much farther down the road. Cues from the body, including the memory banks of the musculoskeletal system, come to us continuously during the day. They can be made more accessible through the practice of relatively simple low-arousal techniques.[3] The point was made above that awareness of environment all too often outweighs self-awareness, and preoccupation with past and future out-balances communication with things as they actually are in the ever-present now. The body provides a convenient matrix, conjoining the outer with the inner world. It is useful to be aware of its messages.

Body Awareness: Messages from Base

Awareness is a composite, comprising many states and stages. The outer world, be it sensory, perceptual, interpersonal, or social, comes to us principally by way of distance receptors. The instruments of sight and sound are still the main sensors by which we navigate through our day. The data conveyed by these sensors — a piece of newsprint, the smile of a man — reach consciousness by way of a succession of instantaneous transactions, astonishing in the selectiveness of their effective and cognitive economy. Gradually, a growing understanding of the staging of these various transactions continues to give us an ever-clearer picture of the way we construct the images of our world. It is increasingly apparent that all perception is monitored against memory stores, and that the gating begins at the outermost edges of the portals of entry — the sensors themselves. There is little doubt that a two-way (centripetal and centrifugal) feedback is continuously playing upon the sensors, and that experience, effective appraisal, and anticipation of the likely outcome (the so-called anticipatory set) all enter into the way we interpret sensory data and prepare our responses.[4] Information furnished through distance receptors is linked to appraisal and planning, and the construction of a cognitive map-in-time. This is not surprising, because distance furnishes the organism time to prepare, swiftly and appropriately, for a congruent response; nor is it strange that in a future-oriented world, with a high load of uncertainty and ambiguity, such cognitive maps should be future-oriented, and that they should engender old and stress-related endocrine, skeletal, and visceromotor responses. These, while appropriate at an earlier stage of evolution, have outlived their usefulness in modern life. Psychosomatic illness provides a good cue to our lack of evolutionary fit.

In a future-oriented society, the home base of the body itself is less familiar. Smell, temperature, and touch are proximate sensors. Enteroceptive signals from deep muscle systems and from viscera share projections to skin areas and related muscle groups that are rarely appreciated, unless they signal distress and alarm. The detailed mosaic of these projections is only just beginning to be worked out. Yet, all the way from the spasm overlying a herniated disc, to the sustained painful contractions of muscle groups around the head and neck and the referred pain of myocardial insufficiency, the non-verbal language of pain is clear.[5] Wilhelm Reich's intuitive concept of muscle armor[6] awaits its quantitative psychophysiology. Biofeedback studies[7] are now beginning to provide relevant data. An impressive body of evidence is gradually linking the relief of pain to techniques furthering both general relaxation and the retraining of specific muscle groups. The specificity in such training is extremely high, extending to the retraining of *single* motor units monitored by microelectrodes in lower motor neuron disease.[8] Similarly, it is evident that so-called involuntary visceral functions have their own learning curves; that gut motility, heart rate[9] and regularity of heartbeat, blood pressure,[10] and peripheral temperature[11] can be beneficially influenced through biofeedback training, a process which proprioception is made instrumentally manifest. Even so, biofeedback (however useful) is viewed by its proponents as a prosthetic training device.

There is, to be sure, quite a distance between the relief of pain and discomfort, and the experience of positive well-being; that territory is relatively untraveled in Western society. The alcohol and tobacco industries, prescription and over-the-counter drugs, and food dependency (and the success of weight reduction enterprises) all attest to the deep dependencies of the average man on chemical prostheses for the relief of anxiety, pain, depression, hostility and anger. These are all negative emotions (though, viewed appropriately, even pain can be seen as a friend) and man appears ready to pay a high price to reduce them. Mere relief of pain and anxiety is, in and of itself, a powerful reinforcement. The highly lucrative alcohol, tobacco, and pharmaceutical industries oblige. The circle of discomfort, dis-ease, and dependency is fostered by an economic cycle, reinforcing dependent states of mind. Drowned by word fallout[12], swamped by products, and stunned by sensory overload (including T.V.), individual autonomy is reduced, and passivity prevails. Like Pirandello's characters, the feeling of being necessary is looking for its authors. All this is obvious, and has been said a thousand times.

But beyond the hoopla of relief of stress and reduction of anxiety, anger, and pain, we again return to the home base of the body. For, while strident or ambiguous in discomfort, dis-ease, and disorder, the body can signal equally clearly when things are going well; when there is ease, comfort, sufficiency, and order. The biological needs of the body ("I'm necessary — use me") and of growth and development ("I renew constantly — challenge me, and expand my capacities") are expressed in various ways: in games, in recreation, in the training of sensormotor skills, indoors and out. Physicians, by and large, are both untrained and unprepared to give expert counsel in these areas. But nothing helps like self-help. Anyone who has engaged a child in an active outdoor game, or has run, or has surfed, will know the peculiar sensation of sensorimotor sharpening and the wonderful feeling of being in touch with one's body. The gates of perception — enteroceptive as well as sensorimotor — can be both open, and focused, in an operation all compact. There is a significant paradox here. While states of well-being can be reached by way of movement and active exercise — running, tennis, squash, swimming, or golf (or, for that matter, disco dancing — more passive avenues, such as sensory awareness[13] or skilled massage, can lead to them also. The sexual dance comprises all elements. Many guides to sensory awareness, to posture and movement, have developed, and hosts of schools, seminars, and workshops are available to return to the alienated body some of its native skills. That a searching awareness industry should be flourishing at the same time a chemical dependency industry, bent on reducing anxiety, thrives, is not without its humor, and attests to the vitality of free enterprise, as well as the balancing forces at work in any economic system. To be sure, mass appeal is a very poor guide. Yet, among a bevy of latter-day dogmas and gurus, there are to be found some important and biologically sound rules, which time will sift, codify, and organize into a coherent body of knowledge. A clearing house of the various approaches, a critical examination of who's who and what's what, is much needed.[14]

Central to the process of body awareness training is learning to attend to the cues the body emits, or the senses convey, and to the contingencies under which bodily sensations are experienced. This proprioceptive attention to cues improves with practice. It is greatly enhanced by careful daily record-keeping, and by an analysis of the days' contingencies in terms of circumstances to which mood and body sensations are related.[15] Furthermore, it is now reasonably established that, as a preparatory step to retraining, such awareness is enhanced by reduction of conscious effort (which is all too often locked into the vigilant scanning of the outer world) and by carefully engaging in states of low arousal (such as autogenic training and meditative states,[16] which allow for a much clearer recognition of signals from within. In these states, the sensory input is deliberately reduced, making for less noise in the detection of enteroceptive and proprioceptive signals. It is, perhaps, also significant that these states are greatly enhanced by the deliberate attention to the function of breathing, the only involuntary function normally under voluntary control. Breathing is slowed, and deepened, and becomes more phrenic-diaphragmatic than intercostal. One wonders, parenthetically, about a possible connection between these practices and the liberation in the brain of naturally produced small molecules (such as the endorphins and related neuropeptides)[17] some of whose sites are congruent with the cells exercising respiratory control. There is, incidentally, one other way of sharpening inner sensory awareness: it is by attempting to observe silence for an extended period, and doing habitual things (whether buttering bread, walking, or biting into an apple) more slowly. A number of religious practices in the East and West have emphasized this simple approach. A practice session of three days, under guidance is recommended as a good learning experience to listening to one's body. Discrimination must be used, however. Obsessionals and hypochondriacs, beware!

Remembering Things Present: Inner Speech, Intention, Will, and Inner Learning

The heart of traditional psychotherapy rests in the bringing into awareness the relation of past history to present events; an appraisal, both in terms of effect and reason, of the genesis of longstanding habits of thought and behavior; and a testing of new insights through enactment in the school of day-to-day living. In this often painful process of inner and interpersonal learning, the recall of repressed memories of distant early childhood looms large. The long period of postnatal maturation and the plasticity of the nervous system in our species make this early period critical in the genesis of models and values, and the parent· figures an immediate family — or their surrogates — still form a most important school in the life of man. Yet much recent thought has stressed the import and positive value of critical phases throughout the life cycle as a whole.[18] Rites of passage, in various forms, mark profound transformations from childhood to adolescence, from adolescence to early adult life, on to the crises of middle age, and thence, by way of other sharp upheavals, to the tranquil harbors of maturity. The life events which commonly accompany these transformations have been codified, and their relative stress quotients assessed.[19] As ego function matures, reactions become more temperate and allowing. There is more centering, more appraisal, and more call upon a caring benevolent will. The mature person is his or her own parent, and the bonding to others is balanced by self-regard and a caring for the loved self.

However, we are not concerned here with therapy, but with day-to-day living. Just as awareness of body signals signify ill-being and well-being, dis-ease and ease, so sensitivity and awareness to ongoing internal symbolic events and their relation to outer situational cues can give one valuable position readings in a complex and continuously changing array of internal transactions. It is often much, much harder to tune into the ongoing present than to project (and avoid) this very present by way of well-traveled trajectories into both past and future. For awareness of things present is often banal and obvious and buried instantly because of such obviousness. But it is the banal and the obvious which form the day. Avoiding the obvious can badly upset internal housekeeping; and dealing with it makes for smoothness, effectiveness, and harmony of operation. The quality, then, is one of inner sensing of events as they occur, and integrating them into day-to-day living. This implies being aware of the inner speech that proceeds continuously within, and of the automatic thoughts it reflects; and drawing cues from related feeling states and bodily sensations.

This is clearly not everybody's game. Carried to the extreme, it results in ruminative obsession and paralysis. But it is also a game which can be learned to be played smoothly and automatically. The above is an elaborate way of stating what is actually quite simple. Spurious self-observation anchored to a particular hypothesis (e.g., infantile trauma, or early cathexes to ambivalent figures in childhood) is apt to be limited in range and limiting in outcome. A habit of self-observation, linking present sensations to immediate antecedents (which may well echo and resonate with older psychological structures), is apt to be as interesting and more productive. It is a way of examining alternatives and instituting change. The practice of self-observation (and self-monitoring) in restructuring assumptions and habits, which (by nothing more serious than default) have come to dominate and to deny the enjoyment of one's day, can be both gratifying and useful. Cognitive therapy[20] is coming into its own in many guises, from the reassessment of vague discomforts, to a clarification of values and priorities (and of congruence between personal time-investment and priorities), the treatment of dependency disorders (including food dependency), and the management of depression.[20] Self-monitoring instruments and devices — forms, cards, charts, and counters — abound, and are designed to further self-reward and to provide incentive as a person navigates through the day and the week. Counting and accounting of events helps; and seeing events in their cognitive, effective, and situational context forms valuable personal training prostheses.

What the author has also found particularly useful is to divide the day into four segments — waking, mid-morning, afternoon, and night — providing a distinct and brief (five to ten minute) review period for the appraisal of each segment, coupled with a more comprehensive whole-day review, focusing, perhaps, on one target aspect at a time. The sense of well-being ("What or whom have I most enjoyed today?" "What has moved me, made me feel better or more hopeful?" "What or who has been toxic, and is to be avoided?") must never, never be let go by default; it is often forgotten because it has not been specifically asked for.

Pervading the above is the cardinal place cognitive appraisal and interpretation in determining effective and visceromotor responsiveness and furthering self-efficacy.[21] This view, supported by strong experimental evidence from the laboratory, outlined elsewhere in this volume, marshals convincing evidence that cognitive structures in this case, expectations of personal efficacy can determine the extent of initiation and duration of coping behavior, and are critical to the acquisition of competence and persistence in a particular task, and its ultimate mastery.

In a curious way, we are witnessing the return of the concepts of intention and will (abused by a rigid Victorian era, and by the blood and iron of World Wars I and II) to practical lifemanship; will, that is, alloyed to a faculty of listening and allowing. This faculty, far from being a demanding, tyrannical quality, emerges as a benificent and integrating force, focusing and fusing deep constructive forces toward optimal development and growth. The school of psychosynthesis,[22] based on cognate premises, has developed a rich array of techniques, using (particularly) imagery, to tap into a person's inner territories and achieve congruence between intention and action. An especially valuable concept has been that of the existence of autonomous subpersonalities (often quite numerous, and mutually contradictory, or even exclusive) in a person, and the development of techniques for their identification and understanding. These techniques appear effective in linking cognitive structures to effect, and monitoring oneself through the confusing babble of internal speech. It is good to know that these approaches are gradually finding wider acceptance, and that the spiritual element of a centering belief in the self (very akin to the Jungian view) is gaining increasing recognition.

The Many in the One: Getting Acquainted with the Persons Within

As the listening to the continuous inner conversation proceeds, a person may, before very long, become aware of the living multiple and ever-changing topology that is him or her. To be sure, the sense of one-ness, of I-ness is comforting; and the executive functions of the ego, if in good working order, guide one safely from task to task. The crisis often comes when an external task, even if well-executed, fails to provide a sense of identity or satisfaction, or when a close relationship falters because of the false premises which inform it. The crises of identity (as we call them) that follow are strange and awesome to behold in the violence of their paradoxes, in the pain, anger, strife, and sadness, and in the sense of waste and futility which they carry in their wake. "Something happened," "He does not know who he is," "She is another person," we say. There is deep truth in such statements. For such crises often signify confrontations between relatively autonomous psychological entities or structures, each having deep (and very different) demand characteristics. They represent other personages within, which may have grown silently at different rates throughout a person's life in response to (or to a lack of) particular challenge or circumstance. They are nourished from various sources, and, with time, they each assume an autonomy of their own, manifesting in dreams and daydreams, fantasies, hobbies, or the fierce frustration and anger of non-achievement. Their genesis in a person's life — the mix of modeling and psychosocial learning which went into their making — does not here concern us. What we wish to emphasize is their autonomy. Appropriately, they have been termed subpersonalities,[23] enacted to various degrees in the private or public stages of our lives, with various degrees of verismilitude. There may, indeed, be quite a cast of characters — the gentle giver, the compulsive care-giver, the acquisitive-taker, the private dreamer-artist, the ruthless manipulator, the public figure, and the practical person-of-affairs. Many of them never see the light of day, and they protest and scream to be heard when they are not. Writers are familiar with the phenomenon: They send these subpersonalities into the world. Most of us are not so well-acquainted with the persons within, and get to know the guests in our taverns only when the noise is too loud to be ignored. It is a matter of simple prudence to spot them beforehand, engage them in conversation, and promote their conversation with one another. Only thus can we determine what and who is compatible with whom; and only thus can we encourage them to do our work for us, conjointly, if possible — and, if this proves impracticable, make them work on a time-sharing basis, identifying their assets and giving their time within the realm of the possible.

There are various approaches to coming to grips with this multiplicity. The uses of imagery and guided daydreams have now been worked out in some detail.[24] Role-playing and role-reversal provide other avenues. Attending to cues in daily life, and, when they occur, keeping appointments with inner demands at appropriate quiet periods of the day may be another approach. Other means are as multiple as one's own creative inventiveness. Yet certain principles inform the process. One is the recognition and respect for the autonomy of these highly organized psychological entities, and the importance of addressing them in a feeling, sentient way in the *present*. A second is great care in attempting premature fusion between incompatibles, or a premature negation of one or another until matters are thoroughly explored. Third is the cultivation of kindly disidentification from tyrannical structures as they recur, and establishment, through practice, of a still inner observer's post in which the huge sway (a sort of gravitational pull) of feelings is noted, but not allowed to overpower this central capacity to observe (this requires much practice). Fourth is the development of a tolerance of ambiguity and incompatibility, and the use of the constructive forces (which may, at times, be hidden in even quite negative experiences or fantasies) by learning to recognize a signal and its obverse. And, finally, a continuous awareness of the hazard of hazards — namely, of the cutting off by denial — must be developed. Implicit in the above is a conscious acceptance of the inner pluralism within, through an awareness of the adaptive and creative role and function of individual components as they are recognized.

Much good can come from such acceptance. Paradoxically, as each is given its place, and as barriers between various subselves are loosened and the rivers of communication begin to flow, the sense of selfhood and fusion, of deeply enhanced personal effectiveness, one-ness, and the feeling of autonomy identity and personal power can be observed to grow in a striking manner. It is moving to note this in a client: The term "guidance" (or self-guidance, or journey) is an entirely appropriate description of the process. The emergent school of psychosynthesis[25] has developed valuable and original approaches for the discrete study of the phenomena seen in such personal changes. Very appropriately, it recognizes the central benevolent function of serious intention and informed will, and reaffirms — as was recognized by Maslow — the deep fear most of us harbor of doing not only our worst, but also our best.[26]

"Time Out": Suggestions for a Pause for Personal Learning

Mention has been made above of the person-in-crisis. It is by now reasonably well known that when seen in practice, such clients do not readily fit established categories, making it hard to do full justice to their needs. Traditional psychotherapy — even limited contract psychotherapy — may not be the method of choice. Experience suggests that despite disabling symptoms (which may variously manifest themselves as panic, diffuse anxiety, depression, and severe somatisation of various kinds), full hospitalization is rarely indicated. There remains the office visit, with the client coping with the daily routine at work and at home as best as he or she can; a combination of intensive office work, psychological homework, and a change in daily routine; the proverbial holiday, with office work before and after; or, if symptoms are severe enough, taking time off and engaging in intensive work with the therapist (who, by now, may be uneasily wondering about hospitalization — *malgré soi*). The modalities have one thing in common: The person undergoing a major life transition, while being pushed and signaled by his symptoms to attend to his or her needs, often does so piecemeal, with time divided unevenly, and inner learning interrupted by counter-productive outer intrusion. However, mental crises, like physical illness, deserve respect. They must be taken seriously and afforded their own good time. It is suggested that setting aside a given and limited time for serious psychological work in a quiet, unobtrusive, unemcumbered environment, (preferably as part of a small group composed of individuals with similar needs) may be an effective and economical way of assisting the person-in-crisis or in transition.

Such needs are seen again and again in a person recovering from unexpected serious illness (such as myocardial infarction, major surgery, or a severe debilitating illness) where a restructuring of goals and lifestyle is desirable, and where convalescence affords a special opportunity for systematic, intensive psychological work and experiential re-learning. Similar needs are encountered in persons engaged in major life changes (such as career change, major crises in marital or family life, retirement, and the crises of aging). A common element is the recognition by the client (or clients) that, to make the process efficient, both a commitment and full-time attention over an agreed and limited period of time are needed, and that personal learning must continue beyond a period of residence, and be carried into daily life. The essence of such a program, named "time out," is to provide a person with the opportunity to examine, in as honest a fashion as possible, the principal forces operating in his or her life to date; to afford an opportunity to view the origins and course of the present crisis; to acquire listening skills with regard to his or her own body, and scanning and analytical skills with regard to contingencies operating in the immediate day-to-day environment (family, friends, work, and the vast array of day-to-day sociocultural demands); to recognize clearly which of these have positive effects and which have negative effects; to appraise realistically the demand characteristics of his or her hidden assets and talents (subpersonalities) and the varying degrees to which these can be satisfied; and to become aware of the negative contingencies, including undesirable habits and dependencies (food, nicotine, alcohol, and chronic pain) which may be at work, eroding day-to-day enjoyment. In short, for the individual to re-examine the hypotheses by which he or she has lived, to put such hypotheses alongside alternative hypotheses, and to acquire, during the full time out engagement, some skills in self-observation, stress reduction, self-regulation, and planning, which are simple and can be readily incorporated into daily life, are unlikely to be lost through non-compliance, and can be monitored in systematic, regular follow-up. Such a psychological program is best combined with a physical health hazard appraisal and recommendations with regard to body fitness, graded exercise, nutrition, and self-management routines, concordant with the results of such an appraisal. The duration of such a program may vary according to condition, needs, and circumstance. As a rule of thumb, it should not be shorter than nine days, or longer than three weeks.

Whatever its duration, the program consists essentially of three phases (of three to seven days each). The first is an exploratory phase of sensing and scanning, in which inner listening is practiced, and sharpening of awareness is enhanced. Such practice is judiciously balanced against other basic skill acquisition. At the end of this phase, a rough topological map of personal assets, goals, and obstacles in achieving goals is available to the client, to be developed further as he or she proceeds. The second phase aims at a deepening of the experience, and the assimilation and synthesis of previous material. Skill training is stepped up, and exercises are designed to show the client's relevance to his or her own personal life circumstances. This could be called a phase of appraisal and personal planning. The third phase is one in which skills are practiced and extended (including exercises of a very practical nature), and the client is prepared for re-entry into daily life, through materials and instructions for home practice and follow-up. This is the phase of testing and re-entry. Throughout the program, there runs, in parallel, a didactic, pedagogic component. This double thread of the pedagogic-didactic and experiential is found to be quite useful. The program will be examined in more detail elsewhere. Below, its essential features are described.

Phase One. As an introductory exercise, the client, either before entering the program or during the early part of phase one, completes a health hazard appraisal questionnaire, undergoes some appropriate psychological testing, and engages in the writing of a personal autobiographical essay. Various formats for writing the essay have been used, some of them coupled with the keeping of a journal.[27] For the purpose of this program, the author has found it useful to invite the client to follow an outline, the flavor of which is given in the introductory paragraphs set out below. It is important that this exercise be a continuous, personal, private, and uninterrupted effort — only thus can the requisite honesty and intensity of work be achieved. If it can be done at home, or in a remote motel room before entering the program, so much the better. However, experience suggests that the flow is enhanced by being in cognate company.

The central message to the client during the autobiography exercise is, quite simply, that there is no place to hide; that the object of the autobiography is to know what can be known. The following initial instructions give the general climate of the exercise:

The purpose of this essay is to give you an opportunity to explore and answer, in writing, the question: "How did I become the person I am?" The gain to you will, in large measure, depend upon the scrupulous honesty with which you pursue this self-enquiry. It is most important, therefore, that you:

1. Report facts as they are, and especially try not to embellish, excuse or disguise unpleasant and unacceptable facts.
2. Be frank with yourself about your own failings as you see them, and equally recognize, without self-diminishment, your assets and achievements.
3. Articulate clearly to yourself the persons and events which influenced your life most, for better or worse.
4. Articulate clearly the rules and values by which you have lived, and any changes that you would hope to achieve in a process of re-evaluation and re-learning.
5. Be as clear as you can be about the events, human relations, and states of mind with which you are most comfortable, as well as those which most disturb or distress you.
6. Be clear about the personal relationships in your life that you have found most nurturing, sustaining, and constructive, even when you were "down."
7. Be clear about personal relations you have found most distressing, disturbing, and draining.
8. Articulate as clearly and realistically as you can what kind of person you would like to be.
9. Articulate clearly the things that give you, or could give you, joy.
10. Define your priorities in terms of job (including its setting), family, friendships, and leisure time activities; and the relative place of public, as opposed to private, recognition of your achievements.
11. Define for yourself the elements which would make a good day for you, and the ways and means of achieving a good day.

The outline that follows is a rough guide to ensure that the topics therein are not omitted by default. You are free to write in any order or style that may suit you. You may wish to consider sections separately, and concentrate on one or two sections at a time. On the other hand, you may wish to write a continuous story. It is suggested that you look over the outline before you begin, and then make, if you wish, an outline of your own, emphasizing the areas that are most important to you. The main thing is to be truthful in telling yourself the story of your life.

This document will be seen only by your therapist and such persons (assigned by your therapist) as are directly working with you. It is privileged communication.

Sections then follow (not reproduced here) covering a range of areas (including: "Personal information: What brings you here?"; "Your family and early life"; "School"; "College"; "Jobs and careers"; "Your social relation and sense of social achievement"; "Your sexual development and attitudes"; "Your courtship, marriage, and children"; "Exercise"; "Your interests, hobbies, and recreation"; "Alcohol and drugs"; "Pain"; "Religious experience, attitude to death and dying"; "Mood and temperament"; and "Your view of yourself and other people's view of you." The client is asked to try to paint a word picture of him/herself: as perceived by him/herself; as perceived by a spouse or companion; as perceived by a best friend; and as perceived by someone the client heartily dislikes. Other areas to be covered are the client's aims and hopes for the future; his or her values and assets; and ways and means of achieving change.

The closing paragraph of instruction reads:

Now return to the introduction of this outline and try to formulate for yourself the things that you value most in your life, and the ways and means by which you think you can achieve them. What are your core values? What are your peripheral values? Remember that the things you consider central to your wellbeing are non-negotiable. Consider your assets and your positive personal traits. Consider the most positive persons and circumstances in your life, and how they can be made to work in your favor. Consider persons and circumstances which are negative, and drain you, and how they may be avoided in the future. Consider your work, job, family. Consider what, realistically, could improve your present circumstances. Consider what could give you a good day. Develop a plan: Think realistically in terms of a timetable and a gradual step-by-step approach. Remember that there is comfort in facts, not in fantasies, and that the best dreams are the possible dreams. You are responsible for your own wellbeing.

Through the completion of this exercise — which can be very meaningful and poignant, the client may begin to acquire a rough map of the terrain, portions of which he or she may be ready to survey in greater depth through the use of relaxation, dream and fantasy work, and guided imagery. These latter techniques are introduced by way of graded exercises, attuned to a person's capacity and readiness to pursue them. At the same time, the client learns some simple, autogenic exercises, and gains familiarity with selfregulation and voluntary control by way of biofeedback (used as a prosthetic tool, rather than as an end). Sensory and body awareness exercises are also introduced at this stage, the overall purpose being to facilitate a gentle loosening of mental spasms, and a safe opening-up of the portals of awareness.

Phase Two. In this phase, the awareness training continues, and more emphasis is placed on a clear recognition of the demand characteristics of various aspects of the personality as it is manifested in the autonomous, and sometimes strident, subpersonalities, within. Vargiu[29] has described the components of identification, acceptance, coordination, utilization, and syntheses (i.e., the establishment of congruence) in work of this kind. A survey of relative hierarchies of priorities (in terms of time the client invests in each in his daily life) clarifies matters of congruence (or lack of it) between aim and practice. In this phase, tentative plans may be emerging for a rearrangement, or a compromise time-sharing in the use of various positive attributes. Distorted relationships to spouse, children, business associates, and friends, may be perceived more clearly, or mourning work may be engaged in for relationships which have outlived their usefulness. At the same time, while awareness training continues (using role-playing, role-reversal, and other in-the-present-tense techniques), some instructional materials are introduced to educate the client in the elements of the self-regulatory process, and in learning skills which may stand him or her in good stead in outside life. These include an exposure to the psychophysiology of coping and stress (including elementary neurochemistry and endocrinology) and its relation to anxiety, insomnia, and depression; the place of cyclic phenomena in the regulation of life events; the relation between life events and coping; the immune response; elements of learning theory and cognitive psychology; and the nature of the restorative processes of healing. There may also be data from experimental and social ecology and epidemiology bearing upon both the failure of competent coping and the enhancement of competence. In all this, the element of personal perception and appraisal is emphasized, enhancing the client's feeling of personal responsibility and personal control. While this is proceeding, there is also some direct exposure to elements of nutrition (first-hand kitchen laboratory experience in the preparation of light, nutritious, and attractive foods); graded active exercise, with emphasis on the psychological factors in performance and their effect on mood; and, if desired, slow-movement modalities which give the body experience in balance and control. There is also the beginning of log-keeping of on-going mental events, contingency analyses of circumstances as they happen; and, if possible, basic training in the gathering, holding, and appraisal of one's dreams.

Phase Three. As the relative constellations and strengths of the various aspects of a person's life emerge, the client may be ready to examine some alternative hypotheses to the one he/she may have lived by, and develop a rationale, articulated plan for a more satisfying and restorative style of life. In this phase, the client is preparing for re-entry. He or she is encouraged to make telephone calls, to check into affairs at home and in the office, and to use the skills acquired in practice runs of all kinds. This involves the creating of a framework of time built into each day, in which the client is available primarily to him/herself. Be it jogging, squash, or tennis, meditation or prayer, journal-keeping, self-monitoring, or the evening review, or weight watching or other habit control, the important element is the acquisition of awareness, and the building of helpful, non-tyrannical routines arrived at by choice, and reinforced by the sheer outcome of their observance. During this phase, too, the client is made familiar with the practices and use of a number of self-observation instruments; is given guidance concerning ancillary training materials which may be commercially available; and is instructed for the follow-up process (and possible future refresher "booster" workshops) which is at the heart of long-term follow-up studies in compliance. The family and work institutions are engaged in this process as allies. This is not always easy, and requires tact, patience, planning, and — above all — gentle persistence.

Follow-Up. Upon discharge, the client is followed by regular telephone contact, follow-up questionnaires (including, if agreed to, one directed to family members, who are asked to share their impressions with the client), letters, tapes, journals, reviews, and the like. The communication is kept easy and encouraging, offering professional service but guarding against anything smacking of dependence. Its message is simply: "It is all your own 'now': Be aware; be responsible."

Summary

Living a good day, one day at a time, is a useful measure of the quality of life. Present-day culture has neglected the day. The abounding hedonic ennui presages the difficulties of a post-industrial age, in which leisure will be a principal product.

It is suggested that inner resources in a person, and capacities for social contact, communication, love, and commitment can be mobilized through training of inner sensing and interpersonal awareness. Aspects of body awareness, listening to inner speech, systematic work with one's subpersonalities, and social contingency analysis are briefly considered and related to concepts of self-efficacy, expectation, awareness, choice, and responsibility.

REFERENCES

1. Knowles, John H. (Ed.), *Doing Better and Feeling Worse: Health in the United States.* W. W. Norton & Co., New York: 1977.
2. Lefcourt, H.M., *Locus of Control: Current Trends in Theory and Research.* Hillside, New Jersey: Lawrence Erlbaum, 1977.
3. Schwarz, G. and Shapiro, D. (Eds.), "Consciousness and Self Regulation," in *Advances in Research and Theory* 2. New York: Plenum Press, 1977.
4. Livingstone, R.B., "Sensory Processing: Perception and Behavior," in *Biological Foundation of Psychiatry,* 1, pp. 47–144, Grenell, R.G. and Gabay, S. (Eds.). New York: Raven Press, 1976.
5. Bakan, D., *Disease, Pain, and Sacrifice Towards a Psychology of Suffering.* University of Chicago Press, p. 129, 1968.
6. Reich, W., *Character Armoring: Selected Writings.* New York: Farrar, Straus, & Giroux, pp. 44–181, 1973.
7. Miller, Neal E., "Biofeedback and Visceral Learning," *Ann. Res. Psychol.* 29: 373–404, 1978.

8. Debacher, Gary and Basmajian, John V., "EMG Feedback Strategies in Rehabilitation of Neuromuscular Disorders," in *Biofeedback and Behavior*, Beatty, Jackson and Legewie, Heiner (Eds.). Nato Conference Series, Series III, Human Factors, New York: Plenum Press, 1976.

9. Engel, Bernard T., "Biofeedback as Treatment for Cardiovascular Disorders: A Critical Review," in *Biofeedback and Behavior*, Beatty, Jackson and Legewie, Heiner (Eds.). Nato Conference Series, Series III, Human Factors, New York: Plenum Press, pp. 395–401, 1976.

10. Schwartz, Gary E., "Biofeedback and Patterning of Autonomic and Central Processes: CNS–Cardiovascular Interactions," in *Biofeedback: Theory and Research*, Schwartz, Gary E. and Beatty, Jackson (Eds.). New York: Academic Press, pp. 183-219, 1977.

11. Taub, Edward, "SELF-Regulation of Human Tissue Temperature," in *Biofeedback: Theory and Research*, Schwartz, Gary E. and Beatty, Jackson (Eds.). New York: Academic Press, pp. 265-300. New York.

12. Elkes, J., "Presidential Address: Word Fallout: Or, on the Hazards of Explanation," in *The Psychopathology of Adolescence*. New York: Grune & Stratton, pp. 118-137, 1970.

13. Brooks, C.V., *Sensory Awareness: The Rediscovery of Experiencing*. New York: Viking Press, 1974.

14. Elkes, J. *Education for Health Enhancement and Behavioral Medicine*, BMA T-233. New York: BMA Publications, 1978.

15. Meichenbaum, D., *Cognitive-Behavior Modification*. New York: Plenum Press, 1977.

16. Luthe, W., *Stress and Self-Regulation: Introduction to the Methods of Autogenic Therapy, A Workshop Manual*. Montreal: International Institute of Stress, 1977.

17. Snyder, S.H., "Opiate Receptor in Normal and Drug Altered Brain Function," *Nature*, pp. 257–262, 1975.

18. Vaillant, G.E., *Adaptation to Life*. Boston: Little, Brown & Co., 1977.

19. Dohrenwend, B.S. and Dohrenwend, B.P., *Stressful Life Events*. New York: John Wiley and Sons, 1974.

20. Beck, A., *Cognitive Therapy and the Emotional Disorders*. New York: International Universities Press, 1976.

21. Bandura, A., "Self-Efficacy: Towards a Unifying Theory of Behavioral Change," *Psychol. Rev.* 84: 191-215, 1977.

22. *Synthesis*. Redwood City, California: The Synthesis Press, 1974.

23. Vargiu, J., "Subpersonalities," in *Synthesis* 1. Redwood City, California: The Synthesis Press, pp. 51-89, 1974.

24. Shorr, J.E., *Psychoimagination Therapy*. New York: Intercontinental Medical Book Corp., 1972.

25. *Synthesis*. Redwood City, California: The Synthesis Press, 1974.

26. Maslow, A., *Neurosis as a Failure of Personal Growth, Humanitas* III: 153-169, 1966.

27. Progoff, Ira, *At a Journal Workshop. The Basic Text and Guide for Using the Intensive Journal*. New York: Dialogue House Library, 1975.

28. Vargiu, J., "Subpersonalities," in *Synthesis* 1. Redwood City, California: The Synthesis Press, pp. 51-89, 1974.

6

The Medical Self-Care Movement: Past, Present, and Future

Keith W. Sehnert, M.D.

School of Public Health, University of Minnesota

One essential element in the perception of health promotion is medical self-care/ self-help. Properly utilized, this element becomes a part of the matrix of the health care process, as lay persons are encouraged to actively function for themselves and their families to prevent, detect, and treat common illnesses and injuries; to promote positive health habits; and to supplement — or, if necessary, to substitute for — professional health care.

Many observers say the medical self-care movement is a "new" phenomenon; others say it has always been a well-established resource. Daniel Weiss, M.D., a professor at the University of Kentucky Medical School, describes self-care as part of the "Dual System" of health care.[1] He has traced it back to ancient Greece and prehistoric times and defines this Dual System as a double level of care offered through the ages, on one level by professionals, the doctor or medicine man, and on another level by ordinary citizens using home remedies and folk medicine.

The mists of prehistoric time, when blown away, reveal the shaman (medicine man) treating people for a fee with his incantations and secret remedies. Those less affluent who accidentally speared themselves while hunting, or who were stricken with illness, had to fend for themselves or seek help from a knowledgeable older member of the tribe.

By 300 B.C. or thereabouts, Hippocrates had helped create in Ancient Greece a professional called "physician." Physicians used observation and logic and developed a training system for those who wanted to enter this new profession. Neophyte physicians took the Hippocratic Oath and pledged certain ethical behavior when they began their practice of medicine.

According to John Scarborough, an expert on medicine in ancient Greece, the new professionals were an elite lot — usually the best educated people in town.[2] Some, such as the mayors of Athens, Sparta, and other city-states, mixed politics with medicine. Physician's fees were high and many could not afford their services. The Greeks, however, were practical folk and ruled that any citizen who couldn't afford to go to a physician could go instead to the agora (market square). There, the ailing and injured made their problems known to their fellow citizens. Self-help advice was offered and usually gratefully accepted.

Helping those who were hurting became a tradition and then a part of Greek law. The law later said that if it was known that any citizen *failed* to give help (and if that particular passerby had the knowledge and experience to help), then the citizen could be sued for all his property. With such a law as that on the books, Greeks had strong motivation to learn and practice self-care skills! (What a far cry from the dilemma facing today's Good Samaritans, who often do not offer help because they fear lawsuits.)

The Dual System persisted throughout the Dark and Middle Ages, through such practitioners as "medical police" (precursors to today's army doctors), folk healers, bone setters, and apothecaries (forerunners to today's pharmacists).

After Colonial America was settled, American merchants and farmers who wanted their sons to become physicians sent them abroad for training at Aberdeen, Edinburgh, and London. This was an expensive undertaking, and the fees the doctors charged on return to the Colonies were high. Therefore, most common people went instead to apothecaries for their care and advice. Early American leaders, such as Cotton Mather, Benjamin Franklin, and Thomas Jefferson, took some training as apothecaries. A popular book used then was John Tennent's *Everyman His Own Doctor: or The Poor Planter's Physician.*[3]

Mr. Jefferson thought the things he learned about handling common ills and injuries so important that, as provost of the University of Virginia, he instituted a self-care/self-help course, making it required for all freshmen.

In more recent times, during the Depression, most people "did for themselves and their families" because they didn't have the money or the transportation for professional help. Older, more experienced individuals in the family provided counsel and help for the ill and injured with an assist from an always ready "Doctor Book."

By the end of World War II, with the advent of higher spendable incomes, the increased availability of health insurance, better communications, all-weather roads, more cars, easier access to doctors and hospitals, and a variety of other social, cultural, and economic influences, people became increasingly dependent upon the professional for health care. The doctor, with new medicines and tools, was supposed to "solve" all the health problems confronting a patient.

This doctor-dependency was accentuated over the years by the experience and training of doctors. Military medicine during World War II, the Korean War, and the Vietnam War favored authoritarian methods: "Take your medicine . . . no questions asked and no answers expected."

America's medical care system thrived as the U.S. entered the 1950's with its Golden Age of Pharmaceuticals: immunizations to control measles, mumps, and polio; tranquilizers for mental ills; and the "Pill" to help family planning.

The Sixties brought Space Age spinoffs and the "marriage" of medicine and engineering. This made possible coronary care units, monitoring of all kinds, and the technology needed for the miracles of transplant surgery. This decade also brought increasing trouble for primary care (the kind of medical care provided by family doctors, pediatricians, general internists, and obstetrician/gynecologists) as older G.P.'s died or retired. Then, after years of neglect, danger alarms were sounding for primary care, and national efforts were started to train more family doctors and allied professionals.

The Seventies found the public with a renewed interest and emphasis on primary care, ushering in a whole new raft of primary care professionals: physician's assistants, nurse practitioners, and paramedics, plus new ways to pay for and deliver primary care (such as Health Maintenance Organizations and Alternative Delivery Systems). Meanwhile, something had happened to Americans—while they weren't looking. The nature of disease seen by health professionals had changed. In the Fifties, the killers and maimers were nature's pathogens: polio, measles, tuberculosis, meningitis, pneumonia, and a wide variety of other infectious diseases. By the Seventies, the enemies were man-made pathogens: the cigarette, the automobile, the gun, air pollution, alcohol, and so on.

Diseases of the 1950's could be controlled or vanquished by washing the hands, covering the nose and mouth, keeping things clean, giving immunizations, taking antibiotics, and following established medical and hygienic programs; but the diseases of the 1970's are, unfortunately, not controlled as easily. New types of "hygiene" were needed. Individuals are "taught" to use the man-made pathogens via advertising. People do not inherently want to smoke or drink alcohol, etc., but are "educated" into it with great skill and at great expense (an example of this expense is a new brand of cigarettes introduced in 1977 by R.J. Reynolds, at a cost of $40 million in *introductory* ads! It will cost that much or more each year to maintain the cigarette's place in the marketplace – paid for by new generations of Americans "taught to enjoy" smoking). The new challenge for us is to help people discard these negative health habits and to replace them with healthy ones.

Most of today's illnesses, injuries, and deaths are directly or indirectly related to lifestyle. The same affluence that brought the all-weather roads, more cars, and better communications also brought high cholesterol, low-fiber diets, decreased physical activity, increased leisure time, increased air pollution, and increased anxiety to be assuaged with tranquilizers and alcohol. Companion changes were greatly increased hospital and medical costs, more super-specialists (and fewer primary care professionals), an increased number of malpractice suits, more potent medicines, and greater reliance by professionals on costly, high-technology equipment for treatment and diagnosis.

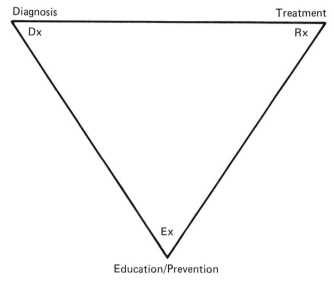

Diagnosis

Treatment

Education/Prevention

Figure 6-1.

The result of all these changes is a movement *away* from what *professionals* can do and toward what *individuals* can do; thus, the medical self-care movement was born, its "parents" being combinations of cultural, social, medical, and economic events.

In the early 1950's, medical students were taught that every doctor-patient visit should have three distinct, equal parts: diagnosis, treatment, and education (as shown in Figure 6-1).

With the assumption that such activities were equally important, it was determined that every dollar spent for health care would be split three ways: 33¢ for each. A recent economic analysis, however, shows that less than 4¢ of each health dollar is spent for education and disease prevention! Substantial increases in money for health education/promotion must be made to put things in balance.

The overloaded primary care system might benefit from such increases. On any given day, 80% of the total demand for health care in America (as shown in Figure 6-2) is for primary care. Studies show that each person requires, on an average throughout life, four such visits per year. But studies show that, in most communities, less than 50% of health professionals are available to deliver such care. This means there is a gap between supply and demand of at least 30%. In rural and inner city areas, overload is much greater.

There is no such overload on services in the secondary and tertiary care sectors. The demand for secondary level care (that is, care associated with the services of community hospitals for conditions requiring operations or more intensive medical treatment) is about 15%. People need such care once every 10 years. Tertiary care is provided by university or other major medical centers

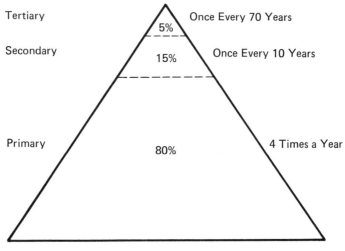

Figure 6-2.

where unusual, complex, life-threatening conditions are treated. Such care is needed only once in 70 years.

Studies of the use of primary care offices show that 30–40% of the visits made to physicians are inappropriate or perhaps even unnecessary. Educational efforts could be made to help decrease such visits. Individuals could be taught how to better use these services. This would help decrease some of the current overload brought on by inappropriate use.

When people are ill or injured, there are three general resources available: professional, community, or individual. During the last three decades, people have been told, "When you get sick, go to your doctor." If that isn't possible, the community offers help through mental health clinics, emergency rooms, immunization services, VD clinics, various counseling and out-patient services, air or water pollution control centers, etc. People seldom think of *themselves* or other non-professionals as proper resources for help. Actually, experience has shown that lay people are capable of handling a third of the common ills, injuries, and emergencies. Patients can become their own "paramedics"! Increasing numbers of people are ready to take this option, and reports show growing interest in classes teaching medical self-care and various do-it-yourself courses.

The Course for Activated Patients (CAP) was first given in Herndon, Virginia in 1970. It was established to provide individuals with skills and experiences that would enable them to take a more active role in their own health care and in that of their families. The initial class was composed primarily of patients receiving their care from a family practice medical group in northern Virginia.[4]

CAP, and a similar program at Georgetown University — the Health Activated Person (HAP), developed by Nowakowski and associates[5] at the School of Nursing — have now been taught to hundreds of persons in metropolitan Washington. Through a series of workshops for program coordinators, sponsored by Georgetown University and later by the Health Activation Network, courses have been taught in over 40 states and in several provinces in Canada. Several thousand individuals have been trained in these related programs.

Typically, the courses are taught in 16 2-hour sessions. Topics covered include: "Your Medicine Chest: Friend or Foe?"; "Listening to Your Body"; "Talking With Your Doctor — Better Communication Pays Off"; "The Dangers of Eating American Style"; "Yoga and You"; and "Here's Hoping You're Coping." The topics are not discrete sessions, but are woven together in a complementary manner that encourages health promotion activities, teaches self-care methods, and emphasizes the benefits of wellness.

Participants learn to look at health not as an absence of disease, but as a way to achieve the energy needed to set and then meet life's goals. Health becomes a necessary resource to do what is wanted in life.

The educational objectives for CAP and similar health activation programs are for individuals taking the course to:

1. Accept more individual responsibility for their own care and for that of their families;
2. Learn the skills of observation, description, and handling common illnesses, injuries, and emergencies;
3. Increase their basic knowledge about health problems; and
4. Learn how to use health care resources/services/insurance/medications more economically and appropriately.

Certain situations and attitudes are necessary for the process of health activation:

1. *Wanting.* Wanting more information about their own health (or someone's in their family) because of personal experience.
2. *Knowing.* Having the capacity for gathering knowledge about the health problems they are likely to face.
3. *Enabling.* Having the technical (blood pressure equipment, thermometers, etc.), educational, and other resources and opportunities for field trips, demonstrations, and so on.
4. *Believing.* Experiencing the feedback from learning experiences that provides self-confidence.

There are five elements interwoven in all the courses so that individuals can learn and then practice the following:

1. *Appropriate use of health care system.* Topics are presented that deal with consumerism as it relates to health care regarding better use of money for insurance/medications, avoiding rip-offs, establishing more realistic ideas about what the system and professionals can deliver, etc.

2. *Compliance/health partnership.* Presentations are made that emphasize the importance of both the professional and the patient in medical regimes for acute and chronic problems. In traditional patient education, much is oriented toward the professional. While CAP's emphasis is on people oriented programs.

3. *Observations/treatment methods.* Health activation provides several "how to" sessions to improve skills of observation about common ills and injuries (when? where? what?) skills needed to describe and record the vital signs (blood pressure, pulse, etc.) and certain clinical events. With such information in hand, treatment methods are undertaken with greater understanding.

4. *Decision-making/increased individual responsibility.* Blended into all sessions is an emphasis on increased individual responsibility, initially for simple health care situations, and later for more complex decisions and actions. Self-care/self-help guide books[6] assist individuals in making observations and appropriate decisions. In the process, persons in the courses move away from an overdependence on professionals and toward a greater dependence on themselves for decisions about health and health care.

5. *Health promotion/self-regulation.* The end result of the above elements is health activation. It increases positive health habits, provides an awareness of wellness, and improves the skill of self-regulation.

These elements of health activation are depicted in Figure 6-3, which shows the interaction of the class sessions and the individual.

The educational experience offered by CAP has been so encouraging that many health professionals have now adopted it for their communities, and versions of it are offered (or will be offered in the future) in most states in the U.S. and provinces in Canada. An organization called the Health Activation Network has been established to help interested professionals and individuals to start and evaluate programs. The motto of the Network is: "Towards a Health Partnership: Individual and Professional Working Together." Headquarters are located in Metropolitan Washington, and information about educational materials and services and a quarterly newspaper can be obtained by writing to Box 923, Vienna, VA 22180. Another source of useful teaching materials can be found in "Medical Self-Care" magazine, Box 717, Inverness, CA 94937.

Beyond the Course for Activated Patients model described here, there are a number of self-care programs at such diverse places as Yale University (under the

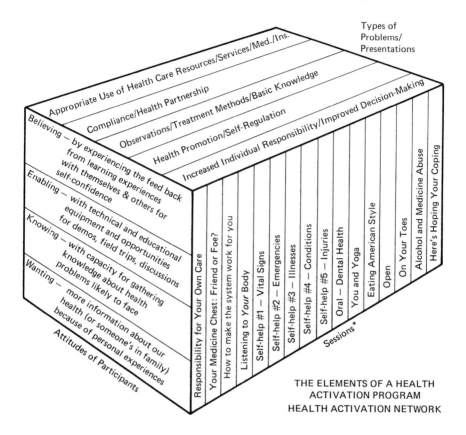

Figure 6-3.

direction of Lowell Levin); the Indian Health Service in Billings, Montana (Ralph Myhre); Minneapolis Health Department, Minneapolis, Minnesota (Al Olson); International Group Plans of Washington, D.C. (Jim Gibbons); the University of Maine, Farmington (Peter Doran); Healthwise, Boise, Idaho (Don Kemper); the University of Nebraska (Betty Young); U.C.L.A. University Extension, Primes Project (Chuck and Mary Ann Lewis); the School of Applied Social Sciences at Case-Western Reserve(Lois Swack and Terry Hokenstad); the Health Skills Association of Dayton, Ohio (Marty Evers); Helping Hand Clinic, St. Paul, Minnesota (Tim Rumsey) and many other academic and health care agencies.

Another sector that should have much future activity in self-care is within American industry. As top executives and their financial staffs have looked at the spiralling health care costs, forward-looking forms such as TRW, a high-technology corporation based in Cleveland; General Mills and Honeywell in Minneapolis; and many other companies across the nation are exploring ways to use health promotion courses and medical self-care.[7]

Medical self-help has been used by people as a health care resource from ancient to modern times. It is likely to extend into the future with an improved level of sophistication and effectiveness because of a number of educational, cultural, social, and economic factors.

Two models of Medical self-care, the Course for Activated Patients (CAP) and the Health Activated Person (HAP), offer skills and options for many persons interested in accepting greater responsibility for their own care and that of their families. These courses, collectively called Health Activation Programs, incorporate the five elements necessary for self-care.

Present trends indicate that an increased number of business corporations, colleges and universities, and health care agencies are developing medical self-help programs to augment primary care. Such efforts should have a positive effect on the future of self-care programs.

REFERENCES

1. Weiss, D., "Who Has Been Responsible for Our Health in the Past? A Workshop: Who is Responsible for Your Health — Your Doctor or You?" Lexington, Kentucky: Kentucky Bureau for Health Services, March 22, 1977.

2. Scarborough, J., *Facets of Hellenic Life*. Boston: Houghton Mifflin, 1976, pp. 212–230.

3. Tennent, J., *Everyman His Own Doctor: or The Poor Planter's Physician, 2nd Edition*. Williamsburg: Printing Office of Colonial Williamsburg, c. 1734.

4. Sehnert, K.W. and Osterweis, M., "The Activated Patient: A Concept for Health Education," *Continuing Education for the Family Physician* **2**, *No. 10*, October 1974.

5. Hamilton, L., "HAP — One Response to Medical Nemesis," *Gerontologist* (in press).

6. Sehnert, K.W. and Eisenberg, H., *How To Be Your Own Doctor — Sometimes*. New York: Grosset and Dunlap, 1975, pp. G1–G128.

7. Sehnert, K.W. and Tillotson, J.K., *A National Health Care Strategy: How Business Can Promote Good Health for Employees and Their Families*. Washington, D.C.: National Chamber Foundation, 1978, p. 1.

7

Health Hazard Appraisal and the Health Care System

John H. Milsum, Sc.D.

Department of Health Care and Epidemiology
and
Director, Division of Health Systems
Health Sciences Center
University of British Columbia

Any *system* — a person, a complete society, or simply an automobile's power steering — must have operational objectives in order to keep working. Further, a system must continually monitor its output performance, in some meaningful terms, to determine how well these objectives are being reached, so that it can then take corrective and optimizing action to reduce any disparities between the desired and the actual performance. In any system which is complex (and certainly, therefore, in the individual human), a whole set of component measures will be necessary to form a meaningful performance criterion. To complicate matters, at least some of these measures will typically be in conflict with others.

Man functionally comprises a large hierarchy of interacting homeostatic systems in which the desired performance level of different systems at one level are set by others at a higher level (as suggested in Figure 7-1). The objectives or desired performance for man's organ systems are relatively easy to establish; for example, the cardiovascular system must maintain a certain cardiac output under given pressure conditions and activity demand. Unfortunately, identifying the objectives becomes increasingly difficult as we move up the hierarchy towards man as a whole system. In this context, Maslow's classification of D-needs (deficiency needs) and B-needs (being needs) provides a useful framework. This Maslovian hierarchy is fundamentally open-ended, since the top is concerned with "various levels of self-actualization." These are presumably not easily included in, nor definable by, the terms of the World Health Organization (WHO) definition of health as "a state of complete physical, mental, and social well-being."

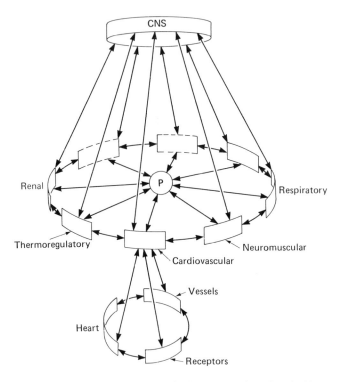

Figure 7-1. The multihierarchical system constituting an organism. Physical interactions between physiological functions are represented by point *P*. (Figure courtesy Academic Press: J.H. Milsum and F.A. Roberge, *Physiological Regulation and Control in Foundations of Mathematical Biology* III, *Supercellular Systems,* Robert Rosen (Ed.). New York, 1973.)

Once we accept that all the feedback control systems in the lower levels of man's hierarchies require objectives for their proper functioning, it becomes even more important to recognize that the higher levels of man's systems controllers (namely, his central nervous system and his psyche) must also have appropriate objectives. Since all of man's subsystems are clearly organized to promote his harmonious functioning as a system, it would seem plausible to expect that health in its full definition would be, at the least, a very important component of harmonious performance at the level of man himself.

The same point may be viewed from a different angle: sickness may be considered a breakdown of the normal harmonious condition of health, due to a strong enough combination of stressful factors acting on the person. In turn, these stressful factors may be highly correlated with the person's perception of a reduced quality in his or her life. In this sense, the integrated amount of sickness across society may represent a measure of reduction in societal quality of life, and thus be conceptually useful for social and political planning.

A problem with the WHO definition of health is that it could be taken to imply that each individual can reasonably expect society to guarantee the conditions for health. However, while it is certainly true that "no man is an island entire of itself," it is equally true and important that each individual be a whole "person," with purposes and objectives appropriate for that person. In this regard, it is worth noting that the word *health* is derived from the Old English word *hāl*, which in turn is cognate with *whole* and *holy*. This implies the integration of body-mind-spirit which has been a central theme throughout human history. Unfortunately, it has become uncomfortable for science to consider the spiritual part, since by its own rules it has essentially nothing to say regarding this matter. On the other hand, since science can apply rigorous methods to those aspects to which it can address itself, its resultant emphasis has been largely upon the body and, more recently, the brain. Thus, by a slow but apparently irrevocable process, medical science has come to look upon man as essentially a machine. McKeown asserts that this has significant implications for medicine, since "the major influences on man's health are behavioral and environmental, rather than the provision of personal medical care."[1] In this vein, Dubos outlined two ideas on health:[2]

1. An approach through a rational way of life, symbolized by the goddess Hygeia.
2. Belief in the physician as healer of the sick, associated with the god Asclepius.

McKeown points out that "since the 17th century at least, the Asclepian approach has been predominant. Philosophically, it derives support from Descartes' concept of the living organism as a machine which might be taken apart and reassembled if its structure and function were fully understood; practically it seemed to find confirmation in the work of Keppler and Harvey and the success of the physical sciences." He continues:

The consequences of this viewpoint are reflected widely in medicine today. Medical education begins with study of the structure and function of the body, continues with the examination of disease processes and ends with clinical instruction on selected sick people. Having regard to the determinants of health, it is as though a training in agriculture ignored limitation of numbers, selective breeding, control of the environment, feeding and care and concentrated on the diagnosis and treatment of sick animals.

The medical services of today are the result of more than a century (three centuries in the case of hospitals) of unplanned development which reflects both the predominant interest in the diagnosis and treatment of acute illness and the relative lack of concern for population measures and the provision of care. Contraceptive advice is only reluctantly accepted as an obligation of health services;

whether to use financial subsidies to make food available to everyone and to influence the kinds of foods that are eaten, is considered to be an economic rather than a medical question; and the control of the physical environment and modification of personal behavior are regarded as subjects of marginal interest which can be relegated to ancillary staff or even removed altogether from medical concern.

The Health Care System

In approaching reconsideration of how best to organize our evolving health care system, a number of different viewpoints may be taken, of which the following three examples are deliberately oversimplified in order to make certain points.

The systems approach is eclectic and multidisciplinary, and consists of a point of view and certain methodology, with the latter being increasingly used in various individual disciplines as well. An elementary attempt at systems analysis certainly suggests strongly that the most important leverage point to consider in trying to bring the costs in our health care system under control, or, more positively, to improve the cost-benefit ratio, would be to increase the proportion of resources given to health promotion and illness prevention. This approach inevitably requires one to consider, as quantitatively as possible, those various costs and benefits in the system which are not easily countable in terms of dollars (e.g., pain, inconvenience, and the value of full health). If such attributes cannot be quantified, then the analysis must be recognized as incomplete. The systems approach also inherently recognizes that the health care system is complex, dynamic, non-linear, and statistical, and that it has multiple feedback and mutually interactive pathways. In such systems, simple interventions seldom have simple expectable outcomes, especially when viewed over a sufficiently long time-scale. For example, while the development of public health measures was clearly essential over the last century, it was done in a way that has resulted in a long-standing, unfortunate lack of integration between public health and personal medical care.

The economist's approach, in principle, is perhaps no different from the above. In practice, it often expected to concentrate upon monetary costs and benefits alone, and to work largely through regression-type models, which are essentially static rather than dynamic. However, econometric modeling, in particular, does consider dynamic aspects. One major problem in analysis is the establishing of a meaningful discount rate, since the outcome of a cost-benefit analysis may be very sensitive to this parameter.[3] The economist's analysis tends to concentrate on man's economic value as a producer, and on the loss to society when he is unavailable for production through illness or death.

The humanistic approach emphasizes the pre-eminent importance of the individual human's "gestalt". Generally, this approach tends to deny that the appropriate attributes for understanding the person's satisfactions and frustrations in the health care system can be quantitatively measurable. This viewpoint would inevitably stress the importance of values, and, consequently, the desirability of helping people to remain healthy.

In approaching the redesign of the health care system, further divisions tend to occur. One viewpoint is that prevention is best pursued through "passive" measures,[4] since man himself is typically not to be trusted with the responsibility for intelligently seeking his own best healthful condition. While, admittedly, the above statement is a simplification, the typical results of this thinking are such measures as good drains, vaccinations, "enriching" additives in food (for example, Vitamin D in milk), and "technological trickery" (for example, that which prevents an individual from starting a car until the seat-belt is buckled). And though almost everyone would accept the first example as being desirable, there would generally be less agreement as we move toward the extreme represented by the last example. Indeed, if we proceed to set up an adversary or competitive situation in order to compel individuals to operate in a way contrary to their normal habits, then they may be stimulated, almost reflexively, to outwit the system. This perverts the individual's normal intention away from promoting his or her own health, and taking responsibility for it, to that of essentially pursuing self-destructive or unnecessarily risky behavior. Such policies could only be effective in the long run if the human were indeed only a passive complex mechanism. The alternative concept for health strategy is that of "active" measures, which stimulate the activity of the person on behalf of his or her health. This involves a tremendous shift of emphasis to educating the public as individuals in terms of understandable, but realistic, models of the nature of health and illness dynamics, with all the complexity implied and discussed above. Thus, for example, it is important to point out the multifactorial nature of illness dynamics, in contrast to the simple cause-effect nature represented by the germ theory, in which an individual almost necessarily succumbs to sickness if attacked by an appropriate agent.

Health Hazard Appraisal

Health Hazard Appraisal (HHA) is an important example of a system which tries to bring together much of the philosophical material so far discussed, but to express it in numerical terms so that the relative importance of different factors can be understood. Furthermore, it is tailored to the individual concerned, focusing on his or her specific health risks. There is, as yet, no convincing evidence that it can achieve a high measure of success in persuading people quickly to embark upon more healthy lifestyles, but preliminary evidence is encouraging. Its primary long-term importance may reside in the fact that it creates a "teachable moment", when a health professional and a client/patient can come together and discuss comprehensively the person's health condition, and the risks to which he or she is being exposed. Possible changes in lifestyle can then be discussed in regard to their potential efficacy, with due respect for the client's present beliefs, reservations, prejudices, etc., in such a way that the decision to contract for change is fundamentally reserved for the client. Further, such frequent repetition of looking at a comprehensive set of risk factors tends to imbue the health professional with a much more urgent sense of the pervasiveness of unhealthy lifestyles and their combined bad effect upon most individuals. An important side-benefit may be that many health professionals will become concerned with improving their own health risks and, hence (ultimately), to become the "exemplars" who can better show the way to their clients. The following excerpt from an anonymous poem seems pertinent here:

> The lectures you deliver
> may be very fine and true
> but I'd rather get my lesson
> by observing what you do.
> For I may misunderstand you
> and the high advice you give,
> But there's no misunderstanding
> how you act and how you live.

HHA was developed at the Methodist Hospital in Indianapolis and is well described in the manual prepared by Robbins and Hall.[5] Since its development in the early sixties, its use has spread widely across North America. However, the proportion of health care professionals in general, and physicians in particular, using it is still very small. Users of HHA have formed the "Society for Prospective Medicine," which holds an annual meeting devoted to discussing developments, experiences and research in the field. This meeting is now in its twelfth year and attracts several hundred participants.

HHA is now typically processed by computer programs, and is offered by many different organizations at a cost which varies considerably, but probably averages around $7 in the U.S.

The HHA Process

The HHA process starts with a questionnaire, currently consisting of about 36 questions in the areas of lifestyle, personal and family medical history, and a limited number of clinical measures. A format used at the University of British Columbia is typical and is reproduced in Figure 7-2. These questions are designed to elicit information for quantification of the person's individual risk factors. The questions are therefore under continual review as epidemiological knowledge changes, and in Canada, for example, it is proposed to modify the set of questions so as to be in accordance with the Canadian experience.

HEALTH
HAZARD
APPRAISAL

Processed by:
Division of Health Systems
Health Sciences Centre
Univ. of BC, Vancouver V6T 1W5

HYGENIA

NAME [| | | | | | | | | | | | | | | | | | | | | | |]
Family   Given   Initial

ADDRESS ——————————

PLEASE RECORD THE MOST APPROPRIATE RESPONSE BY
WRITING THE CODE NUMBER IN THE COLUMN ON THE
RIGHT HAND SIDE OF THE PAGE ——————

or

TO BE COMPLETED BY ALL PARTICIPANTS:

SEX	(1) male (2) female
AGE	(in years)
HEIGHT—without shoes	Ft. Ins.
WEIGHT—IN POUNDS—naked	
FRAME	(1) small (2) medium (3) large
ALCOHOL HABITS (Drinks per week, on average. Include apertifs, wine, beer, etc.)	(1) 41 or more (2) 25-40 (3) 7-24 (4) 3-6 (5) 1-2 (6) stopped (7) never drank
USE OF DRUGS THAT MAY INFLUENCE DRIVING	(1) excess (2) moderate (3) none
SERIOUS DEPRESSION recent, non-menstrual, e.g., disabling	(1) often (2) seldom or never
CURRENT SMOKING HABITS OR HEAVIEST AMOUNT SMOKED IN LAST 5 YEARS (FOR EX-SMOKER, MARK HEAVIEST AMOUNT SMOKED IN YEAR BEFORE QUITTING, EXCEPT AFTER 10 YRS OR MORE NON-SMOKING). (If cigarettes and pipes/cigars, mark only code for cigarettes)	CIGARETTES — (PACKS/DAY) PIPES/CIGARS (#/DAY) NON-SMOKERS (1) 2+ (2) 1 – 2 (5) 5+ or any inhaled (7) do not smoke (3) ½ – 1 (4) ¼ or less (6) 4 or less not inhaled (or have stopped for more than 10 years)
STOPPED SMOKING Mark number of years stopped.* (Mark 0 if still smoking, or non-smoker, or stopped for more than 10 years).	*If stopped less than 1 year mark 1.
MILES DRIVEN PER YEAR (as driver and/or passenger in private motor vehicle) (In thousands of miles)	
SEAT BELT USAGE (percentage of time)	(1) 10% or less (2) 10-24% (3) 25-74% (4) 75-100%
CRIME RECORD	(1) crimes involving (2) crimes with no (3) not possible injury possible injury involved
WEAPONS CARRIED	(1) yes (2) none
EXERCISE PER DAY (1) not much (SEDENTARY) (2) some (LOW MODERATE) (3) fairly active (HIGH MODERATE) (4) very active (VIGOROUS) under 5 flights of stairs 5-15 flights of stairs programmed exercise 4 times/wk. greater than or or or fairly active less than ½ mile of walking ½–1½ miles of walking 15-20 flights of stairs or 1½ miles of walking	
SERIOUS PNEUMONIA (Bacterial)	(1) have had (2) never had
HEART ATTACK PARENTS DIED OF HEART ATTACK PARENTS DIED UNDER AGE 60 NONE OF THESE BEFORE AGE 60 (of other causes), or (4) (1) both parents (2) one parent STILL ALIVE BELOW AGE 60 (3)	
FAMILY HISTORY OF SUICIDE (blood relative)	(1) yes (2) no
FAMILY HISTORY OF DIABETES (blood relative)	(1) yes (2) no
DO YOU HAVE DIABETES?	(1) yes- no treatment (2) yes - under treatment (3) do not have
RECTAL DISORDERS (history of diease other than piles/hemorrhoids	growth: (1) yes (2) no bleeding: (1) yes (2) no
	annual rectal examination (proctosigmoidoscopy) (1) yes (2) no

Figure 7-2. Health hazard appraisal.

TO BE COMPLETED BY FEMALES ONLY: ————————————————— RECORD ALL ANSWERS IN THIS COLUMN ⟶

SOCIAL-ECONOMIC STATUS	(1) low	(2) average	(3) high
JEWISH (Less risk of cervical cancer)	(1) no	(2) yes (if both parents Jewish)	
AGE OF STARTING INTERCOURSE	(1) under 20	(2) 20-25	(3) over 25 or never
PAPSMEAR (1) have not had (2) 1 neg. in 5 yrs (3) 1 neg in 1 yr (4) 3 neg. in 5 yrs or annual			
ABNORMAL VAGINAL BLEEDING IN LAST YEAR (note: not normal menstruation)	(1) yes	(2) no	
FAMILY HISTORY OF BREAST CANCER	(1) Mother or sister had breast cancer. No self exam. (2) Mother or sister had breast cancer but patient examines breasts regularly & has periodic examinations by physician. (3) Neither mother nor sister had breast cancer. No self exam. (4) Neither mother nor sister had breast cancer but patient examines breasts regularly & has periodic examination.		

TO BE COMPLETED BY PARTICIPANT AS MUCH AS POSSIBLE, OR BY PHYSICIAN/NURSE

SYSTOLIC BLOOD PRESSURE* —————————— (in mm.) —————————— DIASTOLIC BLOOD PRESSURE*		
CHOLESTEROL LEVEL*	(1) 280 mg% or over (3) 219 mg% (2) 220-279 mg% or less	Give level if known
RECORD OF EMPHYSEMA OR BRONCHITIS	(1) yes	(2) no
ULCERATIVE COLITIS	(1) Had for 10 years (2) less than 10 years (3) do not have	
CHRONIC RHEUMATIC HEART DISEASE	(1) murmur/no treatment (2) murmur/treatment (3) history/no murmur/or treatment (4) history/no murmur/treatment (5) no history/no murmur	
CHRONIC RHEUMATIC HEART DISEASE (SIGNS OR SYMPTOMS)	(1) no (2) yes	

*LEAVE BLANK IF UNKNOWN. ANALYSIS WILL BE PERFORMED BY ASSUMING NORMAL VALUES.

DATE QUESTIONNAIRE COMPLETED: —————————————————

Figure 7-2. (continued).

It has been found that the questionnaire can be largely self-administered by the client/patient, except for the clinical measures of blood pressures and cholesterol. The average time required is about 10 minutes.

After coding and entry of the questionnaires' answers into the computer, the printout is produced. Again, the format can vary widely among different organizations, and the University of British Columbia's printout shown in Tables 7-1 and 7-2 is fairly typical. This particular printout is for an imaginary, relatively high-risk man of 50 years.

The HHA program is based on the concept of risk, and, in particular, on the risk of mortality over the next 10 years for the individual, compared with an average population for his or her particular sex and, 5-year age group. The first page of the printout (Table 7-1), therefore, lists the top 12 causes of death, ranked in order of importance for this person's age and sex group. In this example, they are headed by heart attack, lung cancer, and stroke. Column 1 prints the risks for this average group in terms of the numbers expected to die per 100,000 people within the next 10 years. (It should be noted that the "top 12"

Table 7-1. Health hazard appraisal (sample) Submitted by "Mr. I.M. Sedentary, Terminal Ave., Fatality Heights." (The risk registry data have been analyzed and the results summarized below as they relate to the 12 most frequent causes of death for males aged 50.

		Chances of Dying per 100,000 Within 10 Years		
Rank	Cause of death	Column 1 Average	Column 2 Appraisal	Column 3 Compliance
1	Heart attack	4456	16977	6327
2	Lung cancer	905	1538	1230
3	Stroke	535	1283	802
4	Cirrhosis of liver	362	724	362
5	Intestinal cancer including rectum	342	855	256
6	Motor vehicle accidents	327	752	359
7	Suicide	316	316	316
8	Chronic bronchitis and emphysema	263	447	312
9	Stomach cancer	227	227	227
10	Cancer of pancreas	183	183	183
11	Diseases of arteries, arteriosclerosis, caps	177	424	265
12	Tumors, lymph, haemo, ex-leukemia	167	167	167
	All other causes	3021	3021	3021
	All causes of death	11281	26914	13827

Given age: 50; Appraised age: 60.9; Compliance age: 52.2.
For height 71 inches and medium frame, 183 lb is approximately 16% overweight. Desirable weight: 157 lb.

Compliance*

Exercise	from	sedentary	to	sedentary exercise program
Smoking	from	still smokes 20+	to	stopped smoking
BP: syst.	from	160 mm	to	127 mm
BP: dias.	from	96 mm	to	86 mm
Alcohol	from	7–24/week	to	3–6/week
Weight	from	183 lb	to	161 lb
Seat-belt	from	10–24%	to	75–100%
Procto. exam	from	not had in past year	to	annual in future

*The compliance chances of dying (column 3) are based upon the assumption that factor(s) are modified as given in table.

Table 7-2. Risk factor analysis—sample material (I.M. Sedentary).

| Contributing Characteristics | Appraisal | | | Compliance | | |
	As Submitted	Actual Risk	Component Risk	As Complied	Applied Risk	Composite Risk
Heart attack						
Blood pressure	160/96	1.3/1.4		127/86	0.9/1.0	
Cholesterol	280+	1.5		280+	1.5	
Diabetes	Not diabetic	1.0		Not diabetic	1.0	
Weight	183	1.0		161	0.9	
Exercise	Sedentary	2.0		Sedentary exercise program	1.0	
Smoking	Still smokes 20+	1.4		Stopped smoking	0.8	
FH/heart	Yes	1.2	3.81	Yes	1.2	1.42
Lung cancer						
Smoking	Still smokes 20+	1.7	1.70	Stopped smoking	1.4	1.36
Cirrhosis of liver						
Alcohol	7–24/week	2.0	2.00	3–6/week	1.0	1.00
Motor vehicle accidents						
Alcohol	7–24/week	2.0		3–6/week	1.0	
Mile/year	13,000	1.3		13,000	1.3	
Seat-belt	10–24%	1.0		75–100%	0.8	
Drug/medication	None	1.0	2.30	None	1.0	1.10
Suicide						
Depression	Seldom or never	1.0		Seldom or never	1.0	
FH/suicide	No	1.0	1.00	No	1.0	1.00

account for some two-thirds to three-quarters of "all causes of death.") The risk from all the other minor causes beyond the first 12 is then listed.

Column 2 presents the individual's appraised figures. The modified chances of dying are determined from the information submitted in the questionnaire, by estimating risk factors as described below. In this particular case, the individual's total risk has been appraised at an almost 27% chance of dying within the next 10 years, compared to a Canadian average for his age and sex of 11%.

Column 3 presents the individual's lesser chances of dying, assuming some improvement of risk factors by complying with a set of prescriptions listed at the foot of the page, under "Compliance." In this case, the individual's chances of dying are reduced from the appraised level of 27% to just under 14%, which, while somewhat above the Canadian average, is nevertheless vastly reduced from the appraised level.

Since experience has suggested that many people find statistics confusing, a second way of presenting the combined risk information has been adopted by HHA; namely, that of presenting the person's condition as represented by three

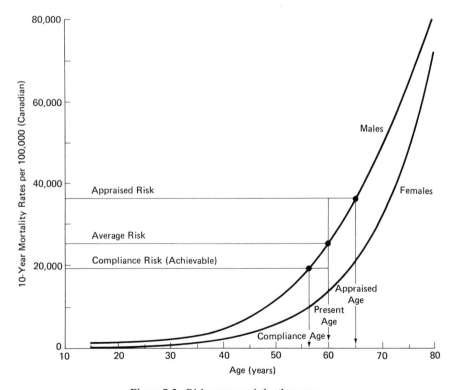

Figure 7-3. Risk curves and the three ages.

ages: given, appraised, and compliance (achievable). The principle behind these ages can best be appreciated by referring to the curve of mortality risk versus age (Figure 7-3). Thus, the person's appraised age is that age at which the person has the same risk as the average person in his age and sex group. It can perhaps suitably be looked upon as the "physiological body" age, and obviously it is desirable to have an appraised age lower than one's given age. In a similar way, as also illustrated in Figure 7-3, the compliance age is that lower risk age which can be reached by complying with the specified health prescriptions for lifestyle change.

At the bottom of Table 7-1, the tabulation under the title "Compliance" lists a number of suggested changes in lifestyle, and possibly also in the levels of blood pressure and cholesterol. It should be emphasized that these suggestions are neither mandatory nor exhaustive. Thus, there may be many further changes which the client might wish to consider in the counseling session with the health professional. Equally, he may be unwilling to undertake some of the major changes suggested in the list; for example, quitting smoking may be unacceptable, but he may be prepared to wear seat-belts.

It should also be noted that the compliance changes do not necessarily suggest full changes to the optimal conditions, since it is assumed that some of these may take much time. For example, it is suggested that exercise go from a sedentary condition to a sedentary exercise program only, with the assumption that when this has been safely achieved, the person may wish to go on to a full exercise program.

The second page of the printout (Table 7-2) contains details on the risk factors. Consider, for example, the risk factors for the patient's major risk of death – heart attack. There are eight component risk factors listed as "Actual Risk" in the printout. The particular numbers which represent the present risk are given in the "Appraisal" column, and for confirmation the answers provided by the person on the questionnaire are reproduced in the column "As Submitted." Note, for example, that under exercise, Mr. Sedentary's sedentary answer results in an "Actual Risk Factor" of 2.0. The eight factors are combined in a complex actuarial form to produce the "Composite (Compo) Risk Factor" for heart attack of 3.81. The "Appraised Risk" of heart attack in Column 2 of Table 7-1 is thus attained by multiplying the "Average Risk" in Column 1 (of 4456) by this factor (of 3.81), to yield the total of 16,977.

The "Compliance Risk Factors" are similarly exhibited in Table 7-2. The "Component Risk Factors" ("Applied Risk") which have been reduced are blood pressures, weight, exercise, and smoking. The resulting "Composite Risk Factor" of 1.42 is still above the national average, which, by definition, is 1, but nevertheless is greatly reduced from the appraised level. This procedure is repeated for many of the individual's top 12, but not usually for all of them. This limitation arises because there are no actuarily sound prescriptions known for all

Table 7-3.   List of all "top 12" causes of death.

Stomach cancer
Intestinal cancer including rectum
Lung cancer
Breast cancer
Cancer of cervix
Cancer of prostate
Cancer of pancreas
Cancer of ovary, tube, broad ligt.
Brain cancer
Leukemia
Tumors lymph, haemo, ex-leukemia
Diabetes
Epilepsy
Chronic rheumatic heart disease
High blood pressure
Heart attack
Other forms of heart disease
Stroke
Diseases of arteries, arteriosclerosis, caps
Pneumonia
Chronic bronchitis and emphysema
Cirrhosis of liver
Congenital anomalies heart, circulatory system
Senility without psychosis
Motor vehicle accidents
Accidental drowning
Air transport accidents
Accidental poisoning
Accidental falls
Accidents caused by fires
Accidents caused by firearms
Suicide
Homicide, etc.

possible "top 12" causes of death. Specifically, the Canadian list of such top 12 currently includes 33 causes (Table 7-3), of which about one-half are considered prescribable. An example of those omitted is accidental drowning, which is one major cause of death in youth, as are some other accidental forms. Unfortunately, it seems neither worthwhile nor possible to make simple prescriptions from which risk factor reductions can be assessed; rather, it can be left to the counselor to make suitable comments about these.

Table 7-4 presents essentially the same information as that given in the previous two tables in a graphical form. Some people prefer this to the tabular form. Again, the main causes of death are printed in descending order, with the

Table 7-4. Appraisal graph—sample material (I.M. Sedentary).

Cause of Death	Percent Risk Related to the Average Condition	Graph

```
                                    0      100%            300              500
                                    +...........+.....+.....+.........+.....+....
                                    +          +                +
                                    +          +                +
Heart attack           380          +---------------HHHHHWEEEEEEEEEESSSSSSS
                                    +--------------HHHHHWEEEEEEEEEESSSSSSSS
                                    +-------------HHHHHWEEEEEEEEEESSSSSSSS
                                    +------------HHHHHWEEEEEEEEEESSSSSSSS
                                    +-----------HHHHHWEEEEEEEEEESSSSSSSS
                                    +----------HHHHHWEEEEEEEEEESSSSSSSS
                                    +---------HHHHHWEEEEEEEEEESSSSSSSS
                                    +--------HHHHHWEEEEEEEEEESSSSSSSS
                                    +-------HHHHHWEEEEEEEEEESSSSSSSS
                                    +------HHHHHWEEEEEEEEEESSSSSSSS
                                    +          +
Lung cancer            169          +-------------SSSS
                                    +-------------SSSS
                                    +-------------SSSS
                                    +          +
Cirrhosis of liver     200          +-------------AAAAAAAAAA
                                    +          +
Intestinal cancer                   +------------PPPPPPP
including rectum       250          +          +
                                    +------------AAAAAAAAAABB
Motor vehicle                       +          +
accidents              229          +-------------
                                    +          +
Suicide                100          +---------
```

Legend

A= Alcohol
B= Seat-belt
D= Diabetes
E = Exercise
H= Blood pressure
M= Drugs/medication
P = Procto. exam
S = Smoking
W= Weight
X= Breast exam
Y= Papsmear
– = Irreducible

"Composite Risk Factor" printed, as a percentage, against each cause. The bars for each cause of death represent by their vertical depth the relative severity of the average risk for this age group and sex, while the horizontal extent represents the individual's appraised risk relative to this average. The lettering in each bar indicates the extent to which the appraised risk can be reduced by adopting that particular lifestyle change, where, for example, S stands for "quitting smoking." The residual dashes (– – –) represent the so-called "irreducible" risk, except that this term may be somewhat misleading. There may indeed be ways to reduce these risks still further, but the extent cannot be readily quantified on the basis of present actuarial knowledge. For example, nutrition and stress reduction are two well-recognized major areas in which it is obviously prudent to counsel improvement whenever possible.

Experience suggests that most health professionals, including physicians, ideally need from 30 minutes to one hour for a relaxed and effective counseling session, at least on the first occasion. It should be emphasized that, during this "teachable moment," it is possible for many diverse subjects to be discussed, whether brought up by the counselor or by the client. While there still is much uncertainty about how best to stimulate behavioral change, it is important that the client be encouraged to enter into some form of "contract" wherein he or she undertakes to make certain changes within certain given time limits. However, these changes must genuinely represent the client's own choice.

It is important to explain to the client that the concept of reduced risk does not necessarily guarantee avoidance of death, or even sickness for a particular individual, but that it would seem prudent to assume this. It is also worth emphasizing that mortality figures represent only a small part of the total disease entity, the tip of an iceberg of morbidity. It may also be helpful to point out that the program is intended to be educational, so that detailed numerical uncertainties or inaccuracies in appraisal estimation are not inherently important; but instead, the important issue is to become aware of how various lifestyle habits are capable of influencing one's health. Further, it should be stressed that, although the prescriptions may appear rather commonplace, and indeed not to be new, these issues keep coming up because they are the important ones. Finally, it should again be emphasized in the counseling that HHA is not primarily a tool to screen for any diseases which may be present in an early clinically-diagnosable stage. Rather, the underlying intention of HHA is to motivate individuals for lifestyle change in those stages when the person's risk of contracting such diseases through imprudent health habits is increasing (Figure 7-4).

The question inevitably arises as to whether HHA is effective as a technique for stimulating healthful lifestyle change. Due to its relatively recent introduction, there are as yet only a few relatively small studies to show this. These are documented especially in the recent annual *Proceedings of the Society for Prospective Medicine.*[6]   Generally, those professionals utilizing HHA are enthusiastic

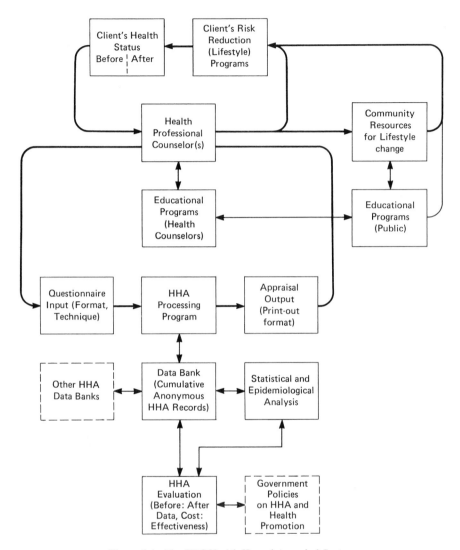

Figure 7-4. The UBC Health Hazard Appraisal System.

about its effectiveness and its potential. Its use seems to be spreading rapidly. While HHA is not presently as comprehensive in its estimation of risks and stimulation for behavioral change as all would like, it does, however, seem to have the innate potential to include within its framework new knowledge as it becomes available, and indeed to stimulate the acquisition of such new knowledge.

In this regard, we have found at the University of British Columbia that HHA provides a core element for developing a system of preventive medicine and health promotion. This involves not only the basic double loop of client/health professional/HHA process, but, in addition:

1. Educational programs for health counselors and the public.
2. Integration with community resources for lifestyle change.
3. Statistical and epidemiological analyses based on a cumulative, anonymous data bank.
4. Evaluation studies on HHA, potentially leading to changes in government policies.
5. Continual updating of risk factors and HHA format.

Concluding Comments

As we struggle to evolve a satisfactory system for the care of health, our intention is necessarily focused increasingly on the underlying nature of health. In many ways, this is a very difficult challenge for the medical sciences, since the interests and the methodologies of medicine have concentrated on the pathology associated with disease. The controversy about the relative priorities for society between acute and preventive care will undoubtedly continue, since so many underlying value judgments are involved, as well as professional territories. Nevertheless, as argued so persuasively by Lalonde,[7] until the scientific community has been able to resolve some of the debates on health-related questions concerning the environment and lifestyle, it appears sufficiently valid for society to take positive action in such lifestyle modifications as suggested by HHA. The underlying philosophy of HHA is to encourage individuals to take successively more responsibility for their own health. Surely, no one can doubt that, ultimately, this will be crucially important to the evolution of a truly healthy society.

REFERENCES

1. McKeown, T., "The Role of Medicine: Dream, Mirage or Nemesis," Blackwells, 1979.
2. Dubos, R., *The Mirage of Health*. New York: Harper, 1959.
3. Laszlo, C.A. and Milsum, J.H., *Cost/Benefit Analysis of Technology in the Health Care System*. San Diego Biomedical Symposium, February 1976.
4. Robertson, L.S., *Whose Behaviour in What Health Marketplace?* Steinhart Conference on "Consumer Behaviour in the Health Marketplace," University of Nebraska, March 1976.
5. Robbins, L.C. and Hall, J., *How to Practice Prospective Medicine*. Indianapolis: Methodist Hospital, 1970.

6. Robbins and Hall, "New Concepts in Health: A New Horizon," *Proceedings of the Twelfth Annual Meeting of the Society for Prospective Medicine.* Indianapolis: Methodist Hospital, 1977.

7. Lalonde, M., *A New Perspective on the Health of Canadians.* Ottawa: Government of Canada, 1974.

8

Behavioral Medicine: A New Perspective in Health Research and Practice

Stephen M. Weiss, Ph.D.

National Institutes of Health
National Heart, Lung, and Blood Institute

Gary E. Schwartz, Ph.D.

Departments of Psychology and Psychiatry
Yale University

The recent shift in emphasis from infectious to chronic diseases as major health problems has been accompanied by a shift from single-cause to multifactorial models of health and illness. These events have paralleled the development of the new field of behavioral medicine. Drawing on the concept of interactive versus parallel approaches to disease prevention and control, it is proposed that research designs which actively integrate the behavioral and biomedical sciences represent a central component of behavioral medicine. The implications of this biobehavioral approach to theory, methods, practice, and training are discussed in this chapter.

Tremendous advances in biomedicine over the past 60 years have forced a continuing reexamination of our perspectives and approaches to the promotion of health and to the prevention and control of disease, resulting in a major shift in research emphasis from the acute infectious diseases to chronic illness. Most of the major viral and bacterial diseases have been conquered or controlled in this country. There are no more polio, tuberculosis, or smallpox epidemics. Measles, mumps, influenza, and pneumonia have lost their capacity to make serious inroads on the nation's health status. The chronic diseases — cardiovascular, pulmonary, neoplastic, cerebrovascular — have become the major source of health concern. Cardiovascular disease in particular, as the nation's number one killer, has become a special area of emphasis in the biomedical research arena. The consequent reallocation of resources and manpower have also called for a "rethinking" of approach – a refocusing of perspective. The search for *the* pathogenic agent (a virus, organ dysfunction, or biochemical substrate), so successful in combating the acute infectious diseases, has failed to come to terms with such health concerns as hypertension, coronary heart disease, cardiac arrythmias, etc. For example, cardiovascular "risk factors" (smoking, hypertension, serum cholesterol) account for less than 50% of the variance associated with myocardial infarction.[1]   Single-factor theories associated with essential hypertension have met with similarly frustrating results.

Clearly, a more comprehensive approach to disease prevention and control is required to comprehend the multifaceted nature of these serious health problems. The impetus for the creation of another perspective has come from several sources. The HEW Forward Plan for Health,[2] the Canadian "LaLonde Report,"[3] and the "Congressional Investigation of the National Institutes of Health"[4] (the Banta Report) have all identified the need for expanded research on the role of behavioral and lifestyle factors in the prevention and control of chronic disease. It is difficult, and perhaps impossible, to fully comprehend the interplay of needs, forces, deficits, and incentives which provide the necessary chemistry to foster the creation of a new field. Yet the conditions under which seminal theory and concepts find maturant environments by definition identify unmet needs in the present state of affairs.

In the formal sense, the birth of behavioral medicine can be dated to the February 1977 Yale Conference on Behavioral Medicine.[5,6] The gestation period, however, extends perhaps to 5000 years ago, to the writings of Homer, Plato, and Aristotle, where one finds speculations remarkably similar to those of today on the relationship between mind and body. In more recent times, such luminaries as Sir William Osler, Claude Bernard, and Walter Cannon, among others, have continued this effort toward a more comprehensive understanding of health and illness. The "labor pains" of behavioral medicine can be dated to the last 40 years, which have witnessed the development of *psychosomatic medicine,* where psychiatry attempted, through psychoanalytic theory, to establish yet another perspective to the mind-body linkage.

This progression of theory, concept, and ideology tended to be regarded with a sometimes jaundiced eye by many of the leading biomedical theorists in each era, yet perhaps less so with each succeeding generation of scientific thought. The weakest link in all of these speculations, however, remained the difficulty in putting into operation such concepts through scientific research, theory, and method acceptable to all the relevant scientific communities. Within the past 10 years, new breakthroughs on the theoretical, conceptual, and technological levels (e.g., biofeedback, the role of the central nervous system in autonomic system mediation, physiologic response to environmental stressors) have dramatized the necessity for reconceptualizing the nature of biological and behavioral interrelationships.

Efforts to broaden the attack on chronic disease problems have identified many "non-traditional" paths for potentially fruitful exploration. Diet, exercise, stress, weight control, smoking behavior, and compliance/adherence strategies, to name a few, have all recently emerged as legitimate areas of research in the prevention and control of chronic disease, as we have tried to come to terms with the potentially deleterious aspects of the American way of life. The role of environmental/behavioral factors as synergistic, catalytic, instigative, modulating, mediating agents in the ultimate physiologic/biochemical/hormonal chain reaction resulting, over time, in organ damage/dysfunction, has become one of the most significant challenges to the biomedical and behavioral research communities.

Most of the early attempts by biomedical and behavioral researchers to independently address these common problems met with less than gratifying results. Too often, more questions were raised than answered. Too often, the biomedical scientists found serious, disqualifying errors or omissions resulting from an insufficient understanding of the biomedicine involved on the part of their behavioral colleagues.

In retrospect, these conditions were the birth attendants of behavioral medicine. Another perspective was in order, to resolve some of the inconsistencies and incongruities resulting from the above state of affairs. It became increasingly obvious that to successfully pursue a multifaceted approach to chronic illness, those with the collective expertise necessary to address the various dimensions of the problems at hand would have to develop better *collaborative* relationships, and become more familiar with one another's language, concepts, and perspectives to successfully initiate joint multipronged attacks on the issues under consideration. Only in this way could one adequately model the combination of "real-life" circumstances which might impinge on the organism—where the *interactive* efforts might result synergistically or catalytically, in a product, the whole of which would be greater than the arithmetic sum of its parts.[7] It has been the search for this "unifying principle" among behavioral and biomedical scientists working on problems of mutual concern which has spawned the concept of "behavioral medicine."

An illustration of the dynamic growth and development of the field, the definition of behavioral medicine developed by the participants during the Yale conference on Behavioral Medicine[5, 6] has already been superseded by a "second generation" definition, promulgated and adopted at the organizational meeting of the Academy of Behavioral Medicine Research, held at the National Academy of Sciences in April 1978. [8] To wit:

Yale Conference Definition: Behavioral Medicine is the field concerned with the development of behavioral science knowledge and techniques relevant to the understanding of physical health and illness and the application of that knowledge and these techniques to prevention, diagnosis, treatment and rehabilitation.

Psychosis, neurosis, and substance abuse are included only insofar as they contribute to physical disorders as an end point.

Academy of Behavioral Medicine Research Definition: Behavioral Medicine is the interdisciplinary field concerned with the development and integration of behavioral and biomedical science knowledge and techniques relevant to the understanding of health and illness and the application of this knowledge and these techniques to prevention, diagnosis, treatment and rehabilitation.

In the 14 months separating these two events, tremendous conceptual development took place, as those directly involved with the form and substance of these issues continued their efforts to eliminate the barriers to more effective collaborative undertakings.

The shift from a parallel to an interactive conceptual model is having significant effects on the language of both the biomedical and the behavioral sciences. We are witnessing the creation of new terms reflecting new fields, both within and between the behavioral and biomedical sciences. Within the biomedical sciences, new fields have emerged which successfully integrate traditional disciplines such as biology, chemistry, neurology, physiology, and endocrinology. Hence, we see the development of biochemistry, neurochemistry, neurophysiology, to mention but a few. These fields have integrated the methods and theories from each of the respective disciplines, and through interactive efforts have generated new theories and data based on the unique information so acquired.

A similar trend is occurring within the behavioral sciences, although the relative infancy of these disciplines provide fewer illustrations. Separate disciplines such as psychology, anthropology, and political science have merged to create new fields such as *psychological anthropology* and *political psychology.* The more complex term, *psychosociocultural,* has been coined to reflect intraindividual characteristics of a person that interact within a social and a cultural milieu. It is important to recognize that even within a single discipline such as psychology, subspecialities that were once seen as antithetical are now being joined. The new area of *cognitive behavior modification,* of special relevance to behavioral medicine, is but one example in which two different traditions are being fruitfully integrated and advanced accordingly.[9]

In light of these developments, the virtual explosion of new terms and fields attempting to integrate the biomedical and behavioral sciences can be better understood and appreciated. The more classic areas of physiological psychology, psychophysiology, and psychosomatic medicine have been augmented by new journals and research societies concerned with biological psychology, neuropsychology, behavioral genetics, health psychology, psychopharmacology, biological psychiatry, and behavioral neurology. Wilson[10] has forcefully written about the need for a new, interactive synthesis, which he terms sociobiology, of which areas such as biological anthropology are seen as one of many components. More complex terms, such as biopsychosocial,[11] psychoneuroendocrinology,[12] and social psychophysiology[13] illustrate the quest for these new, integrative models of health and illness.

The promise and challenge of behavioral medicine is to establish the value of interactive research designs, methods, and theories. Although many researchers have an intuitive sense (if not blind faith) that such models will be fruitful, the long-term significance of such approaches will hinge on the development of theory and data that substantiate the unique contributions of this perspective in addressing critical problems of health and illness. In point of fact, such models already exist, but their true significance is not widely appreciated.

For example, the analysis of variance model demonstrates mathematically how factors A and B may each have little influence on a third factor, C, when examined individually, yet have large (and sometimes opposite) effects when examined concurrently, in interaction with one another. Figure 8-1 demonstrates how main effects of A on C (ignoring B) and of B on C (ignoring A) may show little effect, yet the combined, interactive effect of A and B on C may have dramatic, (and even perhaps *opposite*) effects on C. Thus, specific combinations

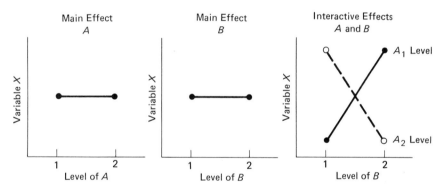

Figure 8-1. Two independent variables, A and B, each at two levels, are examined for their effects on dependent variable X. The particular example is selected to illustrate how in certain sets of data, it is possible for low levels in both A and B (A_1B_1 combination) or high levels in both A and B (A_2B_2 combination) to be associated with low levels of X. However, if A is low but B is high (A_1B_2) or A is high but B is low (A_2B_1), high levels of X may occur. This sort of interaction (a form of the inverted U shaped function for two variables) is not uncommon in behavioral or biomedical data. These interactive effects of A and B on X can be uncovered by graphing the effects on X as a function of both levels of A and B (the interactive effects graph). The important point in this example, illustrated in the graphs depicting the main effects of A and B alone, is that research designs which manipulated only A (ignoring B) or manipulated only B (ignoring A) could come to the erroneous conclusion that A had no effect on X, or B had no effect on X. Interactive biobehavioral research designs that manipulate behavioral and biomedical variables concurrently have the potential to uncover important biobehavioral interactive effects.

or patterns of A and B determine the behavior of C. Clearly, each factor studied alone, with random variance occurring in the other, can lead to oversimplistic and erroneous conclusions regarding the role that each may play in the regulation of C.

Although analyses of variance are widely employed in both the behavioral and the biomedical sciences, the interaction component of the analyses is often viewed as a problem rather than an insight. This is unfortunate. Although one might ideally like to find simple relationships among variables, this is simply not the case when the systems under study become more complex. With each increase in complexity, with each increase in the number of parts comprising the system under study, there is a corresponding increase in the number of interactions among each of the parts that will contribute to the functioning of the system as a whole. The concept of the "whole being greater than the sum of its parts, yet being dependent upon the interactions among the parts for its unique properties" is a basic tenet of systems theory.[7] As Schwartz[14] recently noted, the concept of parts in interaction relates to the notion of emergent properties in all of the sciences, as new phenomena emerge at each level of complexity.

In other words, a standard statistic (the analysis of variance), used in both the biomedical and the behavioral sciences, highlights the concept of interaction which complements more general notions of systems theory and emergent properties. The biologist Von Bertallanfy[7] has clearly indicated how it is not possible to examine parts in isolation if the complex behavior of the system as a whole is to be understood. Placed in more statistical terms, the theory predicts that greater predictability will occur, and that more of the total variance will be accounted for, as the relevant variables are uncovered and investigated in *interaction* with one another.

The potential fruits of interactive research designs are beginning to appear in the biobehavioral literature. The area of hypertension has received extensive biobehavioral consideration,[15] and recent examples illustrate the more general systems issue of combining behavioral and biomedical approaches to this complex, multifactorial problem.[16]

Numerous studies document the role that genetics can play in various central nervous system and peripheral mechanisms involved in the raising of blood pressure.[17] Similarly, various studies document the role that diet, especially sodium intake, plays in the production and maintenance of high blood pressure.[18] It is important to note that even in the field of genetics *per se,* the distinction between genotype and phenotype illustrates the difference between "single" factors versus "multi" factors in the ultimate expression of a genetic trait. Applying this interactive model to hypertension, studies confirm that certain strains of rats, when exposed to high-salt diet, are especially prone to develop hypertension.[19] This type of hypertension clearly is related to the interaction of genetics and diet.

Other studies document the role that psychosocial factors can play in the raising of blood pressure. These studies are typically conducted without regard to the genetic and diet history of the lower animal or person. However, recent studies in lower animals indicate that the effect of psychosocial stress in the promotion of high blood pressure is accentuated if the animals are genetically predisposed to respond to the presence of sodium in the diet.[20] It should be noted that the interpretation of these interactive effects is not currently known, nor is it necessarily straightforward. For example, it is possible that the genetic/salt mechanisms are different from the psychosocial mechanisms, but that these different mechanisms, when occurring in interaction, can have unique emergent properties. On the other hand, it is possible that some aspects of the genetic/salt mechanisms and the psychosocial stress mechanisms are shared in common, and that, through complex positive feedback loops, both sets of mechanisms are similarly accentuated.

Such interactions are of paramount importance to the understanding, treatment, and prevention of high blood pressure in humans. These studies, though in their infancy, point to the potential power and complexity inherent in such an approach. The argument cannot be avoided that inclusion of multiple factors in the design and analysis results in complex conclusions; complex disorders, however, require complex designs and explanations.

It is anticipated that areas of confusion and unreliability in the biobehavioral area will be clarified as interactive theories, methods, and designs are developed. For example, research on personality correlates of essential hypertension is replete with contradictory data and weak findings.[21] However, advances in both the biomedical and behavioral sciences, when appropriately integrated, may make inroads into this confusion. Esler *et al.* have argued that essential hypertension is not a single disorder reflecting a single mechanism, but rather reflects a heterogeneous population of multifactorial disorders.[22] Given the complexity of the cardiovascular system, it is not surprising that numerous processes, in interaction, can all lead to what may at first glance be interpreted as a single problem.[16]

The challenge for future research is to improve our ability to bring to bear state-of-the-art access *in each field* in such a way as to promote interactive designs among them. This will likely occur only if specialists in the relevant disciplines are brought together on a common problem and conduct interactive, multifactorial designs to delineate the interrelationships.

Another example illustrative of interactive research approaches—the current research on coronary prone behavior and coronary heart diseases—finds sophisticated behavioral and biomedical investigators attempting to examine how different patterns of "Type A" behavior are differentially related to different types of coronary heart disease.[23] Again, such findings can only emerge when multifactorial design and statistics include *both the behavioral and the biomedical aspects of the problem.*

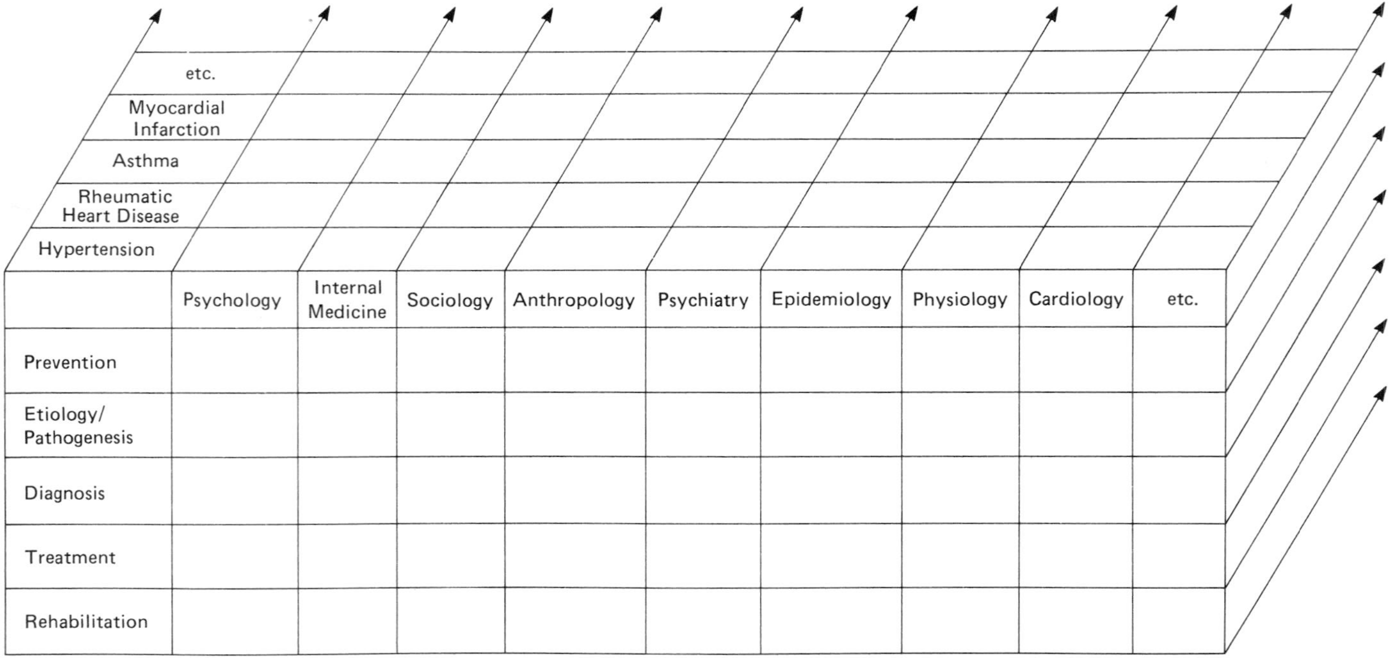
etc.
Myocardial Infarction
Asthma
Rheumatic Heart Disease
Hypertension
Psychology
Internal Medicine
Sociology
Anthropology
Psychiatry
Epidemiology
Physiology
Cardiology
etc.
Prevention
Etiology/ Pathogenesis
Diagnosis
Treatment
Rehabilitation

Figure 8-2.

As illustrated pictorially in the proceedings of the Yale Conference on Behavioral Medicine (see Figure 8-2) one can develop a matrix of various behavioral and biomedical disciplines on one dimension, aspects of the study of disease on a second dimension (from etiology and pathogenesis through treatment and rehabilitation), with types of diseases on the third coordinate. This approach suggests that progress in prevention, diagnosis, treatment, etc., on the diseases in question will depend at least in part on the relevant disciplines attempting to work interactively to account for more of the variance than could be accomplished by parallel efforts. This is not meant to imply that every experiment should include all disciplines, but rather that, whenever possible, researchers should move in the direction of combining two or more "state of science" approaches to come to terms with the problem at hand.

Establishing a fertile environment for the development of such interactive models requires careful examination of the effectiveness of communication within and across the many disciplines involved. Problems currently exist in the use of terminology, where differences in meaning between behavioral and biomedical scientists cause inadvertent misunderstandings.[16] For example, a behavioral scientist might write that operant conditioning had "direct effects" on blood pressure, meaning that the effects were relatively specific to blood pressure when compared with other autonomic nervous system mediated responses. However, for the pharmacologist, the term "direct" has a specific meaning, referring to the site of action of the drug (or agent) on the tissue in question. By this interpretation, operant conditioning of blood pressure must involve a complex set of "indirect effects."

Another inadvertent problem of language concerns the meaning of the term "placebo." To a behavioral scientist, the term "placebo" generally refers to certain nonspecified components of a complex psychological process (using "implied expectancy" and "set" on the parts of the experimenter and the subject). Using this terminology in the biofeedback situation, the subject's expectancies might be labeled as "placebo factors," while the more specific aspects linked to the contingency of the biofeedback would be labeled as "active ingredients." However, to a pharmacologist, the term "placebo" specifically refers to environmental (psychological) factors that are not due to the *direct action* of the drug. From this definition, all behavioral aspects fall under the category of "placebo effects."

Thus, it can be seen that there is a need for behavioral and biomedical scientists to learn the precise meanings of the languages used by each. Our point in mentioning this problem, however, is not only to improve communication, but also to illustrate how new understanding and models may be promoted in the process. For example, in pharmacology, a series of terms is used to refer to different kinds of interactions between combinations of drugs or drug/organism interaction.[16] Pharmacologists explicitly recognize, for example, that drugs can sometimes have *synergistic* effects where the pattern of effects is qualitatively different when the drugs are given in combination than when they are given alone. Not only can behavioral scientists profit from considering these concepts, but more important, they can come to realize how such concepts actually provide a framework for expanding the pharmacologic model to include interactions of behavioral and pharmacologic agents. In other words, the pharmacologic model is not "anti-behavioral," but instead can incorporate concepts from the behavioral sciences in the development of a more comprehensive, *biobehavioral* analysis.

Such collaboration will also, it is hoped, reduce the likelihood of perpetuating current mind/body or behavior/biology dichotomies. For example, Levine, *et al.* recently demonstrated that a sub-group of patients responding to a "placebo" drug were found to show changes in endorphins in the brain.[24] Based on these findings, the authors concluded that such effects were not "placebo" effects, but rather were neurophysiological! This either/or perspective is unfortunate because it fails to recognize that for any "psychological" (e.g., placebo) variable to result in a peripheral "physiological" effect, it must be mediated via the central nervous system. Hence, it is conceptually in error to speak of placebo *versus* physiological effects. One might more profitably speak of behavioral inputs involving neuropsychological processes that modulate, in an interactive sense, peripheral physiological responses.

These issues apply to all aspects of health and illness, from etiology and pathogenesis to treatment and prevention. As noted by Shapiro *et al.,* the concept of "phases" of clinical research in pharmacology can be retranslated into more general terms and thereby be applied to behavioral as well as to biomedical interventions.[25] Using the more general terminology, it then becomes easier to compare and contrast the relative progress made to date in understanding behavioral and biomedical intervention strategies. As mentioned previously, the challenge in behavioral medicine is not simply to study these interventions in isolation, but also to pursue their possible interactions.

Interactive models require multifactorial approaches. This poses several statistical and practical considerations. Typically, one thinks of complex, multifactorial designs involving large numbers of groups and subjects, followed by the collection of masses of data requiring complex interpretations. Fortunately, newer statistical techniques, including multiple regression and multivariate analyses of variance, are being developed to reduce the necessity for doing complete factorial experiments. Modern techniques of pattern recognition and profile analysis, developed by NASA and other agencies, are also being considered applicable to problems associated with behavioral medicine. The challenge is to bring these new techniques of data analysis to bear upon the design and interpretation of interactive behavioral medicine research.

Successful development of the model described above will require multivariate approaches which capitalize upon the potential synergism or catalytic effect of various combinations of biomedical and behavioral variables. Rather than the traditional "either/or" assumptions about the efficacy of behavioral and bio-medical clinical approaches, emphasis must be placed on the most effective combinations of approaches for a given patient to achieve the best clinical result. One interesting aspect of this interactive approach to treatment concerns the various interpretations that are possible regarding which treatment accentuates which. For example, if research were to reveal that combinations of certain drugs and relaxation training results in greater and longer lasting decreases in blood pressure than can be obtained from either treatment alone, two interpreta-tions would be suggested. On the one hand, one might be tempted to conclude that the drugs were potentiating the relaxation effects. Yet, on the other hand, one could equally postulate that the relaxation training was potentiating the drug effects. The latter interpretation may be of particular value because it implies the possibility of reducing the amount of the particular drugs needed, by adding behavioral components as an integral part of the treatment package. The interactive approach, therefore, may provide certain side benefits concerning the extent to which the combination of approaches may improve the quality of care and the promotion of health.

This model will require careful identification of the broad range of biomedi-cal and behavioral research/clinical expertise necessary for such an undertaking to be gathered in such a manner as to ensure *complementarity* of skills within the research or clinical team. The "parallel" efforts described earlier in the in-dependent efforts of biomedical and behavioral scientists must give way to truly interactive undertakings. It will not be sufficient to rely on "occasional consul-tation" or "10% effort" by one discipline group with the other. *Collaborative* effort means just that—a joint venture in quest of solutions to problems shared in common. Only through the combined expertise of the parties involved can meaningful insights acceptable and understandable to all concerned be achieved.

Having proposed such a model begs the question of how this "ideal" may be accomplished. No one discipline receives such orientation in its standard training curriculum. Is a new discipline necessary? We think not. The range of knowl-edge required to comprehend the theory, concepts, and technology associated with the many disciplines contributing to the interdisciplinary field of behavioral medicine suggests an impossible undertaking for any one individual. Further, the very breadth of the field mitigates against any one individual having the in-terest and motivation (even if it were humanly possible) to invest the necessary energy at the various levels and to the various depths required to become truly expert in each area. The barriers to effective collaboration, then, must be bridged through training experiences which allow those from the biomedical disciplines to become conversant with the principles, theories, concepts, and language of the behavioral disciplines—and vice-versa. In the course of such experiences, increased familiarity *among* the behavioral and the biomedical psychologists will become more conversant with the anthropologic perspective, as well as with that of the pharmacologist.

Such research training programs are already underway at various medical schools and universities across the country.[26] The development of complementary programs in clinical training will require similar perspectives to those described above. The clinical "team concept," hardly new to clinical medicine, may be expanded to include relevant biobehavioral expertise. This will have direct implications for expanding the prevention, as well as the treatment, capabilities of the health care system as we know it today.

In the tradition of the ancient Hebrew Passover chant, one might ask: "How is this field different from all other (earlier and alternative) fields psychosomatic medicine, holistic medicine, etc.)?" Perhaps the most cogent difference is the commitment to develop integrative models consistent with the best of biomedical and behavioral research designs at the chosen level of investigation. Review processes will demand excellence from both biomedical and behavioral perspectives; joint expertise in research design and implementation will be the *sine qua non* of behavioral medicine research. Evaluation of the outcomes of such endeavors will be subject to similarly rigorous appraisal. In essence, the necessity for satisfying the criteria established for "both sides of the coin" will encourage a more ready acceptance of findings by the involved research communities, and ultimately by the health care/promotion complex.

As the health establishment is the ultimate recipient of successful outcomes of behavioral medicine research, it is particularly relevant that the development of this offspring of biomedical and behavioral parentage is taking place within the key resource for the nation's biomedical research effort—the National Institutes of Health. This provides the assurance of adequate and competent biomedical, as well as behavioral, review, while facilitating the efficient translation of successful efforts into the relevant sectors of the health care/promotion system. It is encouraging to note the receptivity and continuing commitment demonstrated by the National Institutes of Health to biobehaviorial research through the development of relevant grant review procedures, as well as program activities in selected bureaus, institutes, and divisions. The final judgment concerning the true value of the concept of behavioral medicine will rest in the ability of those adopting this model to contribute more effectively to solutions of the highly complex issues surrounding the prevention and control of chronic disease.

REFERENCES

1. Keys, A., Aravanis, C., Blackburn M., et al. Probability of middle-aged men developing coronary heart disease in five years. Circulation, 1972, 45, 815-828.
2. Forward Plan for Health, FY 1977–81, June 1975 (Publication No. (OS) 76–50024) Washington, D.C.: Department of Health, Education and Welfare.

3. LaLonde, M.A. New Perspective on the Health of Canadians: A Working Document. Ottawa, Canada: Ministry of Health & Welfare, 1974.
4. Banta, D. Investigation of National Institutes of Health. Prepared by staff for use of the Committee on Interstate and Foreign Commerce Subcommittee on Health and Environment, August 1976 (Publication No. 70–661) Washington, D.C.: Department of Health, Education and Welfare.
5. Schwartz, G.E. and Weiss, S.M. Proceedings of the Yale Conference on Behavioral Medicine (Publication No. (NIH) 78–1424). Washington, D.C.: Department of Health, Education and Welfare.
6. Schwartz, G.E. and Weiss, S.M. Yale Conference on Behavioral Medicine: A proposed definition and statement of goals. Journal of Behavioral Medicine, 1978, 1, 3–12.
7. von Bertalanfy, L. General Systems Theory. New York, New York: George Braziller Co., 1966.
8. Schwartz, G.E. and Weiss, S.M. Behavioral Medicine revisited: An amended definition. Journal of Behavioral Medicine, 1978, 3, 249–252.
9. Mahoney, M.J. Reflections on the cognitive learning trend in psychotherapy. American Psychologist, 1977, 32, 5–13.
10. Wilson, E.O. Sociobiology. Cambridge, Mass: Harvard University Press, 1975.
11. Engel, G.L. The need for a new medical model: A challenge for biomedicine. Science, 1977, 196, 129–136.
12. See the Journal "Psychoneuroendocrinology".
13. Schwartz, G.E. and Shapiro, D. Biofeedback and essential hypertension: Current Findings and theoretical concerns. In L. Birk (Ed.) Biofeedback: Behavioral Medicine, New York: Grune and Stratton, 1974.
14. Schwartz, G.E. Disregulation and system theory: A biobehavioral framework for biofeedback and behavioral medicine. In N. Birbaumer and H.D. Kimmel (eds.) Biofeedback and Self-Regulation. Hillsdale, New Jersey, Erlbaum 1979.
15. Weiner, H. Psychobiology and Human Disease. New York: Elsevier, 1977.
16. Schwartz, G.E., Shapiro, A.P., Redmond, D.P., Ferguson, D.C.E., Ragland, D.R. and Weiss, S.M. Behavioral medicine approaches to hypertension: An integrative analysis of theory and research. Journal of Behavioral Medicine, 2, 311–363.
17. Geller, R.G. Report of the Hypertension Task Force-current research and recommendations from the task force subgroups on pediatrics and genetics (Publication No. (NIH) 79–1628). Washington, D.C.: Department of Health, Education and Welfare.
18. Tobian, L., Salt and hypertension. Annals of the New York Academy of Sciences, 1978, 304, 178–197.
19. Dahl, L,K., Heine, M., and Tassinari, L. Role of genetic factors in susceptability to experimental hypertension due to chronic excess salt ingestion. Nature, 1962, 194, 480–482.
20. Friedmann M., and Iwai, J., Dietary sodium, psychic stress and genetic predisposition to experimental hypertension. Proceedings of the Society for Experimental Biology and Medicine, 1977, 296, 405–411.
21. McClelland, D. Inhibited power motivation and high blood pressure in men. Journal of Abnormal Psychology, 1979, 88, 182–190.
22. Esler, M., Julius S., Zweifler, A., Randall, O., Harburg, E., Gardiner, H., and DeQuattro, U. Mild high-renin essential hypertension. New England Journal of Medicine, 1977, 296, 405–411.
23. Jenkins, C.D., Zyzanski, S.J. and Rosenman, R.H. Coronary prone behavior: one pattern or several. Psychosomatic Medicine, 1978, 40, 25–43.
24. Levine, J.D. Gordon N.C., and Fields, H.L. The mechanisms of placebo analgesia, Lancet, 1978, 2, 654–657.

25. Shapiro, A.P., Schwartz, G.E., Ferguson, D.C.E., Behavioral methods in the treatment of hypertension: a review of their clinical status. Annals of Internal Medicine, 1977, 86, 626–636.
26. Weiss, S.M. News and developments: Research training in behavioral medicine. Journal of Behavioral Medicine, 1978, 2, 241–247.

Risks and Prevention

9

Risk Assessment for Disease Prevention

Devra Lee Davis, Ph.D.

Toxic Substances Program
Environmental Law Institute

David P. Rall, M.D. Ph.D.

National Institute of Environmental Health Sciences

with an Appendix on Exposure Assessment Problems
by Brian Magee, M.P.A., M.S.
Environmental Law Institute

The history of public health suggests that successful disease prevention strategies may be devised before the basic mechanisms of diseases have been fully elucidated. It is now generally conceded that during the second half of the nineteenth century, mortality from bacterial diseases was reduced in the developing world almost ten-fold by such public health improvements as improved sanitation, better working conditions and nutrition, and housing improvements.[1] As McKinlay and McKinlay,[2] Rosen,[3] McKeown,[4] Davis and Ng,[5] and others have noted, these improvements in public health constituted a far more significant advance than that introduced by the widespread use of immunization and antibiotics.

Some striking similarities can be detected between the puzzling natures of today's leading causes of death and disease and those of the nineteenth century. Until the turn of this century, infectious diseases caused most sickness and death. Now, as then, although some etiological factors have been identified, the role of predisposing conditions remains in question. Today, chronic degenerative diseases with irreversible, and often slowly debilitating, effects constitute the important mortality problems of cardiovascular disease and cancer; accidents are also leading factors. Morbidity problems include respiratory diseases, circulatory diseases, mental illness, musculoskeletal diseases, and accidents.[6]

While basic mechanisms were not universally understood in the latter part of the nineteenth century, some rather simple, gross observations had been made about the relationship between the environment and infectious diseases. Eckholm[7] suggests that the campfires of prehistoric people undoubtedly caused noticeable pollution. The smoke-filled air inside caves, tents, or homes irritated eyes and encouraged lung and heart disorders. But given the serious threats posed by wild animals and weather, the health toll of this prehistoric air pollution paled in importance. Shakespeare gave literary expression to concern about the air, in *Hamlet*: "This most excellent canopy, the air . . . . why it appears no other thing to me than a foul and pestilent congregation of vapours." Twelve years after *Hamlet's* first production, John Evelyn, in 1616, attempted to relate chronic respiratory disease to air pollution. In his essay, "Smoake of London," he wrote about "the hellish and dismal cloud of 'sea coale'—impure and thick mist accompanied with a fuligious and filthy vapor . . . . corrupting the lungs . . . ."[8] Much later, the English socialists and ministers noted that clean and well-fed people were more healthy;[9] and in 1848, Engels[10] provided a more detailed analysis of the links between some occupations and diseases.

Despite all these observations, some of which were quite meticulous natural histories of occupational and environmental disease, no single view of the underlying causes of these diseases emerged until the late nineteenth century. By this time, substantial improvements in public health had already been achieved. To the extent that today's leading causes of death and sickness are also well studied clinically, although not well understood etiologically, an analogous situation exists. This chapter will argue that while adequate knowledge about basic mechanisms may not be at hand, effective preventive policies for some occupationally and environmentally based diseases may be devised.

Risk Assessment Required for Preventive Policies

Much of the information presented here on the causes of chronic diseases pertains directly to workplace exposures and worker mortality data. This does not imply that general environmental exposures or morbidity data are unimportant, but merely reflects the relative availability of data. In this light, a preoccupation with cancer mortality underestimates the problems of other chronic diseases. Since many of the agents that permeate the workplace are also present in the air and water of heavily industrialized areas, however, worker mortality trends can be viewed as indicators of more generalizable public health problems. And since methods can be developed for reducing exposures to some confirmed carcinogens, the assessment of worker cancer risks should provide important clues for effective prevention strategies. In sum, this chapter focuses on available cancer mortality data while recognizing two needs: that data be developed on other causes of chronic disease and death for workers and the general population,[11] and that such data be used to generate effective disease prevention strategies.

Assessing human health risks in order to restrict or prevent exposures to hazardous substances constitutes one primary prevention policy, akin in its public health impact to improved sanitation and nutrition. With sound health risk evaluations, effective prevention strategies can be created. These strategies will, of course, be further improved when the basic mechanisms of disease are elaborated upon, but such strategies need not await these improvements. If public health policies in the nineteenth century had awaited full scientific confirmation, we might only now be recovering from the effects of polio, diphtheria, whooping cough, and tuberculosis epidemics. Given the recent exponential increase in exposures to manufactured chemicals, most of which have not been evaluated as to health risk, the need to improve our capacity to perform human risk assessment becomes a pressing public health problem.[12]

Any effort to evaluate what proportion of the current disease burden may be linked to environmental and occupational pollutants is itself fraught with risks. Students of environmental health have been confounded for years by the scientific requirement that likely causal links be established between specific environmental pollutants and particular health effects. Because no environmental pollutants occur in isolation from other pollutants, this demand has had the effect of forcing reliance on supposedly definitive laboratory animal studies of single pollutants under highly controlled conditions. Human epidemiological investigations are frequently vulnerable to criticisms that some other variables in addition to the ones being singled out really explain the phenomenon under consideration. Toxicological data from laboratory animals will be faulted in terms of species specificity or homogeneity arguments by some, or because of the numerous assumptions involved in extrapolating from the high dose exposures required for short-lived rodents to the lower doses to which humans are exposed throughout their lifetimes.

Problems of Research Scale. Resource and logistic problems associated with toxicological studies of laboratory animals pose perplexing problems. For instance, manageable sample populations cannot detect increases in toxic events of less than 5-10%. For some health effects, such as mutagenesis and teratogenesis, incidences in the human population of 3 per 1000 or 3 per 10,000 are significant. Obviously, these health effects are not now well studied in whole-body mammalian assays, where only the strongest such effects could be observed. The magnitude of this problem is illustrated by the fact that in assays for environmental toxicants using 1000 animals, each animal is a surrogate for 200,000 people.[13]

Problems of scale occur in epidemiological studies as well. Mack et al.[14] note that in order to detect a doubling of a cancer risk, if only 10% of the members of a population were exposed, one would need to study at least 570 exposed people. For a five-fold increased risk, a baseline of 40 would be required; a baseline of 30 would be required to detect a two-fold risk if half the members of the population were exposed. To put this in perspective, they note that only 1000 new cases of squamous cell carcinoma of the lung occur annually among the entire white male population of Los Angeles County.

In fact, surveys rarely encounter counties where as many as 10% of all people are employed in and exposed to a particular industry. Thus, a 7% increase in lung cancer, if actually due to occupational exposures of the 1-2% of the population employed in that industry, would indicate a risk to workers of 4-8 times that of the general population.[15]   County increases of only 1 or 2 per 100,000 can be quite significant, given the small proportion of workers that may be involved.

Problems of Research Design. As Lalonde[16] and others have documented, public health now reflects a complex interaction between environment, lifestyle, and genetic factors. Toxicological studies of single pollutants necessarily exclude such confounding factors. Epidemiological studies of human populations can embrace some of these multiple factors, but it is rarely possible to devise an epidemiological study which can confirm clear causality—that exposure to substance X causes Y disease, under Z conditions.

Lave and Seskin[17] discuss what an *ideal* study of air pollution and mortality might entail. They note that genetic factors are now difficult to measure conceptually, while data on lifestyle factors such as smoking and nutrition do not generally exist or are poorly measured.

Figure 9-1 provides a path analysis of the air pollution mortality rate model, the arrows indicating the theorized causal links. This path analysis shows that simple correlations between air pollution and mortality reflect numerous influences, including occupation, lifestyle, and genetics. While independent replications of findings under somewhat different conditions will strengthen any hy-

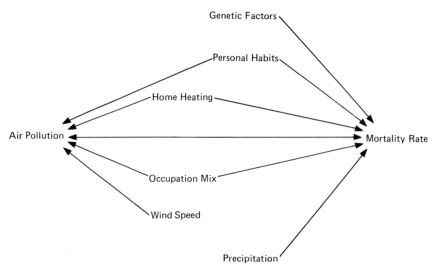

Figure 9-1. Path analysis of the air pollution mortality rate model.[17]

pothesized link between air pollution and mortality, the complex potential interactions will not thereby be eliminated.

One possible solution to this dilemma is a multivariate statistical analysis that controls for the confounding factors.[19] However, this technique is only as good as the data on which it is based, and, for many of the variables in the path model, there are no good data at this time. All of this suggests that expectations for definitive analysis in environmental research may have to be modified.

Problems of Causality. Lave and Seskin suggest that causality may not be a useful concept in investigating the prevention and cure of chronic diseases.

Reduced pulmonary function might arise from a vast number of causes, ranging from acute lung disease and inadequate nutrition to the inhalation of some toxic compound. Whatever the initial cause, the failure of the body to repair the damage may be due to a set of independent factors. Furthermore, the lung damage may become progressive through a third and even larger set of contributing factors, factors including viral infection, occupational exposure, smoking, air pollution, or even one's genetic disposition. What, for example, is the cause of severe dyspnea in a sixty year old asbestos worker who smokes, lives in a large city, comes from an impoverished family, and has never received proper nutrition?[20]

Rall[21] comments on this issue in his review of differences between laboratory animals and humans. "The human population is different . . . .: the mouse doesn't smoke or breath hydrocarbons or sulfur oxides from fossil fuels, doesn't drink, doesn't take medicine, doesn't eat bacon or smoked salmon," while humans obviously do.

Causality cannot be empirically proven, as philosophers of science have often observed. According to Blalock,[22] imputing simple causation entails an artificial isolation or singling out of factors, as though only X explains Y. As Bunge[23] notes, isolation is a simplifying hypothesis rather than a fact. It is indispensable, and even approximately valid in many cases; nevertheless, it is never rigorously true. Thus, isolation is a hypothesis that scientists must make in order to render complex interacting systems explicable in simpler terms.

The Push for Prevention

These caveats notwithstanding, environmental health specialists are now confronted with demands to generate estimates and models of environmentally associated disease. For several years now, federal reports have noted the significance of environment for public health. In 1977, the Second Task Force for Research Planning in Environmental Health Science identified three related characteristics of contemporary public health problems:

1. Further investments in medical treatments and interventions will not yield significant reductions in mortality or morbidity.
2. Prevention of illness and premature death will yield the greatest benefits to society.
3. Therefore, the identification, evaluation, and subsequent modification of the role of environmental factors in causing illness and premature death promise to be critical strategies for the prevention of disease and the promotion of health.

The Task Force concluded that decisions on environmental control significantly affect the quality of our lives and the time and manner of our deaths.

To the extent that specific components of the environment which cause, contribute to, or ameliorate human disease can be identified and altered, means for intervention and control are suggested. Preventive strategy can then be planned. In a society that has been moving steadily toward ever more costly therapeutic approaches, especially those involving hospitalization, preventive approaches may be dictated on economic grounds alone. An even more persuasive force in this direction is the possibility of eliminating or delaying disease and suffering.[24]

Similar sentiments can be noted in the *First Annual Report to Congress of the Task Force on Environmental Cancer, Heart and Lung Disease.*[25] They reported that the risk and occurrence of cancer and heart and lung disease increase with environmental pollution, and, moreover, that current preventive measures are inadequate. The Cancer, Heart and Lung Disease Task Force called for the generation of preventive strategies in order to reduce the health risks of these diseases.

Cancer as a Prevention Priority. Cancer is not the only health problem with which we should be concerned, of course. It has become a key target for preventive actions because data show that many cancers can be linked with our patterns of industrial activity and lifestyle practices. Cancer is also a dread disease that has a great deal of mental and physical pain associated with it. Besides being the second largest cause of death of Americans (as it has been since the 1930's), cancer can strike anyone, regardless of age. More pertinent is that cancer is the leading cause of lost years of productive life prior to age 65. Tables 9-1 and 9-2 taken from a HEW report entitled "Ten Leading Causes of Death in the United States, 1975"[26] indicate the relative importance of the causes of death before age 65.

A recent HEW study[27] considered how best to estimate the proportion of future cancer deaths associated with occupational exposures now and in the future. The study foresees that at least 20% of cancer deaths in this country in

Table 9-1. Ten leading causes of death. (Percentage distribution by cause.
Total population 1+ years of age. U.S.A., 1975.)

Cause	Number of Deaths	Rate per 100,000	Percent of Total
Heart disease	715,472	340.78	38.8
Cancer	365,549	174.11	19.8
Cerebrovascular disease	193,859	92.33	10.5
All other accidents	56,046	26.70	3.0
Influenza and pneumonia	53,456	25.46	2.9
Motor vehicle accidents	45,573	21.71	2.5
Diabetes	35,219	16.78	1.9
Cirrhosis of liver	31,581	15.04	1.7
Arteriosclerosis	28,882	13.76	1.6
Suicide	27,062	12.89	1.5

Table 9-2. Years of potential life lost. (Total population ages 1–64.
U.S.A., 1975.)

Cause	Total Years Lost	Percent Total Years
Cancer	1,802,820	17.5
Heart disease	1,769,180	17.2
Motor vehicle accidents	1,424,823	13.8
All other accidents	1,166,793	11.3
Homicide	621,846	6.0
Suicide	583,751	5.7
Cerebrovascular disease	352,524	3.4
Cirrhosis of liver	320,457	3.1
Influenza and Pneumonia	206,673	2.0
Diabetes	118,119	1.1

the near future may be due to past occupational exposures. It concludes that
reducing occupational exposure offers important opportunities for prevention.
The study describes three caveats in generating estimates of cancer related to
occupational exposures which reflect the general methodological difficulties
noted earlier:

1. First of all, the study concedes that available data are incomplete, both
   for the kinds of substances studied and for the quality of information
   on exposed workers. Rather few potential carcinogenic processes have
   been identified to date; and only infrequently are workers studied from
   time of exposure until their deaths. Thus, if an exposed worker is only
   studied while working, the cancer which develops from this exposure one

year before death at age 62 (a post-retirement age) will not become a data point.

2. Secondly, the fallacy of monocausal explanations for cancer is noted. Rall,[28] Davis,[29] and others have observed that people are never exposed to single carcinogens but to a multitude of potential carcinogens and other toxins. What Albert and Burns[30] point out about low doses is equally true of higher ones; there is an important additional component of risk involving a heightened susceptibility to cancer induction by a variety of agents that would otherwise be relatively innocuous.

3. Finally, the study notes that exposure data are typically weak. It is rarely the case that workers are exposed throughout their entire working lives to the same chemical at similar concentrations. Also, the quality of exposure data is uneven, often having been historically reconstructed.

The HEW report notes that no firm quantification of the risks associated with carcinogens in the workplace can be made, given the state of the art in extrapolating from animals to humans. The report adds, however, that there is no evidence that these risks are substantially less than the risks resulting from exposures in the recent past.

Asbestos: A Case Study in Occupationally Related Cancers. With these qualifications in mind, we present a synopsis of the HEW estimates on asbestos. If only one of the thousands of high-volume chemicals introduced into commerce since the chemical revolution of the 1940's proves to be as hazardous as asbestos, this could sustain rates of occupationally related cancer for decades.

The health hazards of asbestos have been known in the medical literature since the early part of this century. In 1924, Cooke[31] reported on pulmonary fibrosis due to inhalation of asbestos. In 1935, an etiologic link was postulated between asbestosis and lung cancer.[32] The precise history of industry's and government's knowledge of these risks will become clear as a result of current litigation. It seems fair to state now that knowledge of asbestos hazards has been available since the 1940's, although major preventive policies are only now being fully proposed and implemented. Selikoff[32] reports that some 25 million tons of asbestos have been used in this country from 1890 to 1970. During the next 50 years, many of the ships, buildings, locomotives, factories, and automobile parts containing this asbestos will be disposed of, exposing workers and their communities to increased risks.

It has been estimated that between 8 and 11 million workers have been exposed to asbestos in the U.S. since the 1940's. Probably one million of these have already died. About 1.5-2.5 million are presently employed. Of the surviving asbestos workers, 4.5 million worked in shipyards during the 1940's.

Of these and other surviving asbestos workers, about 4 million are believed to have had heavy exposure to asbestos. Between 35 and 44% of heavily exposed workers who have died, have died from cancers, leaving between 65 and 56% of them dying from other causes (most likely heart disease, stroke, and accidents). Although the proportion of deaths due to cancer usually declines with increasing age, these figures may be underestimates of lifetime cancer risks, since most of the workers have not been followed to the end of their lifespans.

Of all workers exposed in the past, between 2 and 2.3 million are expected to die of cancers within the next 30-year period. This creates an annual average of asbestos related cancer deaths of between 58,000 and 75,000. On their own, these numbers constitute between 13 and 18% of all expected cancer deaths in this country, assuming annual totals of 400,000-450,000.

The authors of the HEW report point out that these estimates apply to present and near-future cancer deaths related to past exposures. Insofar as current exposures are reduced, the numbers of asbestos related deaths can be expected to drop. Also, a large proportion of the asbestos related cancers are also related to other exposures, such as smoking and other possible occupational and environmental carcinogens. Finally, the incidence of asbestos related disease is probably understated in mortality data, for several reasons:

1. The major asbestos related cancers of pleural and peritoneal mesothelioma have been classified as lung cancers or as various abdominal cancers in national statistics; some cancer registries have only recently included mesothelioma as a category.
2. Increases in other asbestos related cancers of the stomach or colon would be masked by other long-term trends, usually attributed to dietary or other factors.
3. People dying from heart disease will be classified as heart attack or stroke victims. Although asbestos related disease could have been a contributing cause of death, having weakened the body's defense mechanisms, only single causes of death have been indicated on certificates.
4. The percentage of all deaths routinely autopsied is quite low now; these potential sources of information about contributing causes of death are lost. For example, a recent study has shown that many older men die with undetected prostatic cancers. Although the annual detected incidence of prostate cancer in 70-year-old men is about 200 cases per 10,000 men, or 0.2% annually, routine autopsies of 70-year-old men who had died of other causes revealed microscopic evidence of prostate cancer in 15-20% of the cases.[33] Similarly, if more autopsies were routinely performed, an increase in the incidence of asbestos linked diseases might be detected.

Table 9-3. Twenty-six chemicals or industrial processes associated with cancer induction in humans as identified by the International Agency for Research on Cancer.[34]

Aflatoxins	Cyclophosphamide
4-Aminobiphenyl	Diethylstilbestrol
Arsenic compounds	Hematite mining (? radon)
Asbestos	Isopropyl oils
Auramine (manufacture of)	Melphalan
Benzene	Mustard gas
Benzidine	2-Naphthylamine
Bis(chloromethyl) ether	Nickel (nickel refining)
Cadmium-using industries (possibly	N,N-Bis (2-chloroethyl)-2-naphthylamine
cadmium oxide)	Oxymetholone
Chloramphenicol	Phenacetin
Chloromethyl methyl ether (possibly	Phenytoin
associated with bis(chloromethyl) ether	Soot, tars, and oils
Chromium (chromate-producing industries)	Vinyl chloride

Occupational Exposure to Other Confirmed Human Carcinogens. Epidemiological studies have identified more than 26 substances as carcinogenic to humans (see Table 9-3), and toxicological reviews by the International Association for Research on Cancer, a division of the World Health Organization, have indicated that 221 chemicals have tested positive in animal carcinogenesis experiments (see Table 9-4).[34] To date, every substance known to cause cancer in humans also causes cancer in animals. The majority of these 221 agents can be found in the workplace, but only a small number of them have been regulated as carcinogens. In addition, there are many chemicals to which people are exposed that are suspected to be hazardous to human health, but for which little or no scientific data are available.

In its first two years of activity, the Interagency Testing Committee (established under the authority of the Toxic Substances Control Act to advise the administrator of the EPA) identified 7 individual chemicals and 11 classes of chemicals (each of which includes a number of individual substances) to which thousands of workers have been exposed, but for which little toxicological information is available (see Table 9-5). Many of these same substances were also listed by the Interagency Regulatory Liaison Group in its recent compilation of plans to regulate hazardous materials (see Table 9-6). In some cases, the production of these substances has been steadily rising since the early 1960's, but exposures are too recent to have caused any noticeable epidemiological effects.

Table 9-4. Two hundred twenty-one chemicals found by the International Agency for Research on Cancer to Cause Cancer in Experimental Animals.[34]

Acetamide
Actinomycins
p-Aminoazobenzene
o-Aminoazotoluene
2-Amino-5-(5-nitro-2-furyl)-1, 3, 4-thiadiazole
Amitrole
Aramite
Aurothioglucose
Azaserine
Aziridine
2-(1-Aziridinyl)-ethanol
Aziridyl benzoquinone
Azobenzene
Benz(a)acridine
Benz(c)acridine
Benzo(b)fluoranthene
Benzo(j)fluoranthene
Benzo(a)pyrene
Benzo(e)pyrene
Benzyl chloride
Benzyl violet 4B
Beryllium
Beryllium oxide
Beryllium phosphate
Beryllium sulfate
Beryl ore
BHC (technical grades)
Bis(1-aziridinyl)-morpholinophosphine sulfide
Bis(chloroethyl)ether
1, 2-Bis(chloromethoxy)ethane
1, 4-Bis(chloromethoxymethyl)benzene
Blue VRS
Brilliant blue FCF
1, 4-Butanediol dimethane-sulfonate (Myleran)
β-Butyrolactone
Cadmium chloride
Cadmium power
Cadmium sulfate
Cadmium sulfide
Calcium chromate
Cantharidin
Carbon tetrachloride
Chlorambucil
Chlormadinone acetate
Chlorobenzilate
Chromic chromate
Chrysene
Chrysoidine
Citrus red No. 2
Coumarin
Cycasin
Cyclochlorotine
Daunomycin
DDT
N, N-Diacetylbenzidine

Diallate
4, 4'-Diaminodiphenyl ether
2, 4-Diaminotoluene
Diazomethane
Dibenz(a, h)acridine
Dibenz(a, j)acridine
Dibenz(a, h)anthracene
Dibenzo(c, g)carbazole
Dibenzo(h, rst)pentaphene
Dibenzo(a, e)pyrene
Dibenzo(a, h)pyrene
Dibenzo(a, i)pyrene
Dibenzo(a, j)pyrene
1, 2-Dibromo-3-chloropropane
Dibutylnitrosamine
3, 3'-Dichlorobenzidine
3, 3'-Dichloro-4, 4'-diamino-diphenyl ether
Dieldrin
Diepoxybutane
1, 2-Diethylhydrazine
Diethylnitrosamine
Diethyl sulfate
Dihydrosafrole
Dimethoxane
3, 3'-Dimethoxybenzidine
p-Dimethylaminoazobenzene
trans-2-[(Dimethylamino)methylamino]-5-[2-(5-nitro-2-furyl)vinyl]-1, 3, 4-oxadiazole
3, 3'-Dimethylbenzidine
Dimethylcarbamoylchloride
1, 1-Dimethylhydrazine
1, 2-Dimethylhydrazine
Dimethylnitrosamine
Dimethyl sulfate
1, 4-Dioxane
Dithranol
Epichlorohydrin
1-Epoxyethyl-3, 4-epoxycyclohexane
3, 4-Epoxy-6-methylcyclohexylmethyl-3, 4-epoxy-6-methyl carboxylate
Estradiol mustard
Ethinylestradiol
Ethionamide
Ethylene dibromide
Ethylene sulfide
Ethylenethiourea
Ethyl methane sulfonate
Ethynodiol diacetate
Evans blue
Fast green FCF
2-(2-Formylhydrazino)-4-(5-nitro-2-furyl)thiazole
Glycidaldehyde
Griseofulvin
Guinea green B
Hexamethylphosphoramide
Hycanthone (mesylate)
Hydrazine

Table 9-4 *(continued)*

Indeno (1, 2, 3-cd)pyrene
Iron dextran
Iron dextrin
Isatidine
Isonicotinic acid hydrazide
Isosafrole
Lasiocarpine
Lead acetate
Lead phosphate
Lead subacetate
Light green SF
Lindane
Luteoskyrin
Magenta
Maleic hydrazide
Mannomustine (dihydrochloride)
Medroxyprogesterone acetate
Merphalan
Mestranol
2-Methylaziridine
Methylazoxymethanol acetate
N-Methyl-N, 4-dinitrosoaniline
4, 4'-Methylenebis(2-chloroaniline)
4, 4'-Methylenebis(2-methylaniline)
Methyl iodide
Methyl methanesulfonate
N-Methyl-N-nitro-N-nitrosoguanidine
Methylthiouracil
Metronidazole
Mirex
Mitomycin C
Monocrotaline
Monuron
5-(Morpholinomethyl)-3-[(5-nitrofurfuryli-
  dene)-amino]-2-oxazolidinone
1-Naphthylamine
Native carrageenans
Nickel carbonyl
Nickelocene
Nickel oxide
Nickel powder
Nickel subsulfide
Niridazole
5-Nitroacenaphthene
4-Nitrobiphenyl
1-[(5-Nitrofurfurylidene)amino]-2-
  imidazolidinone
N-[4-(5-Nitro-2-furyl)-2-thiazolyl]-
  acetamide
Nitrogen mustard (hydrochloride)
Nitrogen mustard N-oxide (hydrochloride)
Nitrosoethylurea
Nitrosomethylurea
N-Nitroso-N-methylurethan
Norethisterone
Norethisterone acetate

Norethynodrel
17β-Oestradiol
Oestrone
Oil orange SS
Orange I
Oxazepam
Parasorbic acid
Patulin
Penicillic acid
Phenicarbazide
Phenobarbital sodium
Phenoxybenzamine
N-Phenyl-2-naphthylamine
Polychlorinated biphenyls
Ponceau MX
Ponceau 3R
Potassium bis(2-hydroxyethyl)-dithiocarbamate
Progesterone
Pronetalol hydrochloride
1, 3-Propanesultone
β-Propiolactone
n-Propyl carbamate
Propylene oxide
Propylthiouracil
Pyrimethamine
Quintozene
Retrorsine
Rhodamine B
Rhodamine 6G
Saccharated iron
Safrole
Semicarbazide (hydrochloride)
Sterigmatocystin
Streptozotocin
Strontium chromate
Succinic anhydride
Sudan I
Sudan II
Tannic acid
Terpene polychlorinates
Testosterone
Thioacetamide
4, 4'-Thioaniline
Thiouracil
Thiourea
Trichloroethylene
Triethylene glycoldiglycidyl ether
Tris(aziridinyl)-p-benzoquinone
Tris(1-aziridinyl)-phosphine sulfide
2, 4, 6-Tris(1-aziridinyl)-s-triazine
1, 2, 3-Tris(chloromethoxy)-propane
Trypan blue
Uracil mustard
Urethan
Yellow OB
Zinc chromate hydroxide

Table 9-5. High-priority chemicals for testing and evaluation identified by the first and second reports of the TSCA Interagency Testing Committee.[42]

First report of the ITC:	Second report of the ITC:
Alkyl epoxides	Acrylamide
Alkyl phthalates	Aryl phosphates
Chlorinated benzenes (mono- and di-)	Chlorinated naphthalenes
Chlorinated paraffins	Dichloromethane
Chloromethanes	Halogenated alkyl epoxides
Cresols	Polychlorinated terphenyls
Hexachloro-1, 3-butadiene	Pyridine
Nitrobenzene	1, 1, 1-Trichloroethane
Toluene	
Xylenes	

Given the methodological difficulties indicated earlier, only limited epidemiological data are available on human carcinogens. Even with this reservation, it is worthwhile to consider data on the numbers of workers exposed to various levels of some high-volume carcinogens in addition to asbestos. Epidemiological studies of workers have identified the following substances as carcinogenic to humans: arsenic,[38] benzene,[39] chromium,[40] and nickel.[41] Such studies typically calculate risk ratios, indicating the extent to which exposed workers' risks of contracting some forms of cancer is greater than those of the general population. These risk ratios do not indicate any of the risks associated with the other chronic health effects associated with exposures to these chemicals.

Table 9-6. Twenty-four hazardous materials that two or more interagency regulatory liaison group agencies are planning to regulate and for which development plans have been published.[43]

Acrylonitrile	Diethylstilbestrol
Arsenic	Ethylene dibromide
Asbestos	Ethylene oxide and its residues
Benzene	Lead
Beryllium	Mercury and mercury compounds
Cadmium	Nitrosamines
Chloroform and chlorinated solvents	Ozone
Trichloroethylene (TCE)	PBB's
Perchloroethylene (PCE)	PCB's
Methylchloroform	Radiation
Chlorofluorocarbons (CFC)	Sulfur dioxide
Chromates	Vinyl chloride (VC)
Coke oven emissions	and polyvinyl chloride (PVC)
Dibromochloropropane	Waste disposal to food chain land

Table 9-7. Risk factors associated with workplace exposures to five high-volume confirmed human carcinogens.

Chemical	Target Organs in Humans[a,b]	Other Chronic Health Effects[c,d]	Occupations at Risk[a]	Latency Period for Cancer (years)[a]	Risk Ratios for Cancer[a]	Estimated Number of Workers Exposed Annually
Arsenic	Skin, lung, liver, lymphatic system.	Gastrointestinal disturbances, hyperpigmentation, peripheral neuropathy, hemolytic anemia, dermatitis, bronchitis, nasal system ulceration.	Miners, smelters, insecticide makers and sprayers, chemical workers, oil refiners vintners.	10+	3–8	1,500,000[e]
Asbestos	Lung, pleural and peritoneal mesothelioma gastrointestinal tract.	Asbestosis (pulmonary fibrosis, pleural plaques, and pleural calcification), anorexia, weight loss.	Miners, millers, textile, insulation and shipyard workers.	4–40	1.5–12	1,600,000[f] 2,522,000[g]
Benzene	Bone marrow (leukemia)	Central nervous system and gastrointestinal effects; blood abnormalities (anemia, leukopenia, and thrombocytopenia).	Explosives, benzene and rubber cement workers, distillers, dye users, printers, shoemakers.	6–14	2–3	2,000,000[h] 1,900,000[f]
Chromium	Nasal cavity and sinuses, lung, larynx.	Dermatitis, skin ulceration, nasal system ulceration, bronchitis, bronchopneumia, inflamation of the larynx and liver.	Producers, processors, and users of Cr; acetylene and aniline workers; beachers; glass, pottery, and linoleum workers; battery makers.	5–15	3–4	1,500,000[f] (chromium oxides) 175,000[i] (chromium VI)
Nickel	Nasal cavity and sinuses, lung.	Dermatitis.	Nickel smelters, mixers, and roasters, electrolysis workers.	3–30	5–10 (lung), 100+ (nasal sinuses)	1,400,000[f] (oxides) 25,000[j] (inorganic nickel)

[a]Cole, P. and Goldman, M., in Fraumeni, J. (Ed.), *Persons at High Risk of Cancer*. New York: Academic Press, 1975.

[b]*Occupational Diseases*. Washington, D. C.: U. S. Department of Health, Education, and Welfare, 1977.

[c]Casarett, L. and Doull, J. (Eds.), *Toxicology*. New York: Macmillan, 1975.

[d]Waldbott, G., *Health Effects of Environmental Pollutants*. Saint Louis: C. V. Mosby, 1978.

[e]*Criteria for a Recommended Standard: Occupational Exposure to Inorganic Arsenic*. Rockville, Maryland: National Institute for Occupational Safety and Health, 1975.

[f]*National Occupational Hazard Survey* III. Cincinnati, Ohio: National Institute for Occupational Safety and Health, 1977.

[g]*Asbestos: An Information Resource*. Bethesda, Maryland: National Cancer Institute, 1978.

Table 9-7. *(Continued)*

OSHA Workplace Permissible Exposure Limits (8-hour time weighted average air concentration)[k]	Notes[k]	NIOSH Recommended Standard[l]	Transmitted to OSHA[l]
10 $\mu g/m^3$ (May 1978)	The current standard supersedes the old standard of 500 $\mu g/m^3$ and is presently under litigation.	2 $\mu g/m^3$ 15 min. ceiling)	June 1975
2 fibers/cm^3 (10 fibers/cm^3 ceiling) (June 1972)	A proposal made in November 1975 to lower standard to 15 fibers/cm^3 is pending.	0.1 fibers/cm^3 over 5 μ. (0.5 fibers/cm^3 5 μ. 15 min. ceiling)	Dec. 1976
10 ppm (25 ppm 15 min. ceiling) (1971)	The new standard promulgated in February 1978 of 1 ppm (5 ppm 15 min. ceiling) was vacated by the 5th Circuit Court of Appeals in October 1978.	1 ppm ceiling for 60 min.	July 1974 revised July 1977
chromic acid and chromates: 0.1 mg/m^3 soluble chromium and chromous salts: 0.5 mg/m^3 methyl chromium and insoluble salts: 1 mg/m^3 (1971)	OSHA expects to propose new standards during 1979.	chromic acid: 0.05 mg/m^3 Carcinogenic Cr VI: 0.001 mg/m^3 other Cr VI: 0.025 mg/m^3	July 1973 Dec. 1975
metal and soluble compounds: 1 mg/m^3 (1971)		0.015 mg/m^3	May 1977

[h]*Criteria for a Recommended Standard: Occupational Exposure to Benzene.* Rockville, Maryland: National Institute for Occupational Safety and Health, 1974.

[i]*Criteria for Recommended Standard: Occupational Exposure to Chromium (VI).* Rockville, Maryland: National Institute for Occupational Safety and Health, 1975.

[j]*Criteria for a Recommended Standard: Occupational Exposure to Inorganic Nickel.* Rockville, Maryland: National Institue for Occupational Safety and Health, 1977.

[k]Directorate of Health Standards Programs, Occupational Health and Safety Administration, Department of Labor, Washington, D. C. 20210. Personal communication, 1979.

[l]"Summary of NIOSH Recommendations for Occupational Health Standards." Rockville, Maryland: National Institute for Occupational Safety and Health, 1978 (mimeo).

Table 9-7 shows some relevant characteristics of these substances. More than 12 million workers are annually exposed to at least one of these industrial carcinogens. While Occupational Health and Safety Administration standards have been proposed for several of these, they are not uniformly in effect. And even where standards may be in effect, they may not be effective. This is particularly true where protective clothing and respirators are involved. The epidemiological studies noted above often do not include deaths due to non-cancer, chronic diseases; nor do they generally consider morbidity effects associated with cancer or other diseases.

The most difficult aspect of any effort to assess the risks of exposure to these substances involves efforts to estimate average levels and durations of exposures. The figures indicated in Table 9-7 may be faulted because they derive from the National Occupational Hazard Survey,[44] which asked only how many workers were exposed to a given substance and not at what levels this exposure took place. Thus, these numbers must be regarded cautiously as indicating likely human exposure.

Until exposure assessment methodologies are developed, some surrogate measures will be required, lest the absence of hard numbers lead to a tendency to minimize the significance of exposure problems. One possible measure in this light is offered by data on production and consumption. Table 9-8 summarizes

Table 9-8. Amounts of confirmed human carcinogens potentially available for human exposure, 1940-PRESENT.

Substance, Measure, and Unit	Time Period			
	1940–1949	1950–1959	1960–1969	1970–1976
Asbestos (U. S. apparent consumption, thousands of short tons)	464	742	756	770
Benzene (U. S. production, millions of gallons)	172	286	786	1286
Chromite (U. S. apparent consumption, thousands of short tons)	814	1338	1332	1194
White arsenic (As_2O_3) (U. S. apparent consumption, thousands of short tons)	34	22	Confidential industry data	
	1945–1954	1955–1965	1965–1977	
Nickel (U. S. consumption, thousands of short tons)	91	117	166	

the amounts of confirmed human carcinogens potentially available for human exposure to asbestos, benzene, chromite, and nickel. (Data on arsenic is subject to proprietary restrictions, being domestically produced since 1961 by a single company.)

These last two tables suggest there is reason to expect a sizable increase in some cancer rates in the future due to both workplace and environmental exposures to these few carcinogens. The appendix to this chapter provides further discussion on exposure assessment problems and some more detailed data on domestic production and consumption.

Conclusion

Some individuals who have recently contracted cancer because of an exposure to one of these agents that occurred many years in the past may have been exposed to higher levels than those experienced by workers now. Acceptable levels of some carcinogens in the workplace have certainly been lowered, but at the same time, the production and use of other such agents has been skyrocketing. It is probable that some of the decreases in occupational exposure levels have been offset by the increases in facilities that produce and consume these agents and the concomitant increases in the numbers of exposed workers. Hence, while workers' risks due to a single controlled carcinogen may be less, overall risk may well be greater, due to synergies with other uncontrolled toxic substances. When the risks from these occupations are included with those from asbestos, the overall proportion of cancer now and in the future due to occupational factors comprises at least 20%.

The HEW study uses one well-studied example of occupational carcinogenesis as the basis for estimating general occupational cancer risk associated with six known carcinogens. In light of the rapid growth in chemical testing capacities and requirements related to the Toxic Substances Control Act and other recent environmental legislation, it is reasonable to expect that other such carcinogens and sources of chronic health problems will be identified in the next few years. It should be added that consideration here has been limited to chemical carcinogens alone. The discussion has not included any occupational or medicinal exposure to low-level ionizing radiation, nor likely synergies with naturally occurring hazardous substances.

The numerical estimates in this HEW report have been disputed by some critics, who mistakenly assumed that the purpose of the draft summary was to generate precise predictions. Many of their criticisms stem from the problem of identifying single causes of cancer, because all of the above confirmed carcinogens except benzene have been linked with lung cancer. As Stallones and Downs[45] have recently pointed out, given the present state of knowledge of cancer causation, it is necessary to consider cancer as a multipli-caused disease, for which an unwieldy system of overlapping causes may be necessary. While such a system is open-ended and methodologically difficult, as they note, it offers the best approach at this time. The major point of this chapter, however, was to demonstrate that a major public health disaster can develop while its early manifestations are ignored or lost by being attributed to other factors.

While the precision of the estimates in the HEW report can be disputed, and methodologies for confirming them can be questioned, the overall conclusion stands. Much of cancer today and in the near future can be explained by past occupational exposures. Possibilities for effective preventive policies are clear, although basic mechanisms are not. We are paying the price now for failing to implement these policies earlier.

Appendix: Exposure Assessment Problems

This appendix discusses some of the major methodological difficulties in estimating the nature, level, and duration of human exposure to carcinogens. To assess human exposure, it is necessary to develop information on materials balances, which includes data on environmental transport and fate, and biokinetics, including metabolic transformation. For most substances, such data are not now available. Thus, it is necessary to devise appropriate surrogate measures for exposure in order to set public priorities.

The quantities of cancer-causing chemicals to which humans could be exposed have increased exponentially in the last 20 years. Cancers initiated by exposures to these chemicals do not manifest themselves until appropriate latency periods elapse. Such periods are thought to range from 5 to 40 years. Figure 9-2 shows the production history of some aggregated categories of chemicals known to include carcinogens.

The cancer rate for a given year reflects exposures to carcinogens many years in the past. Exposures occurring since the late 1950's and early 1960's may trigger a great increase in the incidence of human cancer because of the skyrocketing production of chemicals known or suspected of causing cancer, but such an effect might not be evident until the end of this century.

There is no simple way to measure the amount of a carcinogenic chemical to which humans are exposed, either occupationally or environmentally. Routinely collected statistics indicate domestic production and/or domestic consumption. These production measures do not quantify how much of an agent comes into contact with people; rather, they reflect only the amount of a chemical potentially available for exposure. It is reasonable to assume, however, that increased production and use necessitate that more people come into contact with the agent at more different points.

To the extent that production, use, and disposal of a material are associated with risks, domestic production will overestimate the risk in cases where signifi-

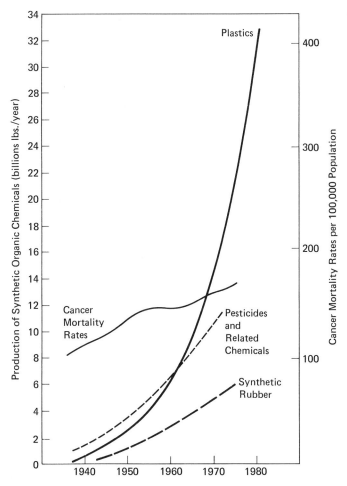

Figure 9-2. Cancer mortality rate and production of chemicals over time.[46]

cant amounts are exported and made no longer available to domestic users. In cases where imports are significant with respect to domestic production, then production will underestimate risk because much of that material used domestically would originate abroad. It would seem, then, that consumption would be a better measure of the potential exposures associated with the production and use of a chemical.

In certain cases, industry data are not available regarding use patterns. In these cases, apparent consumption is reported instead of actual consumption. Generally, this is defined as production plus imports minus exports. Consumption figures, however, are still only surrogates for actual exposure data. They do not include material that was produced domestically and consumed abroad, for instance. If production has a high level of risk associated with it and if exports are high, then the domestic risk will be significantly underestimated. The risk can be doubly underestimated by consumption figures if the material then reenters the country as a finished product. Arsenic, for example, could be produced in the U.S. as As_2O_3 and exported to another country where it is manufactured into an arsenic pesticide. The pesticide could then be shipped back to the U.S. Here, the risks associated with the primary production of the arsenic chemical and the final use of the arsenic product would not be represented in the statistics for apparent consumption. The same would be true even if the actual consumption were measured, because the definition of consumption includes that amount of the material consumed by industry, not by final consumers.

On the other hand, either production or consumption statistics can overestimate the potential exposures if the increased production and use is accompanied with much stricter environmental control measures than were present earlier in time, when production was lower, but exposures per unit total production was higher.

A detailed study of the risks posed by an individual chemical would have to start with production and consumption data and then pursue a serious and complete analysis, taking into account such factors as those mentioned above, and culminating in a consideration of disposal practices and resource recovery possibilities.

Asbestos. Asbestos is the generic name for a group of minerals that exist in fibrous forms. These include chrysotile, crocidolite, amosite, and, to a lesser degree, anthophyllite, tremolite, and actinolite. Commercial asbestos consists primarily of chrysotile, but no particular fibrous form has been demonstrated to be safe.

Because of their unique combination of heat-resistance, anti-corrosion properties, strength, and flexibility, asbestos minerals have a wide variety of uses. They are found in thousands of commercial products, including heat-resistant textiles, reinforced cement, thermal insulation, floor tiles, gaskets, and brake linings.

It is thought that carcinogenic activity derives from the shape and size of the mineral fibers rather than from their chemical nature. Thus, gross weight of asbestos produced and consumed may be an adequate measure of the toxic material potentially available for human exposure.

As reported by the Bureau of Mines, "apparent consumption" is defined as the amount of material sold or used by domestic producers plus imports (unmanufactured) plus stockpile releases (unmanufactured) minus exports and re-exports (unmanufactured). This statistic may slightly underestimate the total amount of material available for exposure to Americans, since manufactured as-

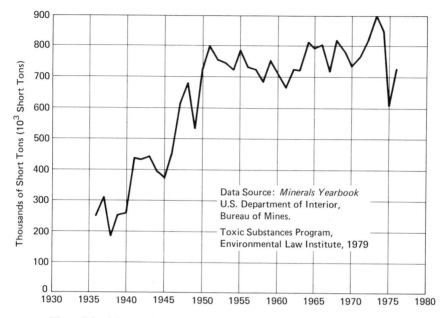

Figure 9-3. Asbestos, U.S. apparent consumption (Thousands of short tons).

bestos products that are imported for consumption are not included. Thus, the thousands of brake linings that enter the country in foreign-made automobiles will present a risk to American auto mechanics, but this asbestos material will not be reflected in the summary statistic (see Figure 9-3).

Chromium. Chromite is the major chromium-containing ore of commercial significance. Chromite is used by the refractory industry to make refractory bricks for lining metallurgical furnaces. In the metallurgical industry, chromite is reduced to metallic chromium, which is used in various stainless steels and chromium alloys. The chemical industry uses chromite to produce dichromate, which is then converted to a variety of chromium chemicals, such as those used as tanning agents, pigments, catalysts, wood preservatives, and plating agents.

Chromium exists primarily in two oxidation states: Cr III and Cr VI. It is the hexavalent (Cr VI) form that is corrosive and highly toxic and has received considerable regulatory attention. The trivalent form has not received such attention because it has generally been thought to be non-toxic. Although it is clear that Cr VI is the more toxic of the two forms, Cr III has been inadequately studied and may also prove to be toxic. All hexavalent chromium is ultimately reduced to the trivalent form, the more stable of the two; but may remain in the very toxic form for long periods of time as airborne particulates or in aqueous solution.

Human exposure to hexavalent chromium is mainly limited to the chemical industry. Most epidemiological information that exists regarding the adverse health effects of Cr VI comes from studies of workers in the industries that produce dichromate from chromite ore. Lung cancer is the most serious health effect noted, but workers have been observed to develop other diseases of the respiratory system and the skin. Few studies have been done on the chromate-using industries, but it is assumed that workers in these industries are also at risk. It is not known whether chromite ore itself should be implicated as a toxic material because the chromium contained therein is primarily in the trivalent state.

Consumption statistics are reported by the Bureau of Mines as actual consumption. In the years 1930–1940, however, no consumption statistic is listed. "Apparent available supply," which is defined as "sales from domestic mines plus imports," is used here as a surrogate for consumption in these years.

The numbers here (see Figure 9-4) represent gross weight of chromium ores and concentrates. The actual chromium content of these ores varies from year to year. Since most of the concern about occupational exposures to chromium centers on the highly carcinogenic hexavalent forms, the total domestic consumption of chromite ore may overestimate the risks presented by chromium. Presentation of just that chromite consumed by the chemical industry would under-

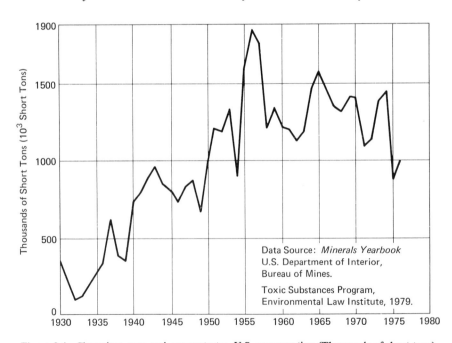

Figure 9-4. Chromite: ores and concentrates, U.S. consumption (Thousands of short tons).

estimate the risks, because many different workers come into contact with the toxic Cr VI as it is converted into, and used as, chromium chemicals. Concern about the risks associated with chromium exposure has to date focused on Cr VI. It may be necessary to expand consideration in the future to Cr III as well.

Benzene. Benzene is a very high-production chemical of great industrial significance. Almost all of the benzene consumed in this country is converted into other chemical products. Workers are exposed to benzene in its central production, as well as during its conversion to other chemicals. Consumers are exposed through numerous sources, including gasoline and household solvents.

The chief health effects associated with exposures to benzene are blood abnormalities, including leukemia. Benzene also acts as a systemic toxin to the central nervous system and the gastrointestinal system.

Prior to 1950, domestic benzene was produced almost exclusively by coke oven operators and coal tar distillers. In recent years, the quantities produced by petroleum refiners have grown such that petroleum is now the major source of domestically produced benzene, accounting for over 95% of production.

These production statistics (see Figures 9-5 and 9-6) include benzene used for blending with motor fuels for the purposes of boosting octane ratings. Total

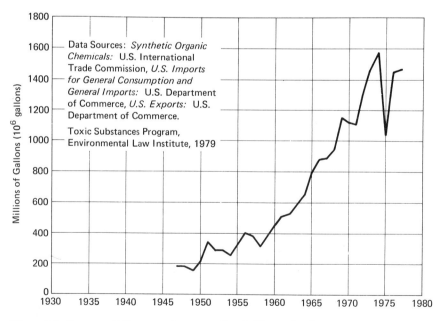

Figure 9-5. Benzene, U.S. apparent consumption (millions of gallons). Includes all grades, including that blended with motor fuels.

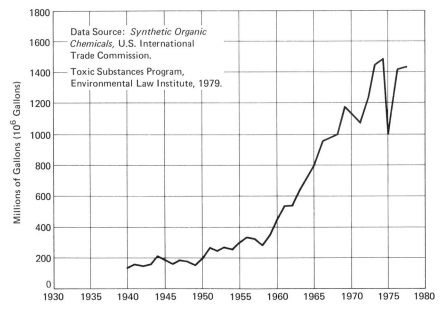

Figure 9-6. Benzene, U.S. production (millions of gallons). Includes all grades, including that blended with motor fuels.

benzene production is slightly under-reported, however, because these figures do not include "other industrial grades" (besides specification grades) produced from coal and coke. This small quantity of benzene amounts to less than 1% of total production.

Apparent consumption is defined here as domestic production plus imports minus exports (both pure and crude).

Nickel. Nickel occurs naturally as either an oxide or a sulfide ore. The nickel is used after being processed either partially to ferronickel or nickel oxide or fully to pure nickel metal. The major use of nickel in the U.S. is in making steel and other alloys. Combined with other metals, nickel provides strength and corrosion-resistance over a wide variety of temperatures. It is thus vital to the iron, steel, and aerospace industries. A large quantity of nickel is also used in electroplating; a lesser amount goes to a variety of chemical and catalytic operations.

Lung and nasal cancer is the primary health risk posed by exposures to nickel. It is thought that respirable particles of nickel, nickel subsulfide and nickel oxide, and nickel carbonyl vapor are the primary nickel species responsible for the induction of cancer. These forms of nickel are associated with all modes of nickel production and utilization.

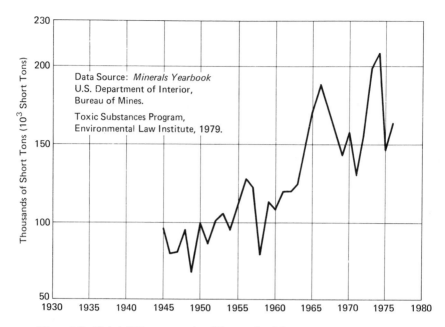

Figure 9-7. Nickel, U.S. consumption (Thousands of short tons, contained nickel).

The consumption data presented here (see Figure 9-7) were collected directly from nickel-consuming industries by the Bureau of Mines through annual surveys, and constitute actual consumption figures. The amount of nickel salts used in the electroplating industries, however, is estimated because of the great number of small businesses involved. This component of nickel consumption is likely to be under-reported by 50%, but in 1976, nickel salts comprised only 1-2% of all nickel consumed.

Since the amount of nickel contained in various products varies greatly, these figures report the actual weight of contained nickel. Excluded from the statistics is all scrap material containing nickel.

Arsenic. The major uses of arsenic are in the production of various pesticides, herbicides, and wood preservatives, and in the glass-making industry as a decolorizing agent. A lesser amount is used in the metallic state by the electronics industry in the preparation of semiconductors.

Most of this arsenic is initially traded as white arsenic. As_2O_3; and then converted into various arsenic chemicals. Since 1960, white arsenic has been produced commercially at only one facility in the U.S. No production figures have been publicly available since that time because of the requirement of government agencies to withhold individual company confidential data.

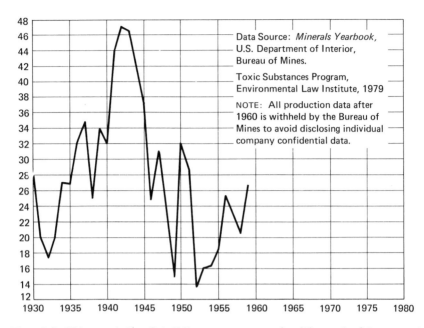

Figure 9-8. White arsenic ($As_2 O_3$), U.S. apparent consumption (Thousands of shorter tons).

Apparent consumption of white arsenic is presented here for the years 1930–1960. It is defined as the amount produced plus that imported minus that exported. Apparent consumption was markedly less in the 1950's than in the 1940's, presumably due to the decreased use of arsenic pesticides in favor of petroleum-based pesticides. There is no way to determine from public documents whether consumption of white arsenic has leveled off or increased over the last 20 years.

In any case, the production and consumption of white arsenic seriously underestimates the amount of carcinogenic arsenic potentially available for human exposure. Arsenic is routinely emitted as a pollutant in the smelting of primary metals: copper, zinc, and lead. It is also present as an impurity in some grades of coal, and thus released during combustion. According to a recent EPA study,[47] the following sources account for the majority of environmental exposures to atmospheric arsenic:

Pesticide manufacture and use: 31.6%
Copper smelting: 29.1
Zinc smelting: 15.0
Glass manufacturing: 6.9
Power plant boilers: 5.3
Lead smelting: 4.1
Cotton ginning: 3.7

Those exposures that result from the commercial utilization of white arsenic account for a sizable fraction of the total (c.40%). It is also likely that these sources of arsenic emmissions also account for a sizable fraction of total occupational exposures. Pesticide manufacturing and use, for instance, results in a large number of worker exposures. Still, the majority of human exposures associated with carcinogenic arsenic are the result of arsenic as an undesirable impurity in the production of metals. The statistics presented here are thus inadequate for the purposes of assessing the total risks to humans posed by arsenic. (See Figure 9-8.)

ACKNOWLEDGMENTS

Brian Magee, Richard D. Morgenstern and Marvin Schneiderman provided invaluable comments. Mary Dearing provided clerical assistance.

REFERENCES

1. Cairns, J., *Cancer: Science and Society.* San Francisco: W.H. Freeman and Co., 1978, p. 151.
2. McKinlay, J.B. and McKinlay, S.M., "The Questionable Contribution of Medical Measures to the Decline of Mortality in the United States in the Twentieth Century," *Milbank Memorial Fund Quarterly* **55**,3: 405–428, 1977.
3. Rosen, G., "The Bacteriological, Immunologic, and Chemotherapeutic Period 1875–1950," *Bulletin of the New York Academy of Medicine* **40, 6:** 483–493, 1964.
4. McKeown, T., *The Modern Rise of Population.* London: Edward Arnold, 1976; and *The Role of Medicine: Dream, Mirage or Nemesis.* London: Nuffield Provincial Hospitals Trust, 1976.
5. Davis, D.L. and Ng, L.K.Y., in this book, Chapter 1.
6. Mushkin, S., "Cost of Disease and Illness in the United States in the Year 2000," *Public Health Reports* **93**, *5:*495–588, September–October, 1978.
7. Eckholm, E., *The Picture of Health.* New York: W.W. Norton and Co., 1977.
8. Wyatt, J.P., "Chronic Lung Disease in Adults," in Lee, D.H.K. (Ed.), *Environmental Factors in Respiratory Disease.* New York: Academic Press, 1972, pp. 120–139.
9. Rosen, "Economic and Social Policy in the Development of Public Health," *Journal of The History of Medicine,* 1953; reprinted in Rosen, *From Medical Police to Social Medicine.* New York: Science History Publications, 1974, pp. 156–200. (Rosen notes that, in the seventeenth century, it was believed to be in the interest of the state to create the largest possible number of healthy and productive subjects. Quantitative studies of public health were developed largely to provide better information on the value of people, especially of those occupational groups esteemed most productive.)
10. Engels, F., *The Conditions of the Working Class in England,* 1848; Henderson, W.O. and Chaloner, W.H. (trs.). Palo Alto: Stanford University Press, 1958.
11. Personal communication, 1979, Sergio Fabro, Director, Maternal-Fetal Medicine Division, Department of Obstetrics and Gynecology, The George Washington University Hospital; Senior Consultant Investigator, National Institute of Environmental Health Sciences, Toxicology Branch, Research, Triangle Park, North Carolina. (One of the most promising areas for development in this regard is that which will provide for the assessment of reproductive effects. A data base indicating subtle behavioral teratological effects, such as mental retardation, and some short-term human effects, such as

fetal wastage, reduced fertility rates, and other reproductive problems, may prove far less expensive to develop and far easier to use in setting public health priorities than the more costly data now available on carcinogenesis.)

12. Weinhouse, S., "Problems in the Assessment of Human Risk of Carcinogenesis by Chemicals," in Hiatt, Watson, and Winsten (Eds.), *Origins of Human Cancer, Book C, Human Risk Assessment.* Cold Spring Harbor Laboratory, 1977, pp. 1307–1310; Rall, D., "Extrapolating Environmental Toxicology; Costs and Benefits of Being Right and Wrong," paper presented to the American Association for the Advancement of Science meetings, New York City, 1975; and Rall, D., "The Role of Laboratory Animal Studies in Estimating Carcinogenic Risks for Man," paper presented to the International Association for Research on Cancer Symposium, "Carcinogenic Risks – Strategies for Intervention," Lyon, France, 1978.

13. Weinhouse, op. cit.

14. Mack, T.M., Pike, M.C., and Casagrane, J.T., "Epidemiologic Methods for Human Risk Assessment," in Hiatt, Watson, and Winsten (Eds.), *Origins of Human Cancer, Book C, Human Risk Assessment.* Cold Spring Harbor Laboratory, 1977, pp. 1749–1764.

15. Blot, W.J., Mason, T.J., Hoover, R., and Fravmeni, J.F., "Cancer by County: Etiologic Implications," in Hiatt, Watson, and Winsten (Eds.), *Origins of Human Cancer, Book A, Incidence of Cancer in Humans.* Cold Spring Harbor Laboratory, 1977, pp. 21–32.

16. Lalonde, M., *A New Perspective on the Health of Canadians: A Working Document.* Ottawa, Canada: Ministry of Health and Welfare, 1974.

17. Lave, L.B., and Seskin, E.P., *Air Pollution and Health.* Baltimore: For Resources for the Future by The Johns Hopkins University Press, 1977.

18. *Ibid.*

19. *Ibid.*

20. *Ibid.*, p. 15.

21. Rall, D., "Thresholds?" *Environmental Health Perspectives* 22:164–165, 1978.

22. Blalock, H.C., *Causal Inferences in Non-Experimental Research.* Chapel Hill: University of North Carolina Press, 1964.

23. Bunge, M., *Causality.* Cleveland: The World Publishing Company, 1963.

24. *Human Health and the Environment: Some Research Needs,* Report of the Second Task Force for Research Planning in Environmental Health Science. Washington, D.C.: U.S. Department of Health, Education, and Welfare, 1977.

25. U.S. Environmental Protection Agency, National Cancer Institute, National Heart, Lung, and Blood Institute, and National Institute of Environmental Health Sciences, *First Annual Report to Congress of the Task Force on Environmental Cancer, Heart and Lung Disease.* Washington, D.C.: U.S. Environmental Protection Agency, 1978.

26. *Ten Leading Causes of Death in the United States, 1975.* Washington, D.C.: U.S. Department of Health, Education, and Welfare, 1978.

27. National Cancer Institute, National Institute of Environmental Health Sciences, and National Institute for Occupational Safety and Health, "Estimates of the Fraction of Cancer in the United States Related to Occupational Factors," 1978, draft paper.

28. Rall, "Thresholds?" *op. cit.*

29. Davis, D., "Multiple Risk Assessment as a Preventive Strategy for Public Health," in Staffa, J. (Ed.), *FDA Symposium on Risk/Benefit Decisions and the Public Health,* 1979.

30. Albert, R. and Burns, F.J., "Carcinogenic Atmospheric Pollutants and the Nature of Low-Level Risks," in Hiatt, Watson, and Winsten (Eds.), *Origins of Human Cancer, Book C, Human Risk Asssessment.* Cold Spring Harbor Laboratory, 1977.

31. Cooke, W.E., "Fibrosis of Lungs Due to Inhalation of Asbestos Dust," *British Medical Journal* 2: 147–152, 1924.

32. Selikoff, I., "Cancer Risk of Asbestos Exposure," in Hiatt, Watson, and Winsten (Eds.), *Origins of Human Cancer, Book C, Human Risk Assessment.* Cold Spring Harbor Laboratory, 1977, pp. 1765-1794.

33. Cairns, J., *Cancer: Science and Society.* San Francisco: W.H. Freeman and Co., 1978, p. 151.

34. Tomatis, L., Agthe, C., Bartsch, H., Huff, J., Montesano, R., Saracci, R., Walker, E., and Wilbourne, J., "Evaluation of the Carcinogenecity of Chemicals: A Review of the IARC Monograph Programme," *Cancer Research* 38:877-885, 1978.

35. *Ibid.*

36. *Ibid.*

37. *Ibid.*

38. Lee, A.M. and Fraumeni, J.F., Jr., "Arsenic and Respiratory Cancer in Men: An Occupational Study," *Journal of the National Cancer Institute* 42:1046-1052, 1969; and Cole, P. and Goldman, M.B., "Occupation," in Fraumeni, J.F., Jr. (Ed.), *Persons at High Risk of Cancer.* New York: Academic Press, 1975. (For an extensive review, see *Medical and Biologic Effects of Pollutants: Arsenic.* Washington, D.C.: NAS, 1977.)

39. Infante, P.F., Rinsky, R.A., Wagoner, J.V., and Young, R.J., "Leukemia in Benzene Workers," *Lancet*, July 9, 1977, pp. 76-78.

40. Enterline, P.E., "Respiratory Cancer Among Chromate Workers," *Journal of Occupational Medicine* 16:523-236, 1974. (For an extensive review, see *Medical and Biologic Effects of Pollutants: Chromium.* Washington, D.C.: NAS, 1974.)

41. Pedersen, E., Hogetveit, A.C., and Andersen, A., "Cancer of the Respiratory Organs Among Workers at a Nickel Refinery in Norway," *International Journal of Cancer* 12:32-41, 1973; Dall, R., Morgan, L.G., and Speiser, F.E., "Cancers of the Lung and Nasal Sinuses in Nickel Workers," *British Journal of Cancer* 24: 623-632, 1970; and Cole and Goldman, *op., cit.* (For an extensive review, see *Medical and Biologic Effects of Pollutants: Nickel* Washington, D.C.: NAS, 1975.)

42. *Initial Report of the TSCA Interagency Testing Committee to the Administrator, Environmental Protection Agency.* Washington, D.C.: 1977; U.S. Environmental Protection Agency and *Second Report of the TSCA Interagency Testing Committee to the Administrator, Environmental Protection Agency.* Washington , D.C.: U.S. Environmental Protection Agency, 1978.

43. *Hazardous Substances: Summary and Full Development Plan.* Washington, D.C.: Interagency Regulatory Group, 1978.

44. *National Occupational Hazard Survey,* **III.** Cincinnati: National Institute for Occupational Health and Safety, 1977.

45. Stallones, R. and Downs, Report to the American Health Industrial Council, unpublished, 1979.

46. Harris, R.H., Page, R.T., and Reiches, N.A., "Carcinogenic Hazards of Organic Chemicals in Drinking Water," in Hiatt, Watson, and Winsten (Eds.), *Origins of Cancer, Book A, Incidence of Cancer in Humans.* Cold Spring Harbor Laboratory, 1977.

47. *Human Exposures to Atmospheric Arsenic.* Washington, D.C.: U.S. Environmental Protection Agency, 1978.

10

Health Risks and Benefits of Nursing or Bottle Feeding: The Limits of Individual Choice

Stephanie Harris

Environmental Defense Fund

Introduction

Promoting individual responsibility for good health practices is but one important component for sound national health policy. It is equally important to ensure environmental and occupational protection against hazardous substances which may cause heart or respiratory disease, or other chronic, irreversible illnesses. The dilemmas confronting potential nursing mothers starkly dramatize the limits of individual responsibility for health promotion and disease prevention. The psychological and early immunological benefits of breast feeding[1] may sometimes now have to be compared with the potential health hazards of contaminated mother's milk or the less nourishing infant formula. Women who have been exposed to pesticides occupationally, environmentally (by living on farms or in forests where extensive pesticides have been used), or nutritionally (by eating foods with high pesticide levels) usually will have levels of contaminants in their breast milk far greater than those in infant formula or in cow's milk. Although many of the most harmful pesticides are now being controlled, their persistence in the environment and their accumulation in body fat is such that contaminants in breast milk will remain a problem for some years to come.

Given this situation, it is not at all clear what to advise potential nursing mothers, most of whom have access neither to testing of their milk supplies nor to adequate information for evaluating health risks and benefits. Public discussion of this issue dates from the past decade. As of this date, the federal government has yet to issue information on the problem.

No sector of the environment remains untouched by the global pollution caused by the family of chemicals called chlorinated hydrocarbons (or organochlorines, "OC's"). This family includes the pesticides: DDT, aldrin, dieldrin, chlordane, heptachlor, benzene hexachloride (BHC), hexachlorobenzene (HCB), endrin, toxaphene, endosulfan, methoxychlor, and pesticidal contaminant tetrachlorodibenzo-*p*-dioxin (TCDD), as well as industrial chemicals such as polychlorinated biphenyls (PCB's) and polybrominated biphenyls (PBB's). Introduction of these chemicals into the environment assures that they will become an integral part of the food chain and, hence, the web of life. The ultimate receptacle of these chemicals, at the very top of the food chain, is the newborn human infant, who has been exposed both in its mother's womb (when the chemicals crossed the placenta and contaminated the fetus) and by the ingestion of its mother's breast milk. The ultimate ramification of this pollution is unknown, although dire predictions can be made.

An individual can take personal action to limit his or her chemical exposure, up to a point, by choosing a "clean" location with pure air and water in which to live, adopting a special diet, and possibly even growing all his or her own food, using organic methods. However, certain chemical exposure is inescapable. Even though DDT has not been used in the U.S. for six years, nearly 100% of animal products as well as 100% of human breast milk samples studied, contain measurable quantities of DDE, the storage product of DDT. Hence, by choosing to live in this modern, industrialized society, an individual is trapped to a certain extent and forced to endure the environmental and personal health consequences.

Following the alarming discovery, in 1950, by Laug *et al.*[2] of DDT in human breast milk, the number of chemicals found in this most basic of all foods continues to mount. Today, there is serious question whether the benefits of nursing an infant outweigh the risks, particularly when some of the more deadly chemicals — TCDD, for example — are present. This chemical legacy is challenging the infant's birthright to the best start in life — its mother's milk — and forcing parents to weigh benefits against risk which were unheard of even a decade ago. The choice is a difficult one, as, to a large extent, it is based upon speculation and hypothesis rather than upon established scientific fact, and it is rare that a clear "right" decision exists. Furthermore, there are no health professionals who can tell parents what the "right" course of action would be, and there is little published information which can help to guide the layperson.

How do these chemicals find their way into breast milk? What risks do they pose? How can these risks be weighed against the benefits of breast feeding? And how can a woman control her lifestyle to minimize the contamination of her body?

Mechanism of Breast Milk Contamination

Environmental Transport. What happens to a pesticide after it is sprayed on a crop? Some types of chemical compounds break down fairly rapidly to less harmful substances. Others are more persistent and can still be found in the environment many years after their initial application. This latter group of chemicals includes the Organochlorines (OC's).

Because the OC's share a similar basic chemical structure, they share many physical and chemical properties. Of greatest importance in this discussion is their persistence — i.e., their ability to remain unchanged for long periods of time. Also of great importance is their fat solubility — a preference for fatty substances rather than aqueous substances.

After these pesticides are released into the environment, they enter the food chain and become an integral part of the web of life. Rains wash soil from the sprayed fields into streams, lakes, and rivers. The pesticides generally adhere to small soil particles and become incorporated into the bottom sediment of the body of water. Small aquatic organisms ingest them, concentrating the OC's in the fat portion of their bodies, then larger organisms ingest the smaller ones, once again concentrating the already magnified pesticide residues, and so it goes up the food chain. The higher an animal is on the food chain, the greater will be the resulting concentration of pesticides. For example, fish can concentrate the level of PCB's in water up to nine million times.[3] Likewise, a greater concentration of OC pesticides could be expected in the fat of cows than on the corn which the cows ingested. It is not surprising, then, to find greater concentrations of OC pesticides in human breast milk than in cows' milk,[4] as human beings are generally at the top of the food chain, concentrating pesticides from ingested animal fats.

The Food and Drug Administration has confirmed this food chain hypothesis by analyzing all of the various food classes for OC pesticides. Their findings, presented in Table 10-1, show clearly that foods of animal origin (meat, fish, poultry, and dairy products) most frequently contain OC pesticides (usually 100% of the time).

Food is not the only means of exposure to pesticides. The transport of pesticides through air can be very significant, particularly in agricultural areas where the pesticide is used on crops, and in homes where the pesticides are applied. For example, chlordane and heptachlor have been banned for most uses but are still allowed for termite control. House dust can be expected to contain chlordane residues. In fact, where pesticides are used for household pest control purposes, house dust becomes the most important source of human exposure.[5]

Industrial chemicals, such as PCB's, are found in all phases of the environment: air, water, and soil. In 1976, the Environmental Protection Agency[6] measured PCB's in 24-hour air samples from Miami, Florida; Jacksonville, Florida; and Fort Collins, Colorado, and found an average of 100 nanograms/cm. Ambient water levels were about 1 part per billion (ppb) PCB's during 1975 and 1976, and an average of 0.02 parts per million (ppm) PCB's were detected in 1434 samples of

Table 10-1. Incidence of chlorinated hydrocarbons in different food classes.

	Meat, Fish, Poultry	Dairy	Potatoes	Grains Cereals	Root Vegetables	Leafy Vegetables	Legumes	Oils and Fats	Fruits
Dieldrin	100%	93%	23%	7%	0	0	0	0	7%
DDE	100%	90%	23%	0	27%	17%	0	13%	0
DDT	33%	93%	27%	10%	0	0	0	13%	0
HCB	13%	10%	7%	0	10%	0	10%	23%	0
BHC	90%	97%	0	7%	0	0	0	0	13%
Heptachlor epoxide	97%	90%	27%	0	0	10%	0	10%	7%

Source: FDA Compliance Program, FY1974, Total Diet Studies (732008).

soil from 12 out of 19 metropolitan areas during 1971-1974. By 1974, as much as 25 ppm PCB's (whole fish, wet weight basis) were detected in Lake Trout in Lake Michigan. The U.S. Department of Interior Fish and Wildlife Service confirmed the seemingly ubiquitous nature of PCB's by identifying them in 90.2% of fresh water fish throughout the U.S. in 1974.[7]

HCB presents an interesting situation as well, since it is a pesticide (fungicide), a contaminant of various pesticides (for example, Dachthal, PCNB), and an air pollutant (a byproduct of chlorination and the production of chlorine). Because of its extreme volatility, it forms a halo around OC factories and solid waste dumps. HCB residues can result on grass growing in the vicinity of these factories, and cows which eat the grass have been quarantined because of excessive HCB residues in their bodies.[8]

Transport of OC into Breast Milk. Once the OC enters the human body, either through ingestion, inhalation, or dermal absorption, it is transported by the blood to the body fat reservoir, where it can remain indefinitely. Two methods of mobilizing the OC are: 1) through weight loss, or 2) through lactation. When a person loses weight, the amount of calories ingested is insufficient to supply the needed calories for energy expended, so the body fat stores are drawn upon to make up the difference. When the body fat is mobilized, it takes with it some OC residues which once again enter the bloodstream. It is during this period of weight reduction that acute toxic effects can be seen. For instance, the soldiers who were exposed to Agent Orange herbicide (and hence its contaminant, TCDD) in Vietnam continued to experience ill effects from their exposure to TCDD as much as ten years later, when they began to lose weight. The classic symptoms of TCDD poisoning began to appear (for example, numbness of extremities, depression, loss of libido, chloracne, birth defects).[9] This is an important factor in doctors' recommendations to pregnant and lactating women not to lose weight, as the amount of OC released into the blood could prove toxic to the fetus or nursing infant.

The second mode of OC mobilization from the body fat is lactation. The body fat reservoir is called upon to provide the energy to create milk and milk fat. The OC is mobilized through the blood stream to the mammary gland, where it is incorporated in the milk fat and then excreted. Hence, lactation is a simple method of ridding the human body of OC residues which have accumulated over a lifetime; however, these residues are then transferred to the innocent nursing infant, and the full ramifications of this transfer are still unknown. It is known that pregnant women have increased metabolic rates which tend to effect greater transfer of the OC's from the maternal blood to the fetal blood,[10] so one would expect to find significant differences in pesticide residues stored in the bodies of women who had been pregnant and lactated and the bodies of men and non-parous women. However, such a study remains to be done.

There is increasing evidence, both in males and in females, to support what can be called a "reservoir buffer hypothesis" of OC storage in the body. An equilibrium of the pesticide in the body fat seems to be established, creating a buffer which prevents significant change in excretion of residues, even when ingestion levels of OC's change. Fries and Marrow[11] have studied this phenomenon in lactating cows. They found that cows fed DDE, PCB, HCB, or PBB reached a steady state of excretion of the chemical in the milk after about 40 days. However, when the animal was given clean feed with no chemical, the level of excretion dropped 50% during 15 days, but then was slower, and the biological half-life was anywhere from 29 to 139 days, depending upon the compound. (This situation is not directly comparable to a lactating woman because it is impossible for her to go on a diet free of DDE.)

For males, with no easy route of excretion, the OC residues can continue to accumulate. Humphrey[12] studied men who ate Lake Michigan fish contaminated with PCB's. The greater the fish consumption, the greater the amount of PCB's in the blood. When the subjects abstained from eating fish for up to 278 days, the level of PCB's in blood showed no appreciable change, and in some cases even increased.

Numerous studies[13] have shown that the longer a woman lactates, the lower the pesticide residues in her breast milk. However, in the short-term, there seems to be no dramatic decrease of pesticide residues. In fact, Curley and Kimbrough[14] noted an increase in total DDT, total BHC, heptachlor epoxide, and dieldrin residues during lactation for the average of subjects over three months, while Quinby[15] followed two subjects over seven months and found variation, but not an appreciable decrease. On the other hand, Page and Harris[16] noted a decrease of DDE and PCB's between the eighth and tenth month of lactation for one nursing subject, while dieldrin, DDT, and heptachlor epoxide diminished after only one month. Kodama and Ota[17] measured the level of PCB's in blood and breast milk during pregnancy and lactation. The average of 46 subjects whose breast milk was studied during 7 months of lactation showed an increase in PCB's between 1 and 3 months, followed by a decrease between 3 and 5 months. The length of time necessary to finally witness a diminution of pesticides from the steady state level will depend upon a variety of factors, including the woman's diet and the amount of the pesticide in equilibrium in the body fat. Hence, each individual will exhibit a unique rate of decline of OC's in breast milk over the course of lactation.

Risks of Organochlorines in Breast Milk for the Nursing Infant

Pesticides. What are the health implications for babies who continuously ingest small amounts of pesticides? The answer to this question deals with two aspects of toxicity: acute (immediate) and chronic (long-term) effects.

Table 10-2. Average daily intake of pesticides by a nursing infant, from 1976 EPA data.

		ACTUAL INTAKE (ug/kg/day)		
PESTICIDE	ADI (ug/kg/day)	AVERAGE	MEDIAN	MAXIMUM
DDE	5	13.8		38.4
Dieldrin	0.1	0.92	0.48	73.8
Heptachlor epoxide	0.5	0.52	0.20	12.3

Some chlorinated hydrocarbon pesticides are very acutely toxic (for example, endrine and dieldrin) while others are much less acutely toxic (for example, DDT). Because of storage in the fat, a toxic dose could accumulate over time. The World Health Organization (WHO) has calculated Acceptable Daily Intake (ADI) levels of pesticides which are believed sufficient to protect adults against chronic poisoning by ingestion of pesticide residues in food. As these numbers are for adults, they are probably higher than a comparable estimate for infants, since the immature livers of infants are less able to detoxify poisons.

As seen in Table 10-2, the amount of pesticides daily ingested in breast milk by babies is shockingly high. In all cases, the amount is equal to or greater than the ADI. In the extreme case, for dieldrin, the level exceeds the ADI by more than 700 times. It is obvious that the potential problem of pesticides in human milk may be substantial.

These data are derived from a study completed by the U.S. Environmental Protection Agency (EPA),[18] in 1976, of the analysis of pesticide residues in the breast milk of 1436 women throughout the country. (This is the largest such study to date.)

Even if these ADI's were sufficient to protect against the subacute health effects caused by the ingestion of pesticides, they are inappropriate for protecting against chronic effects. An ADI cannot be established for a cancer-causing (carcinogenic) chemical because a threshold level for carcinogens cannot at this time be determined. It must therefore be assumed that any amount of a carcinogen presents a risk to health.

DDT, dieldrin, heptachlor epoxide, and BHC have all been shown to cause cancer in test animals.[19] Animal studies suggest that infants are more susceptible to carcinogens than adults,[20] so it can be concluded that the ingestion of seemingly small amounts of carcinogens on a daily basis is potentially a very dangerous situation, although we cannot accurately quantify what the actual risk may be.

In addition to posing a carcinogenic risk, ingestion of these pesticides can produce other chronic effects, including liver damage, nervous system disorders, enzyme induction,[21] fetotoxicity, and other reproductive difficulties.[22]

PCB's. Not only has the toxicity of PCB's been measured in test animals (e.g., rat, mouse, mink, monkey), but human beings have been unwitting guinea pigs. In 1968, over 1000 Japanese, including some pregnant women, were exposed to large doses of PCB's which had inadvertently entered rice oil.[23]   In addition to causing headaches, swelling of eyelids, temporary loss of vision, and many other symptoms, PCB's stored in the fat of pregnant women were transferred through the placenta to the fetuses. As a result, 9 out of 10 of the live-born babies had unusually darkened, grayish skin, and most were born underweight. Findings essentially identical to these were seen in infant non-human primates born to mothers who had been fed diets containing either 2.5 ppm or 5.0 ppm PCB's.[24] To date, a no-effect level for PCB's in any species has not been established.

A follow-up study[25] of these PCB-babies indicates that certain symptoms were abnormally common among these subjects during childhood. These include repeated respiratory infections and abnormalities in the dental and skeletal systems, such as weak teeth and growth retardation. These results are not directly comparable to infants ingesting PCB's in the U.S., because the PCB's ingested by the Japanese babies were probably more highly contaminated by dibenzofurans, a chemical similar to TCDD. The dose of the PCB's for the Japanese babies, however, was slightly *lower* than the average and maximum dose of American babies.

Other effects of exposure to PCB's include porphyria, tumors of the liver, atrophy of the thymus, chloracne (a disabling skin disorder), and learning disabilities.[26]   In addition, recent reports indicate that human beings occupationally exposed to high levels of PCB's have a significantly higher cancer rate than the rest of the population.[27]

Even though a direct comparison of toxicity between humans and monkeys is not possible because of species differences, one can compare the level of PCB's ingested by nursing human infants with that which produced adverse health effects in monkeys. Baby monkeys in which toxicological effects were observed consumed milk contaminated with 16 ppm PCB's on a fat basis. This is equivalent to 64 (μg) PCB's/kg body weight. A human baby consuming milk contaminated with 1.8 ppm PCB's on a fat basis (the average found in the 1976 EPA study) would ingest approximately 10 μg PCB's/kg body weight or about one-sixth of what the monkey received.[28]   In the worst case situation, the baby who consumed 10.6 ppm PCB's in the milk fat (the maximum level found by the EPA) would be receiving a dose of approximately 60 μg PCBs/kg body weight or an amount equal to that received by the baby monkeys. Because of species differences, most regulatory agencies use a safety factor of at least 100 to translate safe levels in animals to a surmised safe level in man. Obviously, such a safety factor does not exist for PCBs. Moreover, even if such a margin of safety did exist, it would offer little reassurance, because, as noted above, for a carcinogen such as PCBs, no level of exposure can be considered safe and without risk.

Looking at all of the data available at the time, the FDA recommended an acceptable daily exposure of 1 μg PCBs/kg body weight/day for infants.[34] Recent data show that this level may actually be too high. However, using this figure one can calculate that an infant should be limited to an intake of approximately 0.17 ppm PCBs in milk fat or one-tenth of what the average American baby is receiving in breast milk.

PBBs. Occurrence: PBBs, used as a flame retardant, were accidentially mixed into the cattle feed in Michigan in 1973 and 1974, thereby causing illness and death among thousands of exposed animals. Farm families who consumed their own dairy and meat products which had been contaminated by PBBs began to complain of illness. There was no question that PBBs were being stored in human tissue after they were detected in human milk. The highest level found in a farm woman's milk was an incredible 92.66 ppm.[30]

Urban consumers of milk and meat were being exposed as well. The Michigan Public Health Department found that 96% of the women from the lower peninsula and 41% of the women from the upper peninsula had detectable residues of PBB's in their milk, ranging from a trace to 0.320 ppm, with a median of 0.068 ppm.[31] The Public Health Department has thus far advised only women from contaminated farms to discontinue nursing. The FDA tolerance for PBB's in cow's milk is 0.3 ppm.

Toxicity: PBB's are five times more biologically active than PCB's.[32] Some of the symptoms of PBB's poisoning are weight loss, fatigue, loss of hair, and aching of joints. Laboratory tests have shown that PBB's are linked to liver degeneration and birth defects.[33] PBB's can cross the placental barrier and accumulate in the liver and fat of the fetus. It is believed that babies do not readily metabolize PBB's, but rather store them in the body fat; consequently, the cumulative effect of ingestion of small doses over time may pose a highly significant risk.

TCDD. Occurrence: Tetrachlorodibenzo-p-dioxin (TCDD) is a byproduct of the synthesis of chemicals from trichlorophenol which occur at very high temperatures. It is present as a contaminant in a number of pesticides (for example, 2, 4, 5-T, Silvex, pentachlorophenol) as well as other products derived from trichlorophenol (for example, hexachlorophene, the disinfectant in some soaps). The EPA has conducted monitoring studies for TCDD in the environment since 1974 and has found it to be present in wildlife collected from areas which have been sprayed with 2, 4, 5-T, as well as in the fat of beef cattle that have grazed on previously treated rangeland. The most controversial part of the EPA study was the finding of TCDD in breast milk. Scientists at Harvard University[34] found TCDD in the milk of 4 of 18 women living in areas of Texas, Missouri, and Oregon that had been sprayed with 2, 4, 5-T. However, they found the

TCDD at levels approaching the detection level (10–40 parts per trillion), and since no other laboratory validated the findings because of insufficient sample quantities remaining, the findings of this study have been severely attacked. Nonetheless, there is little doubt that TCDD is present in breast milk, although the exact amount is under question.

Toxicity: TCDD has been characterized as the most toxic small molecule man has ever created. It is the most potent carcinogen known to man, causing tumors in animals in the parts per trillion (ppt) range[35] (at levels which are comparable to the amount ingested from contaminated beef fat). It is also a powerful teratogen, causing birth defects in test animals.[36] Recently, a group of eight women in Alsea Oregon asked the EPA to investigate the unusual occurrence of miscarriage terminating all of their pregnancies, just following the spraying of the area with 2, 4, 5-T. The EPA verified the high level of miscarriage in the area and found it was associated with the spraying of 2, 4, 5-T. Acute poisoning symptoms with TCDD usually start with chloracne. Other symptoms are severe liver damage, depression, loss of libido, a loss of sensation in the extremeties, nervousness, fatigue, insomnia, vertigo, and death.[37] Because of its extreme toxicity, only a few ppt can cause adverse physiological effects in animals. As it accumulates in the body, it seems that many small doses over time can be more toxic than one large dose;[38] this is precisely the type of exposure which would be experienced by a nursing infant.

Benefits of Breast Feeding

There is an ever-increasing body of scientific literature about the benefits of breast feeding; unfortunately, many of these papers have serious shortcomings. We will discuss some of these studies in the main categories: maternal, psychological, immunological, and anti-allergenic benefits.

Maternal Benefits. Breast-feeding is the natural act to follow childbirth. It stimulates the contraction of the uterus without the necessity of drugs, and thus can prevent hemorrhaging after childbirth. The breasts become engorged with milk, particularly with the stimulation afforded by an infant's sucking, and if breast feeding is not commenced, a drug is administered to dry up the milk. In some cases, this drug is the hormone diethylstilbesterol (DES), a known human carcinogen, which could increase the woman's risk of cancer in later years. Also, there is evidence that the risk of thromboembolism is increased ten-fold if DES is used to suppress lactation.[39]

In addition to these physiological benefits, there are other advantages of breast feeding; namely: no additional cost for the purchase of formula, the ready availability of food for the baby at any time or place, and the ability to immediately satisfy a baby's need for food.

Psychological Benefits. It is almost impossible to quantify the psychological and emotional benefits which may be derived from breast feeding. Is the extra cuddling and skin contact important to the child in developing a feeling of security and trust in the world? Does the mother feel differently toward the infant because she is the sole source of nourishment, just as she was when the baby was *in utero?* Does the ease of feeding (i.e., no bottles to sterilize or formulas to make, no hassles in the middle of the night for a feeding, etc.) help the mother adjust better to her new role? How do the physical and emotional enjoyment of nursing affect the maternal relationship with the infant? We have no hard and fast answers to these questions.

Animal research indicates that lactating females are more resistant to stress, as they seem to have a unique buffering system.[40] Nursing mothers are also free from the mood cycles of ovulation and menstruation.[41] The letdown reflex which initiates lactation, stimulated by the hormone oxytocin, produces a relaxed and pleasurable sensation, thereby enhancing the enjoyment of nursing. Differences in behavior have been observed for nursing and bottle feeding mothers. Mothers are more likely to cuddle, rock, sleep with, and touch their babies than are their bottle feeding counterparts.[42] A great deal of emphasis is currently placed on the importance of skin contact and sensory stimulation of the infant, something which is more easily achieved in a nursing situation. In short, when a woman enjoys nursing her baby, a very close bond is formed between the two partners of the nursing couple. Early bonding takes place, particularly when the woman nurses her child immediately after birth.

Immunological Benefits. Breast feeding provides a smooth transition for the baby from total dependence on its mother for nutrition and immunological protection to its independence. Colostrum (the secretion preceding milk) and breast milk contain many anti-infective properties. Maternal antibodies[43] against various bacteria and viruses E. coli, polio, mumps, influenza, etc.) are present, as well as antistaphylococcal factors.[44] Lysozyme,[45] lactoperoxidase,[46] and lactoferrin[47] are also present, although the actual effect of these factors on babies is as yet unknown. Milk, often thought of as a "living tissue," contains living white cells which not only make antibodies but also can actually engulf and destroy disease-causing bacteria and viruses in the infant.

The intestines of a breast fed infant are inhabited primarily by *lactobacilli,* "harmless" bacteria, while the intestines of the bottle fed baby contain high levels of *E. coli,* potentially disease-causing bacteria.[48] There is a *lactobacillus* promoting factor in human milk, which aids the growth of this bacteria;[49] the bacteria causes an acid environment to develop, which, in turn, discourages the growth of *E. coli.* Breast fed babies are rarely constipated because the curd of breast milk is smaller and more easily digestible than the curd of cow's milk, and breast milk contains proteolytic enzymes,[50] which assist with digestion.

Diseases that are considered chiefly problems for bottle fed babies are neonatal tetany, hypocalcaemia, and hypernaetraemia.[51] Necrotizing enterocolitis also affects bottle fed babies, but solely those who have been born prematurely.[52] Many of these diseases can apparently be avoided if the newborn infant is breast fed for at least the first two weeks of life.

Schaefer[53] has shown an inverse relationship between the incidence of otitis media (ear infection) and the length of time of breast feeding. Nursing had the greatest impact during the first eight months of life, but a further halving of morbidity in children breast fed more than a year suggests that additional breast feeding conveys further benefits. Chronic otitis media can lead to major middle ear and drum destruction, a condition which can persist throughout life.

Finally, a number of studies from England,[54] Canada,[55] and New Zealand[56] conclude that Sudden Infant Death Syndrome (SIDS or "crib death") is rarely found in totally breast fed infants and is most frequently seen in infants artificially fed. However, not all scientists agree that SIDS is more prevalent in artificially fed children.[57] Very few argue that breast feeding is the only factor which influences SIDS; however, it would seem to be one of the variables which plays a role. While many theories exist to explain the correlation between artificial feeding and SIDS (for example, hypersensitivity to cow's milk,[58] poisoning by the endotoxin released by E. coli in the intestines,[59]), none have accumulated enough evidence yet to be scientifically verified.

It is very difficult to perform a well-controlled study comparing either morbidity caused by bacterial or viral agents or mortality for breast fed versus bottle fed babies, but a number of studies have been done in the past — and all have some deficiencies. In 1934, Grulee[60] reported that the overall total mortality for artificially fed babies was 54.8 times that in the totally breast fed group, and 12.3 times that in the partially breast fed group. This study followed over 20,000 babies in a Chicago clinic, primarily of lower socioeconomic background, so that the high mortality rate of the artifically fed babies could be, in part, due to unsanitary conditions in the preparation of the formula and the bottle. Furthermore, the bottle fed babies were receiving boiled, diluted cow's milk with sugar, as the sophisticated formulas of today were not available.

In 1951, Robinson[61] found that not only were mortality and morbidity rates higher for bottle fed than for breast fed babies, but that bottle fed babies also contracted more types of diseases and were sick longer than were breast fed babies.

A very recent study performed by Cunningham[62] is perhaps more relevant to the present situation in the U.S., because formula was fed to the bottle fed babies and a mix of socioeconomic groups were studied. Cunningham found that:

Breast feeding was associated with significantly less illness during the first year, especially if continued beyond 4 1/2 months of age . . . after controlling for parental educational status . . . the difference in significant illness between infants artificially fed and prolonged breast feeders was two- to three-fold.

The benefits were most striking with regard to respiratory illness and gastrointestinal illness.

However, the results of another recent study, by Adebonojo,[63] are in direct conflict and lead the author to conclude that there are "no protective effects from clinical illnesses attributable to colostrum and human milk." In this study, breast fed and formula fed infants from a middle class American community were compared, during the first year of life, for several parameters, including the average number of gastrointestinal disorders, respiratory disorders, and sick check visits. In all respects, breast fed and bottle fed infants were the same.

The Adebonojo study suffers from two deficiencies: 1) the majority of infants were breast fed for only three or four months, while the data on illness covered the first year of life; and 2) it used a small group of children, which makes the study less sensitive to subtle differences between breast fed and bottle fed infants.

Unfortunately, neither of these two recent studies is able to locate a group of infants who were totally breast fed and received no other food, including an occasional bottle, throughout the study period. However, the Cunningham study was far better controlled, and hence his conclusions should be given greater weight than the contradictory evidence of Adebonojo. We can conclude, therefore, that breast feeding, particularly if continued longer than four and one-half months, probably helps to prevent gastrointestinal and respiratory disease.

Anti-allergenic Benefits. The most important factor to be considered with respect to allergies and the choice of feeding method is family history. Allergies seem to be a familial condition.[64] If a parent or sibling has an allergy of any type, the baby is more likely to develop allergies than is the baby with no family history of allergies. Moreover, once an individual is allergic to one substance, other allergies become more common.

It has been estimated that 0.3-7% of the babies in the U.S. develop an allergy to cow's milk.[66] Symptoms of this allergy are vomiting, colic, skin irritation, (dermatitis, hives, or eczema), gastrointestinal infections, respiratory illness, stomach bleeding, growth retardation, and central nervous system damage.

Allergic reaction to milk can be life-threatening for an infant. Severe vomiting and diarrhea are symptomatic of this allergy; if not treated promptly, such a condition can lead to rapid dehydration and death. Some scientists even believe that anaphylactic shock resulting from inhalation of cow's milk could be the cause of "crib death."[67] Indeed, the similarity between the symptoms of hypersensitivity to cow's milk and the symptoms reported in cases of "crib death" is striking.[68]

When there is a family history of allergy, the baby should not be given cow's milk formula from birth. Most pediatricians recommend soy milk formula instead, although there seems to be difference of opinion as to whether soy milk helps to prevent allergies. While Glaser and Johnstone[69] and Johnstone and Duttor[70] showed that babies fed soy milk had a lower incidence of allergies than did babies fed cow's milk, this was later challenged by a study performed by Halpern et al.[71] Therefore, the choice of food for a baby with a family history of allergies would ideally be breast milk, in order to avoid the early introduction of allergens (foreign proteins). Although this may not prevent allergies in the future, it should advantageously affect their onset and severity.

Breast fed babies seem to have a delayed onset and less severe allergy to cow's milk than do babies initially raised on cow's milk formula.[72] This is because: 1) the potential allergen is not introduced into the breast feeding baby's diet until it is older and the intestines are better equipped to cope with the foreign protein; 2) an antibody, secretory immunoglobulin A (IgA), is transmitted to the baby via breast milk and is believed to form a protective paste-like coating on the baby's intestines, thereby preventing the absorption of the foreign protein.[73]

If a baby is fed cow's milk formula and develops an allergy, then it will probably be recommended that a soy milk formula be substituted. However, one study has shown that 30–50% of the children who were allergic to cow's milk developed an allergy to soy milk as well.[74] In such cases, either a meat-base formula or pre-digested milk formula (Nutramigen) can be substituted.

It is clear that when a family history of allergies exists, the importance of breast feeding becomes more evident. Any decision on whether or not to breast feed should take this factor into account.

The Comparison of Risks and Benefits

In comparing the benefits with the risks of breast feeding, we are generally comparing the known with the unknown. Breast milk contains maternal antibodies that are available to the child during the time between birth and the onset of the functioning of the child's own immune system. Presumably, these antibodies help the child fight off disease, but the degree of protection offered remains unclear. When there is a likelihood of allergy because of family history, the onset of the allergy can be delayed and its severity diminished if the child is breast fed. A host of possible diseases (neonatal tetany, hypocalcaemia, hypernaetrae-mia, etc.) can apparently be avoided by breast feeding, even if breast feeding is only for a very limited period of time (two weeks).

The risks, on the other hand, are by and large as yet unproven. No prospective (or retrospective) studies have been completed on breast fed babies in the U.S. to see whether any adverse health effects occur due to the ingestion of chemical contaminants. (An individual might have to be followed for 30 years or more to observe the onset of cancer, a disease with a long latency period, or for a shorter period to observe subchronic effects.) We do know, though, from both human and animal subjects, that the ingestion of PCB's causes various symptoms of acute and chronic poisoning. All of the chlorinated hydrocarbon pesticides found in breast milk cause cancer in test animals, so there is an increased risk of cancer to the nursing infant who is ingesting these chemicals on a daily basis during a particularly susceptible time of life. No scientist has ever been able to determine accurately whether there is a safe level for the ingestion of a carcinogen, so we can only conclude that any amount of a carcinogen poses a hazard.

Breast milk can be analyzed in order to determine the level of contaminants present; however, it is difficult and expensive to have this done by a private laboratory, and the results of the analysis may be difficult to interpret, due to the lack of governmental standards for allowable daily intake of chemicals for infants. If the ADI's of pesticides and PCB's are used to calculate the maximum recommended level of pesticides and PCB's in breast milk, the tolerances for pesticides and PCB's in breast milk on a fat basis become as follows: DDT, 1 ppm (one-third the average DDT level found in 1974); DDE, 1 ppm (one-half the average DDE level found in 1976); dieldrin, 0.02 ppm (one-seventh the average dieldrin level found in 1976); heptachlor epoxide, 0.1 ppm (slightly higher than the average heptachlor epoxide level found in 1976); and PCB's, 0.2 ppm (about one-tenth the average PCB's level found in 1976). It must be understood that the ADI's have been established by using data which today are obsolete, and the ADI's are in reality far too high. Also, they are calculated for adults and not for infants, so the tolerances which are calculated from these ADI's are probably much too high. However, the government has yet to issue more currently calculated ADI's, so these standards, as antiquated as they are, are all we have to guide us. More important, the potential cancer risk caused by the ingestion of the chemicals is not included in this calculation.

ADI's are usually calculated by multiplying the level of the chemical which produced no overt toxicological response in animals by an arbitrary safety factor (1/100th) to take into account species differences. They purport to represent the upper limit of the range of the chemical residues which are safe to ingest. Exposure to chemical residues greater than the ADI might not produce a gross toxicological response but certainly may increase the risk of injury to health. Neither subtle toxicological responses (for example, enzyme or behavioral changes) nor carcinogenicity are accounted for by ADI's. If a woman's milk contains much higher levels than the tolerance limits, she should seriously consider either not breastfeeding at all or just nursing for the first few days so the baby has the benefit of the anti-infective properties of the colostrum. If a woman's milk has around the tolerance level of pesticides, she should carefully weigh the benefits against the risks in order to decide whether or not to breast feed. She might consider nursing for a shorter period of time, or supplementing the breast milk with bottle feedings to reduce the infant's intake of the chemical contaminants.*

Clearly, the benefit-risk calculation will be different for every individual. For instance, if there is a family history of allergies, greater weight should be given to the benefits of breast feeding. However, if a potent carcinogen like TCDD is present in the milk, a woman should give greater weight to the risks of breast feeding and probably not breast feed.

Most publications on this subject suggest that a woman discuss this difficult decision with her doctor. Unfortunately, most doctors are not educated in the field of toxicology of PCB's and pesticides, so, in general, a doctor cannot be considered the ultimate authority. In the final analysis, each parent must make this decision with little assistance.

Ways to Minimize Contaminants in the Diet

Much remains to be known about the mechanism of storage and mobilization of fat-soluble chemicals in the human body. As long as there are some residues remaining in the fat, there will be some residues excreted in the milk. No one knows how long it takes to cleanse the fat stores of all chemical residues, and thus for how long one must eliminate exposure to these chemicals in order to minimize the level of contamination of breast milk.

Diet is probably the major source of PCB's and pesticide exposure for most people without an occupational exposure. It is relatively simple to outline a nutritious diet which minimizes these chemicals. A significant dietary source of PCB's is constituted by those fish which have lived in fresh water for part or all of their lives. Therefore, this is one food which should be avoided. In particular, the fish to avoid are bottom-feeding estuarine fish (i.e., catfish, flounder, sole), Great Lakes fish (salmon, carp), and fatty fish (buffalofish and eels). Ocean fish (i.e., cod, haddock, halibut) are usually free from PCB residues.

The major dietary source of chlorinated hydrocarbon pesticides is food of animal origin (meat, dairy products) and fish, as the pesticide residues are bio-accumulated in the fat over the lifetime of the animals and fish. If meat is to be

---

*Although the levels of contaminants in human breast milk may appear small, they are in fact very significant when the resulting exposure for a nursing infant is compared to that of an adult. For example, the average nursing infant ingests approximately 10 μg PCB's/kg body weight/day. If such a child is nursed for a year and during that year averages, 7.0 kg in weight (about 14 lb), then it will ingest 25.8 mg of PCB's. The average adult, on the other hand, is exposed to only 0.1 μg PCB's/kg body weight/day (about 100-fold less than the nursing infant), and in one year consumes only 2.9 mg PCB's (about one-ninth that amount consumed by the nursing infant). Therefore, the shorter the time or the fewer daily feedings an infant receives of breast milk, the less total amount of PCB's it will ingest. A similar pattern is true for the pesticides found in human milk.

eaten, high-fat meats should be avoided, and from the meat that is eaten, the fat should be removed and the drippings discarded. The better cooked the meat, in general, the lower its fat content. According to the U.S. Department of Agriculture 1976 residue monitoring data for meat, the types of meat in which pesticide residues are most frequently found are beef, veal, chicken, and turkey, while the animals in which residues are least frequently found are sheep, goats, and swine (these studies are on animal fat and may not apply to the meat as eaten; for example, to chicken, which is normally quite lean). Also, grass fed beef should have much lower residues than the usual grain-fed beef. If fish is to be eaten, only deep-sea fish should be chosen (for example, cod and haddock).

Does a totally vegetarian diet really help reduce the chemical contaminants of the milk? A French study published in 1974 focused on the effect of organic versus non-organic foods in the diet but only sampled the milk of primarily vegetarians. The results of the study showed that if 70% or more of the diet contained organic foods (i.e., grown without synthetic chemical pesticides or fertilizers), the pesticide residues in the breast milk were less than one-half those in the median French human milk samples.[75] All of the women who had significantly lower pesticide residues in their milk had been on the diet for six or more years, while those women whose pesticide residues were higher were generally on the diet for three years or less.

Page and Harris[76] found that vegetarians had lower levels of pesticides in their breast milk than did their matched controls. The more high-fat dairy products (cream, cheese, ice cream) included in the diet, the higher the PCB's and pesticides in the breast milk. The longer a woman had lactated, the lower the OC level in her breast milk.

Additional benefits associated with a practice of a low-fat, semi-vegetarian diet are a lowering of dietary fats and cholesterol, which is recommended to prevent heart disease and cancer. Also, a woman will find it easier to regain her figure in the post-partum period if she eats a low-fat diet.

Conclusion

Most of the OC's included in this discussion have been either banned or restricted in use, so that there is little that the government can do to combat the continuing problem of environmental contamination. Individual changes in diet and lifestyle can help to reduce OC exposure but will not eliminate it. Further, it is not known for how long one must lead a "clean" life in order to purge the body of OC's.

Much research remains to be done in this area, both in investigating the mechanism of breast milk contamination and in seeking new strategies for OC reduction in breast milk. Meanwhile, parents are left with a very disquieting choice: whether or not to breast feed an infant, in light of the excessive contamination of this ideal food. With incomplete and contradictory scientific information, and little or no advice from the "experts," the perplexed parent may feel inadequate in deciding how to give an infant the healthiest start in life. Yet this decision could be critical to the continuing health and well-being of the infant, the innocent victim of the Chemical Age.

REFERENCES

1. Motion, Inc., *Breastfeeding: A Special Closeness* (a film). Washington, D.C., 1978.
2. Laug, E.P., Kunse, F.M., and Prickett, C.S., "Occurrence of DDT in Human Fat and Milk," *Arch. Industr. Hyg.* 3:245, 1951.
3. Nisbet, I.C.T., "EPA Criteria Document on PCB's," EPA 440/9-76-021.
4. Bradt, P.T. and Herrenkohl, R.C., "DDT in Human Milk. What determines the Levels?" *The Science of the Total Environment* 6:161-163, 1976.
5. Davies, J.E., Edmundson, W.F., and Raffonelli, A., "The Role of House Dust in Human DDT Pollution," *Am. J. Pub. Health* 65, *1*:53-57, 1975; Warnik, S.C., "Organochlorine Pesticide Levels in Human Serum and Adipose Tissue," Utah-FY 1967-71, *Pest. Monit. J.* 6 *1*:9-13, 1972; and Starr, H.G., Aldrich, F.D., McDougall, W.D., III, and Mounce, L.M., "Contribution of Household Dust to the Human Exposure to Pesticides," *Pest. Monit. J.* 8, *3*:209-212, 1974.
6. U.S. Environmental Protection Agency, PCB data sheets, September 10, 1976, unpublished.
7. Walker, C., *USDI, Testimony Before the DHEW Committee to Coordinate Toxicology and Related Programs*, September 23, 1976.
8. Ruopp, D.J., *Environmental Contamination for Hexachlorobenzene*, U.S., Environmental Protection Agency, Office of Toxic Substances, October 5, 1973, unpublished.
9. Rubin, L. and Davison, A., "Agent Orange: The Effects Remain Long After the "Accidents" are Cleaned Up," *In These Times*, July 19-25, 1978, p. 15.
10. Polishuk, Z.W., Wasserman, M., Wasserman, D., Groner, Y., Lazarovici, S., and Tomatis, L., "Effects of Pregnancy on Storage of Organochlorine Insecticides," *Arch. Env. Health* 20:215-217, 1970.
11. Fries, G.F., Marrow, G.S., Jr., and Gordon, C.H., "Long-Term Studies of Residue Retention and Excretion by Cows Fed a Polychlorinated Biphenyl (Aroclor 1254)," *J. Ag. Food Chem.* 21, *1*:117-21, 1973; Fries, G.F. and Marrow, G.S., "Excretion of Polybrominated Biphenyls into the milk of Cows," *J. Dairy Science* 58:947-951, June 1975; and Fries, G.F. and Marrow, G.S., "Hexachlorobenzene Retention and Excretion by Dairy Cows," *J. Dairy Science* 59:475-480, March 1976.
12. Humphrey, H.E.B., "Evaluation of Changes of the Level of Polychlorinated Biphenyls (PCB) in Human Tissue," Michigan Department of Public Health, unpublished.
13. Savage, E.P. *et al., National Study to Determine Levels of Chlorinated Hydrocarbon Insecticides in Human Milk* I *and* II, 1976, unpublished; Bradt, *op. cit.;* and Page, T., Harris, S., and Balbien, J., "The Role of Vegetarian Diet in Breast-Milk Contamination," paper in progress.
14. Curley, A. and Kimbrough, R., "Chlorinated Hydrocarbon Insecticides in Plasma and Milk of Pregnant and Lactating Women," *Arch. Env. Health* 18:156-164, 1969.
15. Quinby, G.E., Armstrong, J.F., and Durham, W.F., "DDT in Human Milk," *Nature* 207, *4998*:726-728, 1965.

16. Page, *op. cit.*
17. Kodama, H., Ota, H., "Transfer of Polychlorinated Biphenyls to Infants from their Mothers; *Arch. Env. Health 35;* 2:95–100, 1980.
18. Savage, *op. cit.*
19. *IARC Monographs on the Evaluation of Carcinogenic Risk of Chemicals to Man: Some Organochlorine Pesticides 5*, International Agency for Research on Cancer, Lyons, France, 1974.
20. Toth, B., "A Critical Review of Experiments in Chemical Carcinogenesis Using Newborn Animals," *Cancer Res.* 28, 727, 1968.
21. "HEW Secretary's Commission on Pesticides and Their Relationship to Environmental Health Report, "U.S. Department of Health, Education, and Welfare, December 1969.
22. EPA Notice, "Rebuttable Presumption Against Registration and Continued Registration of Pesticides Containing Benzene Hexachloride (BHC)," *Federal Register* 41, 203:46024–46031, October 19, 1976.
23. Kuratsune, M., Yoshimura, T., Matsuzaka, J., and Yamaguchi, A., "Epidemiologic Study on Yusho, A Poisoning Caused by Ingestion of Rice Oil Contaminated with a Commercial Brand of Polychlorinated Biphenyls," *Env. Health Persp.* 1, *119*, 1972; and Kuratsune, M., "An Abstract of Results of Laboratory Examinations of Patients with Yusho and of Animal Experiments," *Env. Health Persp.* 1, *129*, 1972.
24. Allen, J.R., "Response of the Nonhuman Primate to Polychlorinated Biphenyl Exposure," *Federation Proceedings* 34:1675, 1975; Allen, J.R., Carstens, L.A., and Barsotti, D.A., "Residual Effects of Short-term, Low-level Exposure of Nonhuman Primates to Polychlorinated Biphenyls," *Toxicol. Appl. Pharmacol.* 30:440, 1974; Barsotti, D.A. and Allen, J.R., "Effects of Polychlorinated Biphenyls on Reproduction in the Primate," *Federation Proceedings* 34: 338, 1975; and Barsotti, D.A., Marlar, R.J., and Allen, J.R., "Reproductive Dysfunctions in Rhesus Monkeys Exposed to Low Levels of Polychlorinated Biphenyls (Aroclor 1248)," *Food and Cosmetics Toxicology*, in press.
25. Nakayama, K. and Aoki, T., "Hazards of Organic Chlorine Compounds to the Health of Children," *Paediatrician* 6:9–19, 1977.
26. Affidavit of Dr. James R. Allen, before EPA Hearing on Section 307 (A), Proceeding to Establish Toxic Effluent Standards for PCB's, September 1976; Kimbrough, R.D., Squire, R.A., Linder, R.E., Strandberg, J.D., Montali, R.J., and Burse, V.W., "Induction of Liver Tumors in Sherman Strain Female Rats by Polychlorinated Biphenyl Aroclor 1260," in press; and Blumenthal, H., Testimony on PCB's in Paper Food Packaging Materials, available from the Hearing Clerk's Office, FDA, Washington, D.C. (Dockett No. 75 N-0013).
27. Bohn, A.K. Rosenwaike, I., Hermann, N., Grover, P., Stellman, J., and O'Leary, K., "Melanoma After Exposure to PCB's," *New Engl. J. Med.*, August 19, 1976.
28. This is based on the assumptions that baby monkeys weighed 500 g and drank 100cc milk/day, while human babies weighed 6 kg and drank 1000 cc milk/day.
29. Kolbye, A.C., FDA, Testimony before Department of Environmental Conservation, State of New York, November 24, 1975, Albany, p. 9.
30. Press Release, Michigan Department of Public Health, October 15, 1976.
31. *Ibid.*
32. Farber, E.M. and Baker, A., "Microsomal Enzyme Induction by Hexabromobiphenyl," Soc. Toxicol. Meeting, Washington, D.C., March 10–14, 1974.
33. Corbett, T.H. *et al.*, "Toxicity of Polybrominated Biphenyls (Firemaster BP-6) on Rodents," unpublished manuscript, 1975.
34. Baughman, R., Meselson, M., and O'Keefe, P., "Human Milk Monitoring: Preliminary Results for Twenty-seven Samples," Memo to EPA, March 1, 1977.

35. Van Miller, J.P., Lalick, J.J., and Allen, J.R., "Increased Incidence of Neoplasms in Rats Exposed to Low Levels of 2, 3, 7, 8-Tetrachlorodibenzo-p-dioxin," *Chemosphere* 10:625–632, 1977.
36. Courtney, K.D. and Moore, J.A., "Teratology Studies with 2, 4, 5-Trichlorophenoxyacetic Acid and 2, 3, 7, 8-Tetrachlorodibenzo-p-dioxin," *Toxicol. Appl. Pharmacol.* 20:396–403. 1971.
37. Whiteside, T., "The Pendulum and the Toxic Cloud," *New Yorker*, July 25, 1977, pp. 30–55.
38. Allen, J.R., Barsotti, D.A., Van Miller, J.P., Abrahamson, L.J., and Lalich, J.J., "Morphological Changes in Monkeys Consuming a Diet Containing Low Levels of 2, 3, 7, 8-Tetrachlorodibenzo-p-dioxin," *Food and Cosmetics Toxicology* 15,5:401–410, 1977.
39. Daniel, D., Campbell, H., and Turnbull, A., "Puerperal Thromboembolism and Suppression of Lactation," *Lancet* 2:287–289, 1967.
40. Thoman, E.B., Wetzel, A., and Levine, S., "Lactation Prevents Disruption of Temperature Regulation and Suppresses Adrenocortical Activity in Rats," *Commun. Behav. Biol.*, Part A, 2:165, 1968.
41. Cronin, T.J., "Influence of Lactation Upon Ovulation," *Lancet* 2:422, 1968.
42. Newton, N., "Stability of the Family in a Transient Society," in Vaughan, V.C. and Brazelton, T.B. (Eds.), *The Family — Can It Be Saved?* Year Book Medical Publishers, 1976, p. 103.
43. Goldman, A.S. and Smith, C.W., "Host Resistant Factors in Human Milk," *J. Pediatrics* 82, 6:1082–1090, June 1973.
44. Gyorgy, P., "The Uniqueness of Human Milk, Biochemical Aspects," *Am. J. Clin. Nutr.* 24:970, 1971.
45. Goldman, *op. cit.*
46. *Ibid.*
47. *Ibid.*
48. Davies, P.A., "Problems of the Newborn: Feeding," *Br. Med. J.,* November 6, 1971, p. 351.
49. Gyorgy, *op. cit.*
50. Storrs, *op. cit.*
51. Davies, *op. cit.*
52. Jelliffe, D.B., Jelliffe, E.F.P., "Breast is Best," *Lancet,* September 18, 1976, p. 635.
53. Schaefer, O., "Otitis Media and Bottle-Feeding," *Canad. J. Pub. Health* 62:478–489, 1971.
54. Protestas, C.D., Carpenter, R.G., McWeeny, P.M., and Emery, J.L., "Obstetric and Perinatal Histories of Children Who Died Unexpectedly (Cot Death)," *Arch. Dis. Childhd.* 48:835–841, 1973; and Carpenter, R.G. and Shaddick, C.W., "Role of Infection, Suffocation, and Bottle-Feeding in Cot Death," *Br. J. Prev. Soc. Med.* 19:1–7, 1965.
55. Steele, R. and Langworth, J.T., "The Relationship of Antenatal and Postnatal Factors to Sudden Unexpected Death in Infancy," *Canad. Med. Ass. J.* 94:1165-1171, 1966.
56. Tonkin, S., "Epidemiology of SIDS in Auckland, New Zealand," Appendix E-6 *SIDS 1974*, Robinson, R.R. (Ed.). Canadian Foundation for the Study of Infant Deaths, 1974, pp. 169-175.
57. Frogatt, P., Lynas, M.A., and MacKenzie, G., "Epidemiology of SID in Infants ('Cot Death') in Northern Ireland," *Br. J. Prev. Soc. Med.* 25:119-134, 1971.
58. Parish, W.E., Barrett, A.M., Coombs, R.R.A., Gunther, M., and Camps, F.E., "Hypersensitivity to Milk and Sudden Death in Infancy," *Lancet* ii:1106, 1960.
59. Reisinger, R.C., "A Final Mechanism of Cardiac and Respiratory Failure," Appendix P-3 *SIDS 1974*, Robinson, R.R., (Ed.) Canadian Foundation for the Study of Infant Deaths, 1974, pp. 77-82.

60. Grulee, C.G., Sanford, H.N., and Herron, P.H., "Breast and Artificial Feeding: Influence on Morbidity and Mortality of 20,000 Infants," *JAMA 103* 10:735-738, 1934.
61. Robinson, M., "Infant Morbidity and Mortality: A Study of 3266 Infants," *Lancet*, April 7, 1951, pp. 788-794.
62. Cunningham, A.S., "Morbidity in Breast Fed and Artificially Fed Infants, *J. Pediatrics*, May 1977.
63. Adebono, F.O., "Artificial vs. Breast Feeding," *Clin. Pediatrics* 11, *1*:25-29, 1972.
64. Glaser, J. and Johnstone, D.E., "Soy Bean Milk as a Substitute for Mammalian Milk in Early Infancy," *Ann. Allergy* 10, *433*, 1952.
65. Murray, A.B., "Infant Feeding and Respiratory Allergy," *Lancet*, March 6, 1971, p. 497.
66. Jelliffe, D.B. and Jelliffe, E.F.P., "Nutrition and Human Milk," *Postgrad. Med.* 60, *1*:153-156, 1976.
67. Gunther, M., Check, R., Matthews, R.H., Parish, W.E., and Coombs, R.R.A., "The Level of Antibodies to the Protein of Cow's Milk in the Serum of Normal Human Infants," *Immun.* 3, *296*, 1960.
68. Carpenter *et al., op. cit.*
69. Glaser and Johnstone, *op. cit.*
70. Johnstone, D.E. and Dutton, A.M., "Dietary Prophylaxis of Allergic Disease in Children," *New Engl. J. Med.* 274, *715*, 1966.
71. Halpern, S.R., Sellars, W.A., Johnson, R.B., Anderson, D.W., Saperstein, S., and Reisch, J.S., "Development of Childhood Allergy in Infants Fed Breast, Soy, or Cow's Milk," *J. Allergy Clin. Immun.* 51, *3*:139-151, 1973.
72. Gunther, *et. al., op. cit*; Kletter, B., Gery, I., Freier, S., and Davies, A.M., "Immune Responses of Normal Infants to Cow Milk," *Int. Arch. Allergy* 40:667-674, 1971.
73. Jelliffe and Jelliffe, *op. cit.*
74. Gerrard, J.W., Heiner, D.C., Ives, E.J., and Hardy, L.W., "Milk Allergy: Recognition, Natural History and Management," *Clin. Pediatrics* 2:634, 1963.
75. Aubert, C., "Le Lait Maternel," *Nature et Progress* 4:21-29, November-December 1974.
76. Page, *op. cit.*

11

The Emergence of the Workers' Right to Know Health Risks

Vilma Hunt

Office of Health Effects Research
Research and Development
Environmental Protection Agency

Introduction

While traditional and popular accounts have acknowledged occupational risks for hundreds of years, coordinated federal policy to reduce these risks in the U.S. has come into existence only quite recently. This chapter reviews some of the early history of occupational health hazards. Social and political responses in the nineteenth century reveal a laissez-faire approach in America and some effort at systematic control in Europe. Legislation passed in the U.S. over the past decade requires that efforts be taken to reduce risks to the health and safety of workers and that they be informed about occupational hazards. While the legislation is quite explicit, the regulatory development to ensure its implementation has been slow and tortuous, particularly in regard to the free flow of information to workers.

The right to know of hazards in our environment is not a fundamental civil right. Academic investigators have an expectation that scientific enquiry can be pursued without interference and harrassment, at least in the university setting. There is a deeply entrenched tradition that the "open" literature is an insurance against any loss of scientific quality and integrity. It is quite difficult, therefore, to argue within the scientific and medical establishment that truth as it is currently perceived is not directly available to all people for the making of personal decisions. Alice Hamilton[1] wrote early in the century: "It is a question of offering to the poor who need it most the knowledge and the power which have long been the possession of those who need it least."

Hamilton, at the beginning of the twentieth century, never doubted her personal right to know the truth concerning hazards in factories and tenements, even under conditions demanding her own investigatory action. But she was also well aware that she enjoyed the privilege and advantage of her class. As the progressive era gathered momentum in the U.S., Hamilton was a personal link between the medical world of industrial toxicology and the restive working populations already aware that their living and working conditions were intolerable, though they had few resources to understand or change them.

The knowledge, beliefs, and expectations concerning health, disease, and the quality of life that developed during nineteenth century industrialization had to be transmuted as the twentieth century advanced, locked into a technology of increasing complexity. Medical science had developed within a distinct eleemosynary tradition, with its curative emphasis changing only after 1950 into the tax-supported research mode. Debates on the causal relationship between disease and toxic substance exposure tended to be among academic and medical professionals within their own research and clinical domain. With the passage of environmental and occupational health legislation in the 1960's, legislators, regulators, industry, labor, and consumer representatives all became legitimate participants. Experimental and clinical data viewed as adequate for biological research and medical inference were found more often than not to be inappropriate for regulatory decision-making. That is, controversies about the interpretation of data concerning human disease causation were taking on new characteristics and were being argued by a far wider constituency. By the 1970's, the deliberative interactions of government, management, labor, workers, and consumers were enmeshed within a legislative network, with its associated regulations, policies, rights, and responsibilities.

Today, the right to know the identity of toxic substances in the environment and the workplace is being claimed by unions before the National Labor Relations Board and by public interest groups in state and federal courts. In the U.S., in 1979, the legal interpretations are likely to reflect the social expectation that consumers and workers will not be kept ignorant of causes of their ill health and death despite claims by government and industry of national and trade secrets, and effluent innocence.

An examination of the history of industrial society in Europe, particularly in Great Britain, and in the U.S. provides considerable evidence for changes in the expectations of workers and consumers that they be protected from hazards over which they have no direct control.

Folk Knowledge and Industrialization in the Nineteenth Century

How does human experience become incorporated into the applied knowledge of a society? In an earlier time, we depended on folklore based on an oral tradition, which gradually merged into the written word.[2] The history of metal toxicity probably provides the longest written historical record that shows this transition. Evidence for the recognition of lead poisoning is clear in the earliest known illustration of a printing press in Danse Macabre, published in Lyons in

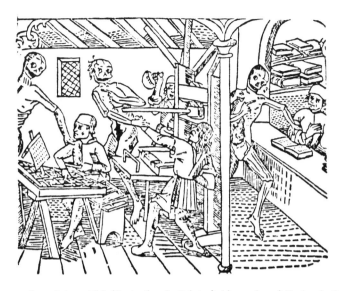

Death among the printers. This illustration in Painter's biography of Caxlon is the earliest known drawing of a printing press. From Danse Macabre, Lyons, 1499. British Museum Cat. 40, cite to Danse Macabre.

1499.[3] Entitled "Death Among the Printers," it depicts the typesetter and printer about to be physically removed by Death, shown as emaciated, not quite skeletal human figures. Agricola's *De Re Metallica*, first published in 1557, was the authoritative scientific source on mining and metallurgy for the next 200 years and was based on field research and observation. Mine safety and health were, in Agricola's view, the responsibility of the experienced foreman. Cause for abandonment of a working mine included poisonous gases and "fierce and murderous demons" — the latter a clear indication that the miner's knowledge or belief was a possible controlling factor in a dangerous work setting.[4] It is not until the early nineteenth century that we find a clear thread of evidence pointing to a recognition of the social disadvantage of those adversely affected by their work environment.[5]

Percival Pott reported scrotal cancer in London chimney sweeps in 1776, the first documented example of occupationally-induced malignancy. Over the next 100 years, middle class do-gooders of England attempted to moderate the excesses of child exploitation in the work force.[6] Protection of the child had become a social issue during a period when perceptions of children and the family were undergoing marked changes in association with the economic stress of industrialization. Thackrah[7] had actively supported the effort to restrict child labor, and described for six- and seven-year-old workers the long hours, lack of sleep, and unventilated, dusty workrooms of the textile mills. The period of the 1830's did not provide a social climate among the people of influence for changing conditions, despite the facts and views like Thackrah's that "the employment of young children in any labour is wrong." It is quite obvious from contemporary reports that the workers knew full well the relationship of their ill health and hunger to the physical and economic conditions of their work. The crusaders were providing the leisured class with explanations for the causes of serious social unrest and the likely influence on the health and integrity of the country's future generations.

Formal reports to government were being translated to a wider public by the literary figures of the time – Blake, Lamb, Browning, Kingsley, and Dickens.* They published poignant poems about crippled children in mills and mines, stories of the dreams and suicides of chimney sweeps and other apprentices. But in England, 100 years were to pass from Potts' original recognition of occupational cancer to the enforced prohibition of chimney sweeping by children, despite legislation in 1814 and 1834. Other European countries had banned the practice many years earlier. Public interest groups formed in many parts of England, calling themselves (for example) "The Society for Superseding the Necessity of Climbing Boys in London" and "The Society for Superseding the Use of Climbing Boys in the Town and Neighborhood of Nottingham." Risk benefit analysis made one of its earliest appearances with the argument of English insurance companies that a change to mechanical sweeping would increase the risk of fire, which was unacceptable.[8]

It was Dickens, the foremost investigative reporter of his time, who attempted to explain, as an eye-witness, the conflicting evidence for owner responsibility and worker misery. In 1869, he described himself as the Uncommercial Traveller, commenting on the street life of London, where he found in one hovel a moribund woman, whose condition was attributed to "the lead, sur. Sure 'tis the leadmills, where the women gets took on at eighteen-pence a day, sur, when they makes application early enough, and is lucky and wanted; and 'tis lead-pisoned she is, sur, and some of them gets lead-pisoned soon, and some of them gets lead-pisoned later, and some, but not many, niver; and 'tis all according to the constitooshun, sur, and some constitooshuns is strong and some is weak and her constitooshun is lead-pisoned, as bad as can be, sur." A daughter in the house was about to apply at the lead mill. "What could she do? Better be ulcerated and paralyzed for 18 pence a day, while it lasted, than see the children starve." Two months later, while on his "beat" again, Dickens came across the lead mills

---

*William Blake's graphic theme of miserable working conditions and death of chimney sweeps in his "Songs of Innocence" (1789) and "Songs of Experience" (1794) was continued by Kingsley in 1863 in "The Water Babies." The life of the chimney sweep has survived as a classic children's story to the present day, with Tom, the little chimney sweep, Mrs. Doasyouwouldbedoneby, and Mrs. Bedonebyasyoudid to become part of the conscience of our industrial society.

and requested entry from the owners, who freely showed him everything he wanted to see. White lead manufacturing processes" . . . are unquestionably inimical to health, the danger arising from inhalation of particles of lead, or from contact between the lead and the touch, or both. Against these dangers, I found good respirators provided (simply made of flannel and muslin, so as to be inexpensively renewed, and in some instances washed with scented soap), and gauntlet gloves, and loose gowns. Everywhere, there was as much fresh air as windows, well-placed and opened, could possibly admit. And it was explained that the precaution of frequently changing the women employed in the worst part of the work (a precaution originating in their own experience or apprehension of its effects) was found salutory." A detailed account of the mill, the work pattern, medical attention, and rest and meal facilities all led him to conclude" . . . it is indubitible that the owners of these leadmills honestly and sedulously try to reduce the dangers of the occupation to the lowest point." He told the owners that they had nothing to conceal and nothing to be blamed for. But he ended his essay with this: "The philosophy of the matter of lead-poisoning and work-people seems to me to have been pretty fairly summed up by the Irishwoman whom I quoted in my former paper. 'Some of them gets lead-pisoned soon, and some of them gets lead-pisoned later, and some, but not many, niver; and 'tis all according to the constitooshun, sur, and some constitooshuns is strong and some is weak.'"[9]

The effects of lead on human health and reproduction were so well known in the nineteenth century that passing references of obvious significance to the general reader appear in the writings of Shaw and Hardy. In Shaw's "Mrs. Warren's Profession," written in 1894, the fear of lead poisoning was used as an excuse for the heroine becoming a prostitute. She described her half-sister who "worked in a whitelead factory twelve hours a day for nine shillings a week, until she died of lead poisoning. She only expected to get her hands a little paralyzed; but she died . . . . The clergyman was always warning me that Lizzie would end up by jumping off the Waterloo Bridge. Poor fool; that was all he knew about it! I was more afraid of the whitelead factory than I was of the river; and so would you have been in my place."[10] The efficacy of lead salts as an abortifacient was part of women's folklore.[11]

Early Regulatory Developments

Chadwick's 1842 "Inquiry into the Sanitary Condition of the Labouring Population of Great Britain" and Helps' 1945 "Essays on the Duties of Employers to the Employed and Means for Improving Worker Health and Comfort" are evidence of the official spread of information to those responsible for the government of the country.[12]

To have drawn so heavily from the nineteenth century British experience does not mean that there was not a comparable experience in the U.S. Social comment on the development of the New England textile industry, particularly in relation to female employment, by European and American observers was ambivalent. There was recognition within the medical profession of the relationship between disease and work. The nascent trade union movement was directly concerned with "the physical and moral injury to women and the competitive menace to men," and, by 1841, a Lowell physician was forced to write "A Vindication of the Character and Condition of the Females in the Lowell Mills."[13] The diffuse influence of writers commenting on working conditions was undoubtedly related to the sectional differences within the U.S. and the state/federal relationships and responsibilities mandated by the Constitution. In contrast, the close relationship between social class, education, and political influence in the small geographic areas of England and of other European countries allowed social commentators more direct impact on their central governments.

An additional reason for the clearer social, political, and medical definition of particular work hazards in England could have been the nineteenth century British obsession with health. Haley[14] argues that it is difficult to ignore the importance of the Victorian concept of health in the intellectual life and popular culture of nineteenth century England. The enthusiasm for sanitation and ventilation, and the cleanliness of the laboring classes, constituted a fundamental basis for both physical and moral goodness in the view of church leaders and writers. They were part of the network (which in the U.S. today might be compared to public interest groups) concerned with making knowledge available and directing influence for societal improvement.

In Chicago and New York, city authorities responsible for tenement-house sanitation and prevention of the spread of contagious diseases via home-manufactured goods also commented on ill effects observed among the family workers themselves.[15] New York City's Board of Health described exposures to lead, arsenic and tobacco.[16] Buck's *Treatise on Hygiene and Public Health*,[17] published in 1879, included a chapter on the hygiene of occupations, but the influence of these reports on national legislation was not comparable to that seen in England and Europe.

The eleemosynary tradition of nineteenth century Europe and Victorian England to a small degree moderated social distress, but it was also part of the social fabric maintaining a paternalistic responsibility from which the patron could all too often absolve himself. The economic and political power of the factory hand was minimal when compared to those who governed them and to those for whom they worked. Americans did have a measure of mobility and independence by comparison. In general, the imminent hazard of injury and death in the mines and mills was accepted as the lot of those who toiled for others. The more insidious poisoning by lead, mercury, arsenic, and phosphorus was also part of that same risk, and we can conclude that, in the nineteenth century, the experience of exposure of workers to those toxic substances produced adverse health effects clearly evident to them.

Technological Change and the Twentieth Century

The turn of the century ushered in a new and complex technology. There was extensive introduction of new organic chemicals following their laboratory synthesis after the 1850's. Marie Curie and others initiated the development of a multitude of uses for ionizing radiation. A new physical and chemical environment never before experienced by workers became more complex as the twentieth century progressed. For most workers exposed to new toxic substances, the significance of a relationship between their health and that chemical environment disappeared from their ken. The long latent period which had to elapse before recognition of the severe onset of chronic diseases, including cancer, was probably the critical element in making the control of toxic work conditions a low-priority goal for management and unions. Ironically, many workers now had more economic power as unions gained strength. But acute economic problems were always present, and, indeed, were an integral part of the covert system of blackmail that successfully kept hazards of the workplace submerged beneath a crazy quilt of machismo, medical ignorance, and suppression of information.

Early Regulatory Developments

On an international level, the development of policies for the reduction of occupational hazards was uneven. Lead, although its adverse effects were well known, was controlled only in some countries. Phosphorus and ionizing radiation control followed a different path.

Lead. By 1898, in England, monthly medical examination of women and young persons working with lead in the British pottery industry became compulsory, and after 1903, examination of adult men became compulsory as well – the employer being responsible for notifying the factory inspector. By the end of the century, in Europe, regulatory efforts to control lead exposure of women, young people, and men were resulting in statistics on the severity and prevalence of lead poisoning. First Germany, than other European countries found the toll of disability and death from lead poisoning to be too high. Rigorous controls to improve unsanitary and dangerous work conditions were imposed with the result that poisoning cases in Germany, for example, were reduced from 21.2% of workers, in 1897, to 9.6%, in 1898, and to 0.97%, in 1912. In contrast, the U.S. by 1912 still had the same prevalence as had Europe 15 years before, and the "lead poisoning evil" was a phrase commonly used in the writing of the time. Alice Hamilton, in her autobiography, recounted her embarrassment at the Fourth International Congress on Occupational Accidents and Diseases in Brussels in

1910, when she could not respond to questions from the participants concerning the rate of lead poisoning by industry and the regulations and compensation system in the U.S. Finally, the chairman dismissed the subject:" 'It is well known that there is no industrial hygiene in the United States. Ca n'existe pas."[18] Alice Hamilton's efforts to make the problem known and to improve conditions in the lead industry, virtually single-handedly, are now part of our history of occupational health.

Phosphorus.   In contrast, the impact of the toxic effects of phosphorus was more direct in societal, economic, and international terms. It is worthwhile to examine the control of phosphorus exposure in some detail. It may have been better regulated because of the immediate physical evidence of its effects and the special groups which sought its control. It stands alone as an unusual instance of effective regulation. Hunter[19] considers the poisoning from white phosphorus to be the greatest tragedy in the whole story of occupational disease. "In 1844," he writes, "twelve years after phosphorus matches were first manufactured, phosphorus necrosis of the jaw was identified and 22 cases were reported from match factories near Vienna. Within a few years practically every civilized country had discovered a new occupational disease." The onset of the disease could be slow, with an average time of five years after first exposure, though susceptible individuals showed symptoms within a few months. The mortality rate for those affected was about 20%, but it was the facial disfigurement, the fetid discharge unendurable to bystanders, and the severe pain over a long period that brought the problem to public attention. Although, as with lead, the symptoms of phosphorus became obvious and well known, there was a more direct effort to reach the workers themselves through social reform and welfare. In 1891, the Salvation Army, as part of its Darkest England Scheme, established a match factory to counteract the use of white phosphorus, underpayment, and economic exploitation of workers. The intent was not only to deal with a toxic substance, but to reform the industry from top to bottom. In General Booth's view, the big match-making companies knew of the cause-effect relationship of phosphorus and the severe necrosis of the jaw, facial deformity, and death, but "callously refused to take any steps to remedy them, making no secret of the fact that they did so because it would have meant lessening the profits which were, in the case of one large firm, no less than 28%."[20] The Darkest England matchboxes soon became a familiar sight throughout England. General Booth's investigator took newsmen and members of parliament on conducted tours of factory workers' homes, showing how the agonized victims glowed in the dark. Britons still preferred "strike anywhere" matches over the new Swedish safety matches, and Booth called for state regulatory intervention. By 1900, public opinion was forcing a change to safe match manufacture, and, by 1908, an Act of Parliament made it illegal to make or sell matches containing white phosphorus after 1910.[21]

In part, the stimulus came from the Berne Conventions of 1906, which included an international prohibition of the manufacture, importation, and sale of matches containing white phosphorus. By 1919, the International Labour Conference of the League of Nations could report the adherence to the Convention of most of the British Empire and Europe.[22] Although not adhering directly to the original Convention, because of constitutional limits, the U.S., in 1912, passed the Esch-Hughes Act, which prohibited importation and exportation of white phosphorus matches, and levied a prohibitive tax on manufacture. Following the 1919 Conference, Japan, India, and China were exhorted to prohibit the use of white phosphorus, and, by 1923, had registered their agreement to adhere to the Berne Convention with the League of Nations. The activism of religious organizations was of considerable importance in what appears to have been a continual international effort, from the 1890 Salvation Army intervention in England to the efforts of the Industrial Committee of the National Christian Council of China in the 1920's.[23]

The legislative action in the U.S. followed reports in 1910 by the U.S. Department of Commerce and Labor on phosphorus poisoning in the match industry and pressure from the American Association for Labor Legislation and similar groups, at a time when potential federal intervention for the public health was under intense examination in the Congress. The hearings, in 1910 and 1911, before the House Committee on Interstate and Foreign Commerce were dealing primarily with bills to establish a national department of health, but included specific reference to phosphorus poisoning in match manufacture. The House Ways and Means Committee also heard testimony on white phosphorus matches in 1910 and 1911. The U.S. Bureau of Labor had reported earlier on women and children in the match industry in 1902, and the 1910 study dealt with 15 of the 16 match factories in the U.S. There were 3591 persons employed – 2024 men, 1253 women, and 314 children under 16 years of age (121 boys and 193 girls), with 65% of them working with direct exposure to phosphorus. However, 95% of the women and 83% of the children worked in phosphorus processes, so most of the women and children were at high risk. Phosphorus necrosis had been diagnosed in 150 workers, 4 of whom had died of the disease.[24]

Patents for a safe match manufacturing process had been granted in Europe and the U.S. in 1898. The Diamond Match Company purchased the U.S. rights in 1900 for $100,000, but found that although successful in Europe, the matches were unsatisfactory under the climatic conditions of the North American continent. The Diamond Match Company adapted the formula to U.S. conditions and allowed the use of the patent to all its competitors in 1911. The Esch-Hughes Act was passed the next year.

The activism of religious organizations and public interest groups to control phosphorus poisoning and to ban a product throughout the world may well be unique in our experience with toxic substances. The original recognition of illness in 1844 had eventually lead to the first ban on manufacture in Finland in 1872. The efforts of the Salvation Army on behalf of England's working poor were no doubt viewed as an appropriate responsibility by a Victorian society now identifying women and child workers as particularly vulnerable and in need of protection. By the end of the century, European countries, including Great Britain and her colonies, were developing a regulatory base to limit exposure of women and young persons (as they were called at that time) under 16 or 18, to most of the known toxic substances being used in manufacture. As a result, work conditions were often improved for adult men as well.

It is not easy to explain the sustained concentration on the elimination of white phosphorus in the face of opposition from those concerned with international trade, wars, and fluctuating economic conditions. The visible severity of "phossy jaw" in contrast to the slower and more ambiguous symptoms of lead poisoning and other occupational diseases could be invoked, or the growth of a social sensibility that the future of the human race might be better assured if women and children were protected.[25]

Ionizing Radiation.   For the last three-quarters of a century, workers in dangerous trades (as Alice Hamilton and other called them) have suffered disease and death, in part because medical knowledge was not adequate to identify the relationship between a toxic substance and illness, and in part because information about a known relationship was suppressed.

The most notorious example of this century so far is the experience of the young girls and women who were first exposed to the radioactive elements radium and mesothorium as they painted luminous paint on watch dials during World War I in a New Jersey factory of the U.S. Radium Corporation. In 1922, the first of many cases of radium poisoning was diagnosed. The Consumer's League of New Jersey became the advocate for the victims, having received a request from the New Jersey Department of Health to contribute "their excellent research skills." The League had been established in Boston 25 years before "to educate public opinion and to endeavor to direct its force as to promote better working conditions," and had maintained an active concern for the female workforce, particularly. The membership throughout the country included women who were at the forefront of campaigns concerned with child labor, maternal and infant mortality, and wages and hours of work for women — Alice Hamilton, Crystal Eastman, Elizabeth Butler, M. Katherine Wiley, Florence Kelley, and others. The Consumer League's national success in generating massive publicity around examples of industrial accidents and disease gave them the experience to help the radium dial painters in their long and expensive civil court procedures. The company management had had no foreknowledge that their work conditions would result in fatal disease. But when information was made available by Dr. Cecil Drinker of the Harvard Medical School, as a consultant to the company in 1924, the company submitted an altered form of his report to the Health Department of New Jersey, stating that "every girl was in perfect condition." A report from a second expert, the medical officer from the Standard Oil Company, concluded on examination of one woman that she had "no more trouble with her teeth than anyone who neglected her teeth." As a result, the investigation by the state authorities was delayed a full year, by which time women were in the final months of a fatal disease, osteogenic sarcoma. In the meantime, the Consumer's League had provided enough evidence to the U.S. Department of Labor to launch a thorough investigation of the incidence of jaw necrosis in the radium industry, and the New Jersey legislature, in 1926, amended its Workmen's Compensation law to add radium poisoning to its list of nine compensable occupational diseases. But compensation for the disability could only be awarded if radium necrosis developed within one year of terminating the occupational exposure, and the new law did not cover the women who had been exposed to radium before its passage. These women filed a civil suit against the U.S. Radium Corporation that resulted in a year-long trial with national and international publicity. The case was settled out of court, with each woman receiving $10,000 per year pension and all past and future medical expenses. The women's lawyer agreed never again to be involved in a similar suit! The Consumer's League, with the help of Alice Hamilton, and publicity by Walter Lippman at the *New York World,* then pressured the U.S. Public Health Service to hold a conference of industry, scientists, the government, and the public, to ensure full analysis of the experience. That knowledge has been invaluable in the establishing of radiation exposure standards to the present day — yet no workers' compensation award has ever been made in New Jersey for radium poisoning because of the requirement to file a claim within one year of exposure. The U.S. Radium Corporation moved to New York City and then to Bloomsburg, Pennsylvania, where problems of building decontamination and worker exposure persisted up to at least 1969.[26]

A detailed examination of the radium dial painter experience shows virtually all the characteristics of subsequent episodes of serious occupational disease in the dangerous trades. The next nationally publicized scandal was the finding of fatal silicosis in a high proportion of the workers at a Union Carbide subsidiary in West Virginia. In 1930, drilling was begun for a three-mile tunnel at Gauley Bridge, West Virginia, through almost pure silica, with inadequate worker protection. Congressional Committee hearings six years later established that the number of deaths could not be accurately determined because of secret burial of victims to avoid autopsy evidence of an occupational disease.

In the 1970's, a series of highly publicized episodes of obvious occupational disease had a common thread — the long-term exposure to excessive and hazardous levels of toxic chemicals. These working conditions were sufficient to cause severe effects on the reproductive system, in the case of exposure to dibromochloropropane, severe neurological symptoms due to exposure to the pesticides leptophos and Kepone, and lung cancer due to inhalation of bischlormethylether. In each case, the suspicions of the workers themselves initiated the evaluation of the adverse changes they experienced, which led to medical evaluation and confirmation.[27]

Extensive litigation has now been initiated against asbestos manufacturers by shipyard workers and others exposed to asbestos in shipyards and on construction sites during, and since, World War II. Charges have been made that, although the health hazard of asbestos exposure was known to corporate doctors, the workers themselves were not informed. The U.S. House Committee on Education and Labor, Subcommittee on Compensation, Health, and Safety has had to consider how the compensation system could be improved to assure benefits in a timely manner to disabled or ill workers, which presupposes that the worker is aware of the exposure and of the relationship of asbestos to the illness. Federal legislation is being proposed to provide compensation for workers with asbestos-related diseases, and it is likely that controversy will continue as to who should pay the compensation — the federal government, employers, suppliers of asbestos products, or tobacco producers. The problem of liability for diseases of long latency has been further complicated by the workers' ignorance of their exposure experiences.

A similar dilemma confronts the Department of Defense. It has been impossible to establish the radiation exposure history of army personnel who participated in nuclear bomb tests in the 1950's. The wider significance of the secrecy or ineptitude is that the continuing evaluation of the effects of low levels of ionizing radiation on human populations is markedly impaired. Suspicion that the occupational standard for radiation exposure does not provide an adequate margin of safety cannot be readily confirmed or refuted by that experience. Individuals have been denied disability benefits by the Veteran's Administration because no record of individual radiation exposure was available, although average levels had been estimated for the participants in the test army exercise.

The long litany of disasters in this century is in marked contrast with the sophisticated advances in medicine, chemistry, physics, and engineering. One response to the obvious discrepancies has been the increase in the regulatory responsibility taken on by the federal government.[28] We have at last found the toll of disability and death to be too high.

The Federal Role in the Right to Know

The social and physical damage associated with coal mining has been known for centuries, particularly by miners themselves — a partial explanation for the earlier regulatory development and compensation programs in contrast to other occupational hazards.

In the U.S., a change in the federal role in terms of occupational health came with the passage of the Coal Mine Health and Safety Act of 1969. The current outlay of $67 million per month to 365,000 individuals for payments to those disabled by black lung disease and to their dependents is the integrated societal payment for generations of illness and death resulting from inadequate control of the mine environment. For most of that time, even into the seventies, a miner's right to know that his lungs had been adversely affected was not necessarily acknowledged by mine owners and physicians. When the legislation was first enacted, Pennsylvania received a far larger proportion of benefits than all the rest of the coal mining states because of its history of diagnosing the disease, acknowledging its relationship to coal mining, and providing monetary compensation. It has taken some years for miners in other states to reach the same level of coverage, a condition directly influenced by the knowledge they acquired concerning the cause of their lung disease.[29]

The Occupational Safety and Health Act of 1970 (PL 91-596) contains several important provisions. The use of labels or other appropriate forms of warning are prescribed "as are necessary to insure that employees are apprised of all hazards to which they are exposed, relevant symptoms and appropriate emergency treatment, and proper conditions and precautions of safe use or exposure." The Secretary of Labor "shall also issue regulations requiring that employers, through posting of notices or other appropriate means, keep their employees informed of their protections and obligations under this Act, including the provisions of applicable standards." Employers must maintain accurate records of employee exposures to potentially toxic materials or harmful agents which are required to be monitored or measured and employees or their representatives must have the opportunity to observe the monitoring or measuring and to have access to the records. Each employee or former employee must have access to those records which indicate his or her own exposure to toxic materials or harmful physical agents. Employers are required to promptly notify any employee who has been or is being exposed in concentrations or at levels which exceed those prescribed by an applicable occupational safety and health standard and employees who have been exposed are to be informed of the corrective action being taken.

A far more complex set of requirements has been incorporated into the Toxic Substances Control Act (PL 94-469) to ensure that information is conveyed to the Environmental Protection Agency and to the public. The Congress found that among the many chemical substances and mixtures which are constantly being developed and produced, there are some whose manufacture, processing, distribution in commerce, use, or disposal may present an unreasonable risk of injury to health or the environment. "It is the policy of the United States that adequate data should be developed with respect to the effect of chemical substances and mixtures on health and the environment and that the development of such data should be the responsibility of those who manufacture and those who process such chemical substances and mixtures." Submission of data to the Administrator of the Environmental Protection Agency is part of the information network which is intended to ensure that chemicals of unknown toxicity cannot become a public health hazard. It is appropriate to note that the requirements placed on the manufacturers and the Administrator of the EPA are based on the assumption that a firm foundation of interlocking responsibilities is now in place. That foundation depends upon long-standing federal administrative procedures involving publication of notices in the Federal Register and the close surveillance of those notices by unions and public interest groups, who have participated in the development of the current climate of social regulation. That the public (including workers) does not ordinarily know the contents of the Federal Register is assumed. But it is also assumed that the public's representatives and advocates now have a sophisticated understanding of environmental and occupational health effects, as well as the legal competence to initiate countervailing influences when needed, to protect the individual and the public.

The protracted procedures for the promulgation of regulations for these two complex acts are still in progress in early 1979.

The Occupational Safety and Health Administration has only in 1978 and 1979 revised and proposed regulations and rules to permit worker access to the employer's log of job-related injuries and illnesses at the employee's workplace, where there are 11 or more employees. Proposed rules require employers to preserve medical and toxic exposure records for the duration of the worker's employment plus five years, unless longer periods are specified in particular standards. Affected employees and their designated representatives or physicians would have access to medical records. In order to prevent premature destruction of records before the rulemaking procedure was completed, an immediately effective rule was issued in 1978 to preserve those records covered by the proposal. Confidentiality of medical information and the patient-doctor relationship are sensitive issues still under discussion. Trade secrets have also been a central concern of management, where exposure data must be revealed.

Eula Bingham, Assistant Labor Secretary, has stated that the goals of occupational safety and health "are not adequately served if employers do not fully share available information with their employees. Lack of such information has too often meant that occupational diseases and methods of reducing exposures have been disregarded, and employees have been unable to protect themselves or insist that their employers provide adequate protection. Increased awareness of workplace risk also should make it more likely that prescribed work and personal hygiene practices, including the wearing of respirators and protective clothing, will be diligently followed."[30]

The long delay since the passage of the Occupational Safety and Health Act of 1970 has resulted in more attention being paid by unions to health and safety provisions in their contracts. A 1978 survey of collective bargaining negotiations and contracts estimated that there were safety and health clauses in 87% of the manufacturing sector agreements and 73% of the non-manufacturing agreements. The clauses appear in all mining, chemical, rubber, paper, and fabricated metal contracts. Four industries, however, showed a lower percentage of these provisions — apparel at 44%, retail at 48%, services at 44%, and insurance and finance at 29%. These are all female-intensive industries. A wide variety of issues concerned with physical examinations, employee responsibilities, hazardous work, inspections, and investigations are covered in the contracts examined, each one individual to the industry and union negotiating. It can be expected that, with the close to parallel development of federal rulemaking and negotiated contracts concerning safety and health, there is a basic premise that workers should know the hazards of work and their impact on them.[31]

A more difficult problem is the development of a worker notification and information program for workers who may have been exposed to hazardous conditions in the past without their knowledge or understanding. The National Cancer Institute of the U.S. Department of Health, Education, and Welfare is now developing protocols to ensure that workers, ex-workers, and, where appropriate, their families are being or have been informed when exposed to job-related risks which may cause cancer (particularly asbestos).

A national right-to-know movement has been launched by the Philadelphia Area Project on Occupational Safety and Health, with a coordinated effort to establish the right to know through union grievance procedures, arbitration, publicity, and other tactics. The program includes a strong worker education component to provide occupational health information on hazardous work conditions.

Conclusion

Progress toward the development of employer/employee responsibilities for maintaining a safe work environment has been hampered throughout the twentieth century. One important factor has been the isolation of workers from information about the hazards which could cause illness and death many years after exposure. The conclusion of a symposium on public information in the prevention of occupational cancer in 1976 was that such information cannot ethically be withheld from workers.[32]

Sissela Bok's discussion of lying and the moral choices in public and private life is not restricted to intentionally deceptive statements, but also includes intentionally misleading activities. The efforts of workers and their representatives to learn the truth about their workplace conditions and the effects on their health has uncovered both "ignorant truthfulness" and equally harmful "educated deception."[33]

Federal regulation of industry may be part of the solution. However, the critical pressure to ensure some measure of success will come from the active participation of workers and their advocates. The right to know, like acknowledged civil rights, must be exercised if the relationship between work conditions and worker health are to be in positive balance in the future.

REFERENCES

1. Hamilton, A., *Poverty and Birth Control.* American Birth Control League, 1929.
2. Ramazzini, B., *Diseases of Workers.* Translated from the Latin text by Wilmer C. Wright, De Morbis Arti ficum of 1713. New York: Hafner, 1964.
3. Painter, G.D., *William Caxton: A Biography.* London: Chatto and Windus, 1976.
4. Agricola, G., *De Re Metallica.* Translated by H.C. Hoover and L.H. Hoover, *Mining Magazine.* London, 1912.
5. Gaskell, P., *The Manufacturing Population of England, Its Moral, Social and Physical Conditions and the Changes Which Have Arisen from the Use of Steam Machinery.* London: Baldwin & Cradock, 1833; and Engels, F., *The Condition of the Working Class in England.* Translated by W.O. Henderson and W.H. Chaloner. Palo Alto: Stanford University Press, 1968.
6. Hunter, D., *The Diseases of Occupations, 5th Ed.* Boston: Little, Brown, 1975.
7. Thackrah, C.T., *The Effects of Arts, Trades and Professions, and of Civic States and Habits of Living, on Health and Longevity.* London and Leeds, 1832.
8. Hunter, *op. cit.*
9. Dickens, C., *All the Year Round New Series* 1,:13, 15; *13,* December 19, 1869; and *35,* February 27, 1869.
10. Shaw, G.B., *"Mrs. Warren's Profession."* 1894.
11. Karlog, O. and Moller, K.O., "Three Cases of Acute Lead Poisoning," *Acta Pharm. et Tox.* 15:8, 1958.
12. Chadwick, C., *Inquiry into the Sanitary Condition of the Laboring Population of Great Britain,* 1842; and Helps, A., *The Claims of Labor: An Essay on the Duties of the Employers to the Employed and Essay on the Means of Improving the Health and Increasing the Comfort of the Laboring Classes.* London: William Pickering, 1845.
13. Literary attention was even less. Rebecca Davis' story, "Life in the Ironmills," was published in the *Atlantic Monthly* in 1861 and has been viewed as the earliest recognition and criticism of the adverse environmental impact of industrialization on the American continent and its people. In her next story, "Margaret Howth," she wrote of a child crippled in a cotton mill. Davis' influence was short-lived and her social message, so admired by the Transcendentalists of Boston, did not travel far. The story itself was "lost" for over 100 years, its significance realized again by Tillie Olsen, who discussed the possible reasons for its obscurity following the national recognition its author received. (Olson, T., *Biographical Interpretation of "Life in the Iron Mills."* Old Westbury: Feminist Press, 1972.)
14. Haley, B., *The Healthy Body and Victorian Culture.* Cambridge: Harvard University Press, 1978.
15. Rosen, G., "Early Studies of Occupational Health in New York City in the 1870's," *American Journal of Public Health* 67:100-1102, 1977.
16. Reports of Board of Health. New York: 1872-1873.
17. Buck, A.H. (Ed.), *A Treatise on Hygiene and Public Health.* New York: William Wood, 1879.
18. Hamilton, A., *Exploring the Dangerous Trades.* Boston: Little, Brown, 1943.
19. Hunter, *op. cit.*
20. Sandall, R., *The History of the Salvation Army, Volume III, 1883-1953: Social Reform and Welfare.* New York: Nelson & Sons, 1955.

21. Collier, R., *The General Next to God, The Story of William and the Salvation Army.* New York: Dutton, 1965.
22. League of Nations., "Report on the Employment of Women and Children and the Berne Conventions of 1906." Report 3, International Labour Conference, Washington. London: Harrison and Sons, 1919.
23. Maitland, C.T., "Phosphorus Poisoning in Match Factories in China with Brief Observations on the General Conditions of Labour Found." Report to the Industrial Committee of the National Christian Council of China. *The China Journal of Science and Arts* 3, 2, 3, February and March 1925.
24. U.S. Bureau of Labor, Bulletin #86, Bureau of Labor Statistics, Washington, D.C., 1910.
25. Hunt, V.R., *Work and the Health of Women.* Cleveland: CRC Press, 1979, Chapter 8.
26. Baron, S.L., "Watches, Workers and the Awakening World, A Case Study in the History of Occupational Medicine in America." Undergraduate Thesis, Harvard University, 1977; and Hunt, *op. cit.*
27. Figueroa, W.G., Raszkowskis, R., and Weiss, W., "Lung Cancer in Chlormethyl Methyl Ether Workers," *New England Journal of Medicine* 288:1096–1097, and Randall, S. and Solomon, S.D., *Building 6.* Boston: Little, Brown, 1977.
28. Davis, D.L., and Rall, D., Chapter 9 in this book.
29. Kerr, L.E., "Informing the Worker – An Assessment in Proceedings of a Symposium, Public Information in the Prevention of Occupational Cancer." Washington, D.C.: National Academy of Sciences, December 1976.
30. Bingham, E., Quoted in *Occupational Safety and Health Reporter,* 1978, p. 235.
31. *Occupational Safety and Health Reporter*, September 14, 1978, p. 464.
32. Kerr, *op. cit.*
33. Bok, *Lying: Moral Choice in Public and Private Life.* New York: Pantheon Books, 1978.

12

Determining Unreasonable Risk*

J. Clarence Davies, Ph.D.

Sam Gusman, Ph.D.

Frances Irwin, M.A.

The Conservation Foundation

With an Appendix on Federal Statutory Directives by
Gregory S. Wetstone, J.D.
Environmental Law Institute

For most of the federal statutes controlling hazardous substances, conflicting values must be considered in reaching regulatory decisions. The language of the Toxic Substances Control Act (TSCA) makes it quite clear that opposing values must be taken into consideration when the Environmental Protection Agency (EPA) determines what constitutes an unreasonable risk. The final decision of whether the risk posed by a chemical is unreasonable must be based on a trade-off between health and environmental protection, on the one hand, and the benefits of the specific chemical, on the other.

Even if the language of TSCA did not require it, trade-offs would still have to be made to determine what risks are unreasonable. It has been argued that consideration of the economic benefits of a chemical serves only as an excuse "to avoid taking action which is necessary or desirable in order to truly protect the health of the public or the integrity of the environment."[1] Such an argument is usually based either on the premise that some values (for example, human life) are absolute, or that formal techniques of cost-benefit analysis obscure or distort factors that should be considered in making decisions. The notion that health, or, more specifically, human life, is an absolute value that should override any

---

*This is an edited version of a larger issue report published by the Conservation Foundation, 1717 Massachusetts Avenue, N.W., Washington, D.C. 20036.

196

consideration of other values is ethically appealing, but it is not very useful in establishing public policy, since there are other things people value besides health, and there are not sufficient resources to both maximize health values and achieve the other things that society values.

Cost-benefit Analysis

Cost-benefit analysis originally referred to a specific analytical technique developed by economists. For the purpose of this discussion, it is useful to distinguish among what we will call one-value, two-value, and multi-value cost-benefit analyses.

One-value Analysis. One-value analysis is the classic economist's cost-benefit technique. In its simplest terms, it entails expressing all the major costs and benefits of a proposed action in dollars so that the overall value of the action can be expressed in a single quantitative term, the ratio of costs to benefits. The technique has been applied most widely, and reached its greatest level of sophistication, in the analysis of water resource projects.

The obvious disadvantage of one-value cost-benefit analysis is that elements of great importance to the decision — in the case of toxic substances, the *most* important elements — are not bought and sold in the marketplace and therefore cannot be accurately assigned a dollar value.

Two-value Analysis. Some economists concede that certain important elements, such as human life, should not be reduced to dollar terms. They have tried to retain the advantages of traditional cost-benefit analysis by reducing the decision to two dimensions, one expressed in dollar terms and the other not.

Robert Dorfman's essay on "Methods of Policy Analysis,"[2] written for the National Research Council, provides an illustrative format of a quantitative policy analysis which includes several monetary (i.e., expressed in dollar terms) and several non-monetary elements. When he turns to the question of making a decision among several alternatives, he directs the reader to "assume that all important non-monetary benefits associated with the different alternatives can be expressed in a common unit such as lives saved."[3]

The problem, of course, is that, in most cases, the assumption cannot be made. Many elements are relevant to the decision — recreation, aesthetics, injuries, damage to the environment — that cannot be subsumed under the category of lives saved.

Multi-value Analysis. If the analysis involves three or more irreducible elements, the most obvious advantage of traditional cost-benefit analysis — the ability to show by numbers which alternative is "best" — is lost. Nevertheless, the usefulness of the general cost-benefit approach is not totally lost. The general concept of casting a decision in the context of trading off competing values remains valid. Traditional cost-benefit analysis has produced a variety of techniques for quantifying such values.

Cost-effectiveness Analysis

Whereas cost-benefit analysis is designed to ascertain what goal or standard or level of control is preferable, cost-effectiveness analysis takes the goal as given and is designed to ascertain what method is most efficient for reaching the goal. If cost-effectiveness analysis is to be useful, however, the goals to be achieved must be expressed quite specifically. It is not sufficient to say that the goal is to minimize the number of injuries; one must specify exactly how many injuries one is willing to tolerate. Although it may be helpful in choosing among alternative regulatory techniques once the decision about level of control has been made, cost-effectiveness analysis still suffers from many of the same problems of inability to quantify and aggregate that are presented by cost-benefit analysis.

Decision Analysis

Decision analysis combines the techniques of systems analysis and statistical decision theory to provide a collection of methods to quantify and define uncertainty about values and other aspects of decisions that are usually not quantified. It differs from cost-benefit and cost-effectiveness in that it is not a technique for arriving at a decision; i.e., the application of decision analysis does not result in defining one alternative course of action as preferable to another. Rather, it makes the process of decision-making more formal, explicit, and unequivocal. The EPA has begun to explore using decision analysis methods, notably in the establishment of an air quality standard for ozone.[4]

Other Approaches

The difficulty of applying formal analytical methods to the control of toxic substances has led to the development of other approaches which avoid the necessity of explicitly balancing competing values. The most widely used of these is to require the application of the best available or best practicable control technology. The major difficulty with this approach is that, in theory, application of best technology tells the decision-maker nothing about either the costs or the benefits of his decision. In reality, the costs will usually be known, and, at least under TSCA, will be considered in the decision. But the benefits often are not known, and the minimum level of benefits needed may not be attained even under the best technology, or they may be attainable using considerably less than the best technology.

Another related problem with technology-based standards is that they tend to conceal the trade-offs being made by the decision-maker. What constitutes the "best available" technology is rarely clear, and when, as under TSCA, economics must be considered, the choice becomes even less clear. In fact, the decision-maker is forced to trade off costs and benefits, but the technology-based facade of the decision tends to conceal the nature of the trade-offs and how the balance was struck.

The TSCA context makes the technology-based solution particularly inappropriate for three reasons. First, the law requires that a broad variety of factors must be considered in regulatory decisions, so there is no escape from the necessity for balancing competing values. Second, the range of regulatory controls available under TSCA is much broader than under, for example, the Clean Air Act or the Water Pollution Control Act. There is no reason to rely only on technological controls when a variety of alternatives, ranging from labeling to banning, are available. Third, TSCA deals with substances which could pose major risks to health and the environment. The margin for error may be very small.

Specification of Alternatives and Stages of Analysis

In the analysis done to determine whether a chemical poses an unreasonable risk, it is of crucial importance to be very specific about what is being analyzed. The analysis of unreasonable risk cannot be separated from the analysis of alternative methods of controlling the chemical. This is because risk is the product of inherent toxicity and exposure, and exposure is determined by the controls (voluntary or regulatory) placed on the chemical. The application of controls to chemicals is the process of making unreasonable risks reasonable. The use to which a chemical is put is one kind of control, as TSCA specifically recognizes by authorizing use limitations as one kind of regulatory measure which the EPA can impose.

The determination of unreasonable risk begins with an analysis of the inherent toxicity of the chemical. "Risk," in this context, is defined as the biological or ecological effects that a chemical produces at given levels of exposure. The determination of such risk is, at least in theory, a scientific process. But the inadequate state of scientific knowledge is such that even this stage of the process is subject to political disputes over such questions as the validity of extrapolations from animal tests to humans or the shape of the dose-response curve at low doses. Despite these controversies, it is important to retain the distinction between the essentially scientific question of "risk" and the political/economic/philosophical question of "unreasonableness."

The way in which the results of the risk analysis are reported and incorporated in the analysis of regulatory alternatives is of crucial importance. The whole nature and impact of the program will be greatly influenced, for example, by whether a chemical is considered as simply a carcinogen or whether one also considers the extent to which its carcinogenic action has been verified, the potency of its carcinogenic activity, and its synergistic or antagonistic relationship to other chemicals.

Once the inherent toxicity of a chemical is ascertained, the toxicity must be juxtaposed with existing or proposed controls to determine risk. But even before this stage, controls and toxicity must be considered together to some extent, because the controls will affect the type and extent of toxicity testing necessary, as the debate over testing requirements for new chemicals has made clear. To the extent that toxicity testing is tailored to controls, the EPA will have to utilize its significant new use authority to ensure that the adequacy of testing matches the degree of exposure.

Assuming adequate toxicity data, the first of two critical stages in determining unreasonable risk is *comparison of risk posed by the chemical under alternative assumptions about the controls (including use) to be applied to the chemical.* The second critical stage is *comparing risk with the costs of alternative regulatory measures.*

It is necessary to address a question that has produced some confusion during discussions of unreasonable risk. If we use the general paradigm of unreasonable risk being a trade-off between costs and benefits, then one must be careful to specify what is being analyzed. There are basically two options. The analysis can be focused on the costs and benefits of *the chemical,* given alternative regulations. If this is the focus, then the costs are such factors as deaths and injuries caused by use of the chemical, and benefits are such factors as the contribution of the chemical to the GNP, the balance of trade, etc. Alternatively, one can focus on the costs and benefits of alternative *regulations,* in which case the costs are such factors as lost markets or employment, the cost of applying control technology, or the cost of government and industry time spent complying with the regulation. The benefits would be reduction in damage to health or the environment. The elements considered in either case are the same, but which elements are considered costs and which are labeled benefits are opposites. We focus on the alternative regulations approach because it more closely approximates the choice faced by a regulatory agency.

Once the range of risks associated with different controls has been determined, the need for regulatory action by the EPA must be evaluated. It is useful in this context to divide chemicals into three groups:

1. Some chemicals, because of their inherent characteristics or because of controls that will be applied by the user, clearly do not require regulatory action. An example would be chemicals that can only be used as intermediates.[5]
2. Some chemicals will require regulatory action, but not under TSCA. The two most likely situations are chemicals occasionally released to the environment, and chemicals that may pose an occupational risk.

3. Some chemicals potentially should be regulated under Section 6 of TSCA, although such chemicals will most likely have to be regulated under other statutes as well.

For many (perhaps most) chemicals, it will not be clear from a simple examination of the available data to which category the chemical belongs. It will be necessary to do at least a preliminary analysis of *the degree of risk compared with the cost of regulation under alternative regulatory assumptions.* It is hoped that the EPA will have the resources to conduct such a preliminary analysis for all new chemicals that require it. A priority-setting mechanism will have to be established for selecting already commercialized chemicals to be analyzed.

If the preliminary analysis indicates that regulation under TSCA may be required, a more thorough analysis should be performed. If the preliminary analysis shows that the chemical should be regulated, but not under TSCA, then appropriate steps will have to be taken to ensure such action.

It is a well-established principle of economics that the analysis of alternative actions should be based on the marginal or incremental benefits to be gained from the incremental costs incurred. If the costs of Option A are $100 and the costs of Option B are $110, the analysis should focus on what benefits are obtained for the incremental $10, not on the total costs of each option, nor on the total benefits. This basic point is often neglected in the analysis of proposed regulations. It will be more difficult to apply this principle to TSCA than to the Clean Air or Clean Water Acts because the large variety of possible regulatory actions under TSCA do not form a continuum. It is harder to incrementally compare banning, use restrictions, quantity limitation, and labeling than to compare various degrees of emission controls.

Costs and Benefits of Quantification

We have been assuming that it is desirable to quantify as many of the elements of a regulatory analysis as possible. Quantification is not an end-in-itself but is rather a means of clarifying the reasoning behind a regulatory decision.

There are at least two possible disadvantages to being clear and explicit. First, the amount of conflict and controversy over a proposal or decision may be increased if the basis on which a decision is made is clearly revealed. Second, quantification may result in the decision-maker slighting those elements that cannot be quantified, such as aesthetic value, effects on innovation, or the political impact of a decision.

The concern that some unquantified values will be slighted if the analysis is quantified to the maximum extent possible may have some validity. However, as long as the final decision is determined through the judgment of a decision-maker, with his or her own values and biases, unquantified values may receive excessive attention as often as not. Also, it is not clear that the unquantified values lie more on one side of the cost-benefit calculus than the other. The suffering attendant on a human death is unquantified, but so is the impact on technological innovation.

Finally, it should be noted that quantification should extend to the degree of uncertainty surrounding the data used in the decision analysis. Most of the information used in TSCA decisions is highly uncertain. If the EPA is to be explicit about the basis for its decision, it should explicitly indicate how reliable the data it has utilized are.

Priority-setting—What to Regulate

The initial decision with respect to collecting information for TSCA regulation is choosing which chemicals should have priority for being considered for possible regulatory action. Because all new chemicals will be reviewed by the EPA to some extent, and because information will be provided in premanufacturing notices, the major problem concerns existing chemicals. The TSCA inventory contains about 45,000 compounds. EPA resources (and perhaps those of the private sector, as well) are sufficient to collect detailed information on somewhere between 0.1% and 1% of these compounds each year. How should the EPA select the one chemical in a thousand or a hundred to be investigated?

The Interagency Testing Committee (ITC), established by TSCA to select chemicals for further testing, has developed a methodology for assigning priorities. The ITC methodology basically involves two stages. The first involves scoring chemicals for degree of human and environmental exposure. The exposure scoring is based on the quantity of the chemical produced annually, the amount released into the environment, the number of individuals exposed and the duration of their exposure, and the extent of general population exposure. In the second stage, chemicals are scored with regard to cancer, genetic effects, birth defects, acute toxicity, other toxicity, bioaccumulation, and ecological effects. Scores are either numerical (0, 1, 2, or 3) or by letter (x, xx, or xxx). A number indicates that tests results are available; the number's value indicates the degree the effect was confirmed or the dose level at which it was found. A letter indicates need for further testing; the number of "x's" expresses the numerical score which might be expected after testing. Substances are ranked for each effect and for total effects.

One difficulty with the ITC methodology is that it considers the risk of the chemical *in toto*. Because it fails to distinguish among different uses of the chemical, its use in different geographical areas, or the potential impact of a wide variety of regulatory options, it implicitly assumes that the only regulatory option available under TSCA is a total ban. This approach is economical in terms of resources expended to collect information, but may overlook situations where regulatory action could have the greatest pay-off.

Predictability of Targets

It has been argued that the selection of chemicals for regulation should not be done too systematically or predictably because, if the chemical industry can predict which chemicals will be subject to regulation, it will tend not to exercise voluntary controls over the vast majority of chemicals that will not be regulated.

Industry representatives strongly dispute this line of reasoning. They argue that the more the EPA's priorities are predictable, the greater will be the degree of voluntary compliance. If the industry does not know what the EPA considers an unreasonable risk, it becomes much more difficult to voluntarily take steps to eliminate such risks.

The differences between these two lines of argument are based on several assumptions. The randomness argument assumes that what chemicals pose an unreasonable risk should be clear to the manufacturer, or at least clear enough to provide a basis for a high degree of self-regulation. The industry argument assumes that what the EPA will choose to consider an unreasonable risk may not be the same as what the industry would consider an unreasonable risk, and therefore clear guidance and predictability are needed. On this point, past experience supports the industry's contention.

Another contrasting assumption relates to the extent to which manufacturers themselves are faced with a priority-setting problem. The randomness argument assumes that a manufacturer can adequately determine and control the risk from his entire product line. On the surface, this is a reasonable assumption, and it finds legal support in the liability laws. However, with respect to existing chemicals, large manufacturers face the same problem of priorities as does the EPA. Toxicity data on existing chemicals are likely to be inadequate, and resources to obtain better data are severely limited. Choices must be made to determine which chemicals should be reviewed. If the EPA does not provide guidance, the industry itself devises methods for choosing priorities. The more random the EPA's priority-setting process is, the more resources consumed by actions that may have lower net benefits to society than other actions that could have been taken. This is true by definition if we assume that a predictable and systematic process can be established which will identify the regulatory targets that will yield the greatest net benefits. The EPA's goal should be to strive for the most predictable and systematic priority-setting process possible.

Use of Categories

Consideration of chemicals in categories or groups, rather than individually, has been a matter of intense debate. The debate centers on the need to consider categories of chemicals, rather than individual chemicals, in order to get the most effect from the limited resources available.

The category that has received the most attention consists of chemicals called carcinogens. The criteria for definitively deciding that a chemical is a carcinogen in the context of the science of toxicology may, in the view of many, be impossibly demanding in terms of governmental regulation. A toxicologist may need "dead bodies" before concluding definitively that Chemical x is a carcinogen. Rather than waiting for the bodies, the regulator may accept lesser proof, such as tests on rats. The regulator thus uses a different operational definition of a carcinogen than does the scientist. The difference in definitions need not lead to a dispute over either science or regulation if the interested parties can recognize the difference in the two contexts.

The Universe of Relevant Factors

Some of the specific factors which need to be taken into account in assessing unreasonable risk are stated more or less explicitly in TSCA. For example, the administrator is required by Section 6(c) to consider the following factors before prohibiting or regulating commerce in, or particular uses of, a chemical substance or mixture: Effects on health and the environment; magnitude of the exposure of human beings and the environment; benefits for various uses; availability of substitutes for such uses; reasonably ascertainable economic consequences; the national economy; small business; technological innovation; the environment; and public health. It is important to note that, for many of these items, it would be necessary for the EPA to know which segments of society are affected. Benefits to manufacturers and processors would have to be distinguished from benefits to consumers and society. Risks to workers would have to be differentiated from risks to consumers or the general public.

Political factors also make a difference; for example, whether unemployment caused by a regulation will occur in the district of a freshman congressman who has no relationship to the regulating agency, or in the district of the chairman of the committee that controls appropriations for the agency. Some have urged that such political factors be explicitly identified in the regulatory analysis. It seems certain that the decision-maker's staff will identify such factors for him, but it also seems unrealistic to ask the agency to identify these factors in the *Federal Register* or to somehow weigh or measure political factors with health, environmental protection, or economic costs. Insofar as the analysis deals clearly and explicitly with non-political factors, it is likely that the influence of politics will be reduced.

Availability of Information

Much information needed to make sound regulatory decisions under TSCA will be either unavailable or unknown. Exposure assessment, for example, is much more primitive than toxicology. Our tools for ascertaining how much, and in what way, segments of the population are exposed to a particular chemical are inadequate.

It is often assumed that the economic information used in determining unreasonable risk is more precise than the scientific information on toxicity. This assumption may be false. The estimated economic costs of regulation may be unreasonably high because they are based on inflated information supplied by the industry to be regulated, or because the EPA systematically underestimates the ability of the private sector to adjust to regulatory intrusions into the market.[6] The projected estimates may be unreasonably low because the EPA has an incentive to make them low. In the absence of analysis of past decisions, it is impossible to know how accurate the economic projections have been or in which direction they err, but the margin of error in the economic information used to make decisions may be greater than the margin of error in the risk-related information.

The obstacles to obtaining valid information will, in some respects, be greater for new chemicals than for existing ones. There is the obvious difficulty that data concerning exposure, economic benefits, employment, etc., will be based largely on speculation rather than on empirical information. The toxicity data will depend almost entirely on testing done by the manufacturer, who, by the time a pre-manufacturing notification is submitted, will have a strong stake in the future marketing of the chemical.

Analysis of Information

The very large amount of information relevant to regulating a chemical and the heterogeneity of the data make it impossible for anyone to reach decisions based on the universe of raw data. Somehow, the information must be analyzed and synthesized. It would be preferable if the analysis could be made systematic and predictable.

Uniqueness Versus Consistency

Decision-makers frequently argue that each regulatory decision poses a unique set of problems and involves consideration of a unique data base. To some degree, this is unquestionably true. There are, however, major disadvantages to considering each decision as unique. Thinking may be excessively influenced by short-term considerations, such as newspaper coverage or a telephone call from a congressional staff person. In any case, the decision is likely to appear "political" to outside observers. Institutional learning within the agency is minimized, so that the lessons learned in making one decision are not carried over to the next. The regulated parties find it impossible to predict what the agency considers important or how it really defines unreasonable risk, and voluntary compliance therefore becomes difficult. All of these difficulties could be ameliorated if the agency attempted to put its decision analysis on a more systematic and predictable basis.

The EPA's Current Risk Analysis System

The EPA Office of Toxic Substances has begun a commendable effort to put the risk assessment phase of regulation on a more systematic basis. The current process involves three stages. The first is hazard assessment, which is a preliminary look at what is known about the risks posed by a given chemical. If available information is inadequate, the hazard assessment stage may result in the agency promulgating a rule under Section 8(a) of TSCA in an effort to obtain additional information. A "Phase I review," which is a more detailed assessment of the risks, based on all available information, forms the second stage. A "Phase II review," a full risk assessment and analysis of the potential for regulatory action, is the final stage.

Information on the economic impacts of proposed regulation is not analyzed until the Phase II review, but to proceed to Phase II there must be reasonably good evidence of serious risks posed by the chemical. By that time, it is almost certain the agency will regulate the chemical. The agency's resources to do full risk analyses are limited, and its performance is judged, in part, by how much regulating it does. Therefore, it cannot afford to invest too many resources in analyses that do not produce regulatory action.

Consolidation of Factors for Decision-maker

The responsible decision-maker requires concise descriptions of the costs and benefits of regulatory actions. One possible format for such a description is shown in Table 12-1. There are, however, three dimensions to analyzing TSCA regulations that greatly complicate the analysis and presentation of the information in Table 12-1: uses, the distribution of costs and benefits, and the availability of substitute chemicals.

It should be noted that Items 1, 2, 3, and 8, under "Health and Environmental Effects" in Table 12-1 will not change for the different regulatory options. Regulation cannot change the inherent toxicity of a chemical; it can only change the patterns of exposure to the chemical. Thus, the information about inherent toxicity could be included only in the separate risk analysis prepared by the EPA, not in the regulatory option format of Table 12-1.

An alternative method would be development of a hazard index to combine both types of information. There are many difficulties in formulating such an index, but if a reliable one could be developed, it would be very useful.

Table 12-1. Illustrative format for display of information (for regulatory options 0, I, II, and III, where 0 is the "no action" regulatory option).

Health and environmental effects	Regulatory Options			
	0	I	II	III
1. Nature of the effect.				
2. Probability that effect is real.				
3. Severity of the effect.				
4. Nature and size of the population or system at risk.				
5. Intensity of exposure (amount and duration of exposure).				
6. Probability of occurrence of the effect in this population.				
7. Amounts of substance entering the environment.				
8. Persistence of the substance in the environment.				

Note: Repeat 1 through 6 for each separate kind of effect, and 4 through 6 for each separate population or system at risk. Consider effects resulting from commercial use of the substances as well as substitutes. Effects of concern (Item 1) may be quite diverse; for example, cancer, birth defects, genetic effects, other chronic human health effects, acute health effects, damage to ecosystems which adversely affect agriculture, recreation, aesthetics, survival of species, etc. Populations at risk (Item 4) may be persons exposed in their place of employment, consumers of the substance for a particular use, residents in a particular location, future generations, etc.

Costs of regulation	Regulatory Options			
	0	I	II	III
1. Uses.				
a. Description of the use.				
b. Nature of the benefit derived from the use.				
c. Nature of the benefit of the substance in the use, in comparison with substitutes.				
2. Direct economic effects.				
a. Manufacturer.				
b. Net change in employment.				
c. Government expenditures.				
3. Indirect economic effects.				
a. Customers and suppliers.				
b. International trade.				
4. Changes in industrial structure.				
a. Effects on innovation.				
b. Effects on small business.				

Quantification of Factors

The factors relevant to regulatory decisions are measured in a variety of very different units — dollars, lives lost, sick days, etc. Although the final decision will not be made by numerically counting up the costs and benefits, it would be of immense help to the decision-maker if the different units could be made commensurable so that they could be aggregated and compared in some systematic way.

The traditional way in which the disparate units have been made commensurate and aggregated is by translating non-dollar elements into dollars. However, for some of the most important elements in health and safety regulations, such as health effects, it has not been possible to obtain dollar equivalents that command any general agreement. Furthermore, expressing all the elements in dollars has moral and political overtones that are unacceptable to many who are involved in the decision-making process. Perhaps it is time to consider an alternative.

If we accept the subjectivity of the dollar values attached to non-marketable factors such as lives, then perhaps we should accept a subjectively established rating system. Instead of translating all factors into dollars, each quantified element (including dollars) would simply be multiplied by a numerical rating factor designed to indicate that element's importance relative to other factors. Tables 12-2, 12-3, and 12-4 provide a highly simplified illustration of how such an analysis would work.

Table 12-2. Raw data.

	Do Nothing (Option 0)	Regulatory Option I	Regulatory Option II
Benefits			
Lives lost	100	40	0
Biological index of diversity	27	34	63
Costs			
$ Costs to manufacturer	0	$5 million	$20 million
Number of jobs lost	0	100	600

Table 12-3. Weighting factors.

Factor	Weight
Lives lost	100
Biological index of diversity	5
$ Costs to manufacturer	10^{-5}
Number of jobs lost	5

Table 12-4. Multiple value calculation of costs and benefits.

	Option I	Option II
Lives lost	(60) (100) = 6000	(100) (100) = 10,000
Biological index of diversity	(7) (5) = 35	(36) (5) = 180
Total benefits	6035	10,180
$ Costs to manufacturer	(5,000,000) (10^{-5}) = 50	(20,000,000) (10^{-5}) = 200
Number of jobs lost	(100) (5) = 500	(600) (5) = 3000
Total costs	550	3200

Table 12-2 is simply the basic information collected for the analysis. In any actual decision, more than four factors would be involved, but the illustration is limited to four to keep things simple. The rating factors shown in Table 12-3 were also chosen arbitrarily and only for illustrative purposes. In the context of actual decision-making, the choice and value or rating factors is obviously the critical step in the analysis.

The calculations in Table 12-4 are not complicated. Option I would save 60 lives (40 lives lost, compared to the baseline case of 100 lives lost), and the 60 is multiplied by the rating factor of 100, for a value of 6000. The biological index of diversity would improve by 7 (34, compared to the baseline of 27), and this is multiplied by the rating factor of 5 to produce a value of 35. The two benefit factors are added to produce a total benefits value of Option I of 6035. The comparative analysis of the different options would proceed as in a standard cost-benefit analysis.

There are undoubtedly many refinements that can be incorporated into this basic approach. For example, the application of the rating system really does two things: it transforms the raw data into comparable magnitudes so that they can be aggregated, and it also indicates the relative importance of each of the factors. Because it is difficult for most people to intuitively compare a rating of 100 with one of 10^{-5}, a two-step process in which the raw numbers were first translated into comparable magnitudes (dollars expressed in millions, to be more comparable with lives, for example) could be used, and then, as a second step, rating values indicating relative importance could be applied.

It could be argued that this non-monetary approach is simply a subterfuge for using dollars. But it is more than this. It has the merit of explicitly showing that the relative importance attached to the factors in the decision is a subjective matter. Perhaps more important, it brings the analysis of decision trade-offs back to fundamentals. The EPA is not a business firm or a Corps of Engineers. In the health and safety context, arguments about the discount rate and the dollar value of lives have tended to obscure the fundamental need for some method, however basic, of systematizing and making explicit the trade-offs that every decision-maker must make. Perhaps it is time to focus on this need as a starting point to construct a method of analysis more appropriate to regulatory requirements.

The Final Decision

The last stages of determining unreasonable risk involve the Administrator of the EPA, the Assistant Administrator for Toxic Substances, and perhaps one or two other high-level officials evaluating the evidence and analysis, sorting through their own personal values, perhaps testing the political winds, and then coming to a conclusion. It is definitely not a process that can be subjected to tidy rules or guidelines. However, there are certain practices that can help to assure rational, democratic, and workable decisions.

Weighing Costs and Benefits. As we have tried to make clear, the information on costs and benefits that will be provided to the decision-makers will not dictate a particular course of action.* There is no absolutely objective way to rationalize a given decision. The final decision is a matter of judgment, not science or mathematics.

The exercise of judgment may be assisted by an improved understanding of the types of decisions that must be made. Only very recently have scholars begun to get some perspective on societal decisions of the type discussed in this chapter. How to deal with situations that have a low probability of posing a very high risk, how to treat information that is surrounded by a high degree of uncertainty, and how much of what types of risk society is willing to bear are all subjects of active current interest that will — it is hoped — shed light on determining unreasonable risk under TSCA.[7]

Distributive Questions. The major aspect of unreasonable risk decisions not adequately covered in the analysis of costs and benefits is the question of how the costs and benefits are distributed. Harold Lasswell has defined politics as the determination of "who gets what, when, and how." In this sense, regulatory decisions under TSCA are essentially political decisions. Four dimensions of the distribution of costs and benefits are particularly important: geographical distribution, distribution among social classes, distribution over time, and distribution among levels of government.

---

*In one important sense, high-ranking decision-makers will be constrained. As Andrew has succinctly stated: "Most administrative decision processes in fact consist of extended series of decision points, each of which constrains those that follow. At each of these points values are brought to bear, implicitly if not explicitly." (Andrew, Richard N.L. and Waits, Mary Jo, *Environmental Values in Public Decisions.* Ann Arbor: University of Michigan, 1978, p. 16.)

Geographical Distribution. The geographical aspects of how costs and benefits of regulatory decisions are distributed is, if anything, likely to be given excessive importance in the U.S. because of the election process. If a decision will result in a New Jersey plant being closed, it is little consolation to the New Jersey congressional delegation that the workers will find employment elsewhere and that the productive value of the plant will be put to work elsewhere, especially if elsewhere is in some other state.

Distribution Among Classes. There are two aspects of distribution among classes. The first involves the effects of a decision on different income classes. This has been a major question in some environmentally-related policy areas, notably energy, but is not likely to be a salient feature of toxic substances decisions. Toxic substances decisions do not have a major impact on redistributing income among economic classes, and any progressive or regressive effect on income distribution is overshadowed by considerations of public health and environmental balance.

The second aspect involves distribution among workers, consumers, and the general public. The problems presented by this aspect are as much legal as distributive. Each of these three segments of the public are covered by different laws — workers by OSHA, consumers by CPSA and related Acts, and the general public by the Clean Air and Water Acts, RCRA, and the Safe Drinking Water Act. Thus, the regulatory alternatives considered and the information received under the authority of TSCA will have to be viewed in light of which segments of the community are at risk.

Distribution Over Time. A given amount of benefit is worth more if it is obtained now than if it is obtained sometime in the future. But many TSCA decisions are made to avoid future risks: risks to people who may not have been born. Thus, the problem of how to discount future benefits, a problem which has plagued much cost-benefit analysis, is also a problem for TSCA decisions.

Levels of Government. Far more than most environmental statutes, TSCA authorizes regulatory actions that are entirely within the ability and jurisdiction of the federal government. But because regulatory decisions under TSCA will inevitably involve recommendations for regulatory action under other statutes, and because these other statutes are often heavily dependent on state and local governments for successful implementation, it will be necessary to consider the abilities, resources, and priorities of these other governmental levels. The analysis of any regulatory alternative should include a detailed consideration of how the regulatory action will be implemented. It is likely also that most major toxic chemical problems will fall under the jurisdiction of several different federal statutes in addition to TSCA. Costs and benefits will be considered separately for each separate statute, and this may well distort the results of the analysis. David D. Doniger[8] has observed that, "Fragmented analysis tends to overstate the benefits of a substance or to understate its risks." As Doniger and others have pointed out, an aggressive interpretation of TSCA would allow the EPA to conduct a unified analysis of all the risks and benefits of a chemical, thereby eliminating the analytical distortion caused by the fragmented jurisdiction over toxic substances.

Openness and Access. Both to implement democratic principles of participation and to facilitate the quality and integrity of the decision-making process, it is important that this process be as open and accessible to interested parties as possible. (The ways in which this can be done have been described in detail elsewhere.[9]) The first two years of TSCA implementation seem to indicate that the EPA fully recognizes the need for meaningful participation by the interested public.

The final decision among regulatory alternatives is not, and should not, be truly final. Any governmental decision should be open for reconsideration, especially in a rapidly evolving field such as toxic substances. But reconsideration and change are not easy for those who have invested time, resources, and perhaps political capital in the original decision. Participation by the public can help to bring about such change.

Appendix: Federal Authority Directives Concerning Hazardous Materials*

In the effort to deal with toxic environmental contaminants, Congress has passed a diverse assortment of legislative measures. At present, a toxin entering our environment might be subject to control under no less than 14 different statutes which parcel out authority among the Environmental Protection Agency, the Department of Transportation, the Food and Drug Administration, the Consumer Product Safety Commission, the Occupational Safety and Health Administration, and the Nuclear Regulatory Commission.** While these measures offer a variety

---

*This appendix was prepared by Gregory S. Wetstone, assisted by Mary Dearing, Laura Hedal, Brian Magee, Tina Williams, and Elizabeth Wirtz of the Toxic Substances Program, Environmental Law Institute.
**A toxin entering our environment might be dealt with under the Federal Environmental Pesticide Control Act, the Safe Drinking Water Act, the Federal Food, Drug, and Cosmetic Act, the Clean Air Act, the Federal Water Pollution Control Act, the Marine Protection Research and Sanctuaries Act, the Atomic Energy Act, the Federal Hazardous Substances Act, the Consumer Product Safety Act, the Poison Prevention Packaging Act, the Occupational Safety and Health Act, the Resource Conservation and Recovery Act, or the Toxic Substances Control Act. The Federal Meat Inspection Act, 21 USC § 60 et seq., the Egg Products Inspection Act, 21 USC § 1031 et seq., and the Poultry Products Inspection Act, 21 USC § 451 et seq. are also concerned with the regulation of toxins.

of approaches to toxic substances-related problems, they are in many respects fundamentally similar. All are intended to grant the respective government agencies sufficient authority and direction to take effective regulatory action. All should therefore provide guidance as to how the agencies should proceed in moving from legislative goals to specific realities through regulatory actions. As the accompanying chart of 12 toxic substance-related statutes indicates, in providing this direction, many of these measures present the agencies with criteria which base the regulatory decision on an evaluation of whether the health or environmental effects associated with a particular substance or activity are "reasonable."

In general, determining reasonableness in this context requires an evaluation of the risks to public health or the environment posed by the substance or activity in question. In many cases, this evaluation of risks – often very difficult to identify, detect, and quantify – must be contrasted with an assessment of the social and economic costs of the regulation under consideration.* The agencies are normally confronted with a broad assortment of potentially relevant factors to take into account in such a determination. Before a decision on "reasonableness" may be reached, it is necessary to determine which factors should be considered, what importance should be attached to each, how conflicting priorities should be resolved, and how the diffuse, uncertain, and/or unquantifiable scientific and technical information which may lie at the heart of the issue should be dealt with.

The existence of these broad questions of policy invariably associated with the determinations of "reasonableness" in these statutes suggests that the nature and specificity of the direction which the statutes in this area furnish to the agencies is of crucial importance. Some measures offer no guidance on these fundamental decision-making issues beyond the direction to avoid "unreasonable" risks or effects. Others address the problems associated with translating vague statutory guidance into regulatory action by providing, with varying degrees of specificity, indications of what factors are relevant and where the priorities should lie. Table 12-5 is intended to offer some insight concerning the manner in which the major legislative efforts in the toxics area deal with these issues.

For each of the 12 statutes examined in this table, the provisions which most directly address the manner in which the agency is to proceed in reaching a decision on whether to regulate are quoted or paraphrased in the row headed "directive." The lower row provides a brief comment on the specificity of the legislative guidance. With some minor exceptions, the measures fit into five categories, which lie along a continuum in terms of the specificity of the statutory direction.

---

*Though the process of assessing reasonableness involves a weighing of costs and benefits, the approach and the methodology are very different from those involved in formal economic "cost-benefit" analysis.

Table 12-5. Federal statutory directives concerning hazardous materials.

	FEDERAL INSECTICIDE, FUNGICIDE AND RODENTICIDE ACT		CONSUMER PRODUCT SAFETY ACT	TOXIC SUBSTANCES CONTROL ACT	FEDERAL FOOD, DRUG AND COSMETIC ACT						OCCUPATIONAL SAFETY AND HEALTH ACT
STATUTE	7 U.S.C. § 136a (1947, as amended 1972) Pesticide Registration	§ 136d(b) (1972, as amended 1975) Cancellation of Change in Classification	15 U.S.C. §§ 2056(a), 2058(b) (1972, as amended 1976)	15 U.S.C. § 2605 (1976)	21 U.S.C. § 346 (1938) Tolerances for Poisons in Food	§ 346a(b) (1938) Pesticide Tolerances	§ 348(c)(5)(1938) Food Additives	§ 348(c)(3)(A) (1938, as amended 1962) Carcinogens in Food (Delaney Clause)	§ 355(d) (1938, as amended 1962) Drug Products	§ 360b(d)(2)(1968) Animal Drug Products	29 U.S.C. § 655(b)(5)(1970) Occupation Exposure to Toxic Substances
DIRECTIVE	Register pesticides which, in addition to other requirements, will not cause "unreasonable adverse effects on the environment" (§ 136a(c)(5)(C)(D)). The term refers to "any unreasonable risks to man or the environment taking into account the economic, social, and environmental costs and benefits of the use of any pesticide" (§ 136(bb)).	If a pesticide or its labeling does not comply with this subchapter or generally causes unreasonable risk of adverse effects on the environment, cancel or change the classification or hold a hearing to see if either of these actions are necessary. Take into account: the impact of the proposed action on production and prices of agricultural commodities, retail food prices, and otherwise on the agricultural commodity.	The commission is to establish such standards as are reasonably necessary to prevent or reduce an unreasonable risk of injury to health or safety associated with a consumer product (§ 2056(a)). Consider relevant available product data including the results of research, development, testing, and investigation activities conducted generally. Also consider and take into account the special needs of elderly and handicapped persons to the extent to which such persons may be adversely affected (§ 2058(b)).	Take action if a substance "presents or will present an unreasonable risk of injury to health or the environment." Consider: the effects of such substance for various uses and the availability of substitutes for such uses; and the reasonably ascertainable economic consequences of the rule, after consideration of the effect on the national economy, small business, technological innovation, the environment, and public health.	Take into account the extent to which the use of such substance is required or cannot be avoided in the production of each article, and the other ways in which the consumer may be affected by the same or other poisonous or deleterious substances.	Regulate the use of pesticides on agricultural commodities to the extent necessary to protect the public health. Give appropriate consideration, among other factors, 1) to the necessity for the production of an adequate, wholesome, and economical food supply; 2) to the other ways in which the consumer may be affected by the same pesticide chemical or by other related substances that are poisonous or deleterious; and 3) to the opinion submitted with a certification of usefulness.	In assessing the safety of a food additive, consider among other relevant factors: the probable consumption of the additive and of any substance formed in or on food because of the use of the additive; the cumulative effect of such additive in the diet of man or animals, taking into account any chemically or pharmacologically related substance(s) in such diet; and safety factors which in the opinion of experts qualified by scientific training and experience to evaluate the safety of food additives are generally recognized as appropriate for the use of animal experimentation data.	No additives found to induce cancer in man or animals shall be deemed safe.	Approve a drug if it is safe for use under the conditions prescribed, recommended, or suggested in the proposed labeling and it is shown to have the effect it purports or is represented to heave.	Consider among other relevant factors: 1) the probable consumption of such drug and of any substance of any substance formed in or on food because of the use of such drug, 2) the cumulative effect on man or animal of such drug, 3) safety factors which in the opinion of experts are appropriate for the use prescribed, recommended, or suggested in the proposed labeling are reasonably certain to be followed in practice.	Set the standard which "most adequately insures to the greatest extent feasible . . . that no employee will suffer material impairment of health or functional capacity."
AGENCY	EPA	EPA	CPSC	EPA	FDA	FDA	FDA	FDA	FDA	FDA	OSHA
Specifity of Guidance Directing Agency in Evaluating Relevant Decisional Factors	General guidance id-ntifying types of relevant considerations.	General guidance identifying types of relevant considerations.	A list of relevant factors is provided; no priorities are provided.	A list of relevant factors is provided; no priorities are provided.	A list of relevant factors is provided; no priorities are provided.	A list of relevant factors is provided; no priorities are provided.	A list of relevant factors is provided; no priorities are provided.	Decision based on single factual and/or policy finding.	A list of relevant factors is provided; no priorities are provided.	A list of relevant factors is provided; no priorities are provided.	Guidance in weighing considerations is provided.

Table 12-5. (Continued)

	FEDERAL WATER POLLUTION CONTROL ACT	MARINE PROTECTION RESEARCH AND SANCTUARIES ACT	SAFE DRINKING WATER ACT	NATIONAL ENVIRONMENTAL POLICY ACT	RESOURCE CONSERVATION AND RECOVERY ACT	CLEAN AIR ACT				HAZARDOUS MATERIALS TRANSPORTATION ACT
STATUTE	33 U.S.C. §§ 1314 (b)(1), 1314(b)(2) (1972) Best Practicable Technology; Best Available Technology Effluent Limitations	33 U.S.C. § 1412 (1972, as amended 1974) Ocean Dumping	42 U.S.C. §§ 300g-1(a)(2), 300g-5(a) (1974) Drinking Water Contaminants.	42 U.S.C. § 4321 et. seq. (1969)	42 U.S.C. §§ 6921a, 6922, 6923(a) (1976) Generators and Transporters of Hazardous Waste	42 U.S.C. §§ 7408, 7409 (1970, as amended 1977) National Ambient Air Quality Standards	§ 7410 (1970, as amended 1977) SIP Approval	§ 7411 (1970, as amended 1977) New Source Performance Standards	§ 7412 (1970) National Emissions Standards for Hazardous Air Pollution	49 U.S.C. § 1801 et. seq. (1975)
DIRECTIVE	*Listing:* Maintain a list of toxic pollutants taking into account the toxicity of the pollutant, its persistence, degradability, the usual or potential presence of the affected organisms in any waters, the importance of the affected organisms, and the nature and extent of the effect of the toxic pollutant on such organisms. In his discretion the administrator may publish more stringent (than BAT) effluent limits at the level which (s)he determines provides an "ample margin of safety." (§ 1314 (a) (4)). *Standard Setting:* Total costs, age of equipment and facilities, processes involved, engineering aspects, environmental factors, and energy requirements are to be taken into account in assessing Best Practicable Technology and Best Available Technology *Dupont v. Train* (4th Cir. 1976) among others held that no exact cost benefit analysis is required.	Issue permits allowing ocean dumping only where such dumping will not "unreasonably degrade or endanger human health, welfare, or amenities, or the marine environment, ecological systems, or economic potentialities." Consider, though not exclusively: the need for the proposed dumping; the effect on human health and welfare, including economic, esthetic and recreational values; and the effect on fisheries resources, plankton, fish, shellfish, wildlife, shore lines and beaches; and the effect on marine ecosystems, particularly with respect to several specified.	Protect health to the extent feasible using technology, treatment techniques and other means, which the administrator determines are "generally available" (§ 1412 (a) (2)).(A state with enforcement responsibility may exempt a public water system upon finding that due to compelling factors (including economics) the state is unable to comply and that the exemption will not result in an "unreasonable risk" to health.) (§ 1416(a)).	Federal agencies are required to assess the expected effect of a proposed action on the environment and to evaluate possible alternatives to the action. In *Calvert Cliffs Coordinating Committee v. AEC* D.C. Cir. 1971) the D.C. Court of Appeals interpreted NEPA to require a "balancing analysis" in which economic and social benefits are to be weighed against environmental costs.	*Listing:* Develop criteria for identifying and listing hazardous wastes "taking into account toxicity, persistence, and degradability in nature, potential for accumulation in tissue, and other related factors such as flammability, corrosiveness, and other hazardous characteristics." (§ 3001) *Standard Setting:* Set standards for hazardous waste transporters and generators "as may be necessary to protect human health and the environment." (§§ 3002, 3003)	*Listing:* Maintain a list of air pollutants which in the administrator's judgment cause or contribute to air pollution which may be reasonably anticipated to endanger public health or welfare. (§ 108 (a) (1) (A)) *Standard Setting:* Set standards to "protect the public health allowing an adequate margin of safety."	The factors to be considered, listed in § 110 (a) (2), involve the effectiveness, efficiency, procedural fairness of the SIP. *Union Electric v. EPA* (U.S. 1976) held that § 110 (a) (2) bars consideration of economic or technical feasibility.	Standards are based on the level of technology which has been "adequately demonstrated." Consider the costs of compliance as well as any non-air quality health and environmental impacts, and energy requirements. *Portland Cement v. Ruckelshaus* (C.A.D.C. 1973) held that a cost-benefit analysis is not required.	*Listing:* Maintain a list of hazardous air pollutants for which the administrator intends to establish an emissions standard. *Standard Setting:* Once a substance is placed on the list the administrator is to prescribed an emissions standard at a level which in his judgment "provides an ample margin of safety to protect the public health" barring a finding that the pollutant is "clearly not hazardous."	Upon a finding that transportation of a particular quantity and form of material in commerce may pose an *unreasonable risk* to health and safety of property (§ 1803) the secretary may regulate any aspect of the transportation of such "hazardous materials" as he deems necessary or appropriate (§ 1804).
AGENCY	EPA	EPA	EPA	ALL GOVERNMENT AGENCIES	EPA	EPA	EPA	EPA	EPA	DOT
Specifying of Guidance Directing Agency in Evaluating Relevant Decisional Factors	A list of relevant factors is provided; no priorities are provided.	A list of relevant factors is provided; no priorities are provided.	§ 1416 *Exemptions:* no guidance (beyond reasonableness). § 1412: guidance in weighting considerations is provided.	General guidance identifying types of relevant considerations.	*Listing and Standard Setting:* A list of relevant factors is provided; no priorities are provided. *Standard Setting:* Decision based on single factual and/or policy finding.	A list of relevant factors is provided; no priorities are provided.	General guidance identifying types of relevant considerations.	A list of relevant factors is provided; no priorities are provided.	*Listing:* no guidance (beyond reasonableness). *Standard Setting:* Decision is based on single factual and/or policy finding.	No guidance (beyond reasonableness).

This table was produced as part of an on-going study at the Environmental Law Institute examining the attributes of the various legislative approaches to the control of toxic substances which is supported by a development grant from the Andrew W. Mellon Foundation.

The legislation can be classified into the following categories:

1. Those measures which offer no guidance to the agency beyond the direction to eliminate risks or effects which are "unreasonable."
2. Those which offer general guidance as to the types of considerations which are relevant, directing the agency to consider (for example) environmental, social, or economic factors.
3. Those which outline more specifically the relevant factors, providing a list of relevant considerations, but offering no indications of where the priorities lie.
4. Those which offer guidance on the issue as to which considerations merit higher priority.
5. Those measures which require that the decision be based on a single factual or policy finding, usually concerning whether a given substance or activity endangers the public health. This type of directive does not directly require an assessment of reasonableness. However, because these factual/policy matters often lie in areas of scientific uncertainty, it does not necessarily follow that the limitation to consideration of a single factor significantly narrows agency discretion.

Health protection is no longer an absolute value. To an increasing extent, federal laws and regulations have required that protection of human health be balanced against the economic impacts of the protection measures. The problem has been posed most sharply in the debates over whether the U.S. can afford national health insurance. But on another level, the trade-offs in health protection measures must be made for the establishment of particular standards for toxic chemicals. Such trade-offs between health protection and economics pose a multitude of difficult problems.

REFERENCES

1. Zimmerman, Burke K., "Risk-Benefit Analysis: The Cop-Out of Governmental Regulation," *Trial,* February 1978, p.44.
2. National Research Council, *Decision Making in the Environmental Protection Agency, Vol.* IIb, *Selected Working Papers*, pp. 82–97.

3. *Ibid.*, p. 89.
4. EPA Office of Air Quality Planning and Standards, "A Method for Assessing the Health Risks Associated with Alternative Air Quality Standards for Ozone," draft, July 1978.
5. For the complete TSCA definition, see *Federal Register* 42, *247*:64576, December 23, 1977.
6. National Academy of Sciences, "Decision Making for Regulating Chemicals in the Environment," p. 13.
7. Page, R. Talbot, "A Generic View of Toxic Chemicals and Similar Risks," *Ecology Law Quarterly* 7, *2*:207–244.
8. Doniger, David D., "Some Observations on Balancing," prepared for the Conservation Foundation Conference on Unreasonable Risk, p. 16. (See also Doniger, Liroff, and Dean, "An Analysis of Past Federal Efforts to Control Toxic Substances," Report of the Environmental Law Institute to CEQ, July 1978, pp. 45–63.
9. National Academy of Sciences, *op. cit.*, pp. 4, 5, 23–31.

13

Incentives for Health Promotion: The Governments Role

Eugene C. Nelson, D.Sc.

Adam M. Keller
Community and Family Medicine
Dartmouth Medical School

Michael Zubkoff
Community and Family Medicine
Dartmouth Medical School
Amos Tuck School of Business Administration
Dartmouth College

This volume is based on the proposition that, to improve its effectiveness, our national health policy and the health system that flows from it must strike a better balance between promoting wellness and treating illness.* The Fogarty Task Force on Health Promotion and Consumer Health Education[1] came to this conclusion:

To many, it appears that therapeutic medicine, important as it is, may have reached a point of diminishing returns. The 12–15 percent increase that we are

---

*Effectiveness of any nation's health system at improving the health status of the population depends on carefully adjusting health resource commitments to the society's cultural patterns, level of industrialization, level of personal socioeconomic status, and changing epidemiological profile (i.e., rates of death, disease, and disability by cause). Based on this type of analysis, McDermott[2] identifies four phases in the development of an effective health system for societies ranging from underdeveloped to fully industrialized. The first stage is a non-medicine phase, where the greatest potential for improvements in health status can be realized by measures aimed at improving household sanitation, while the last phase is continuing health services, where personal health services are most effective.

adding to our 100 billion-dollar health care bill each year — even the portion that is not consumed by inflation — apparently has only a marginal utility.

The purpose of this chapter is to discuss the government's role in providing incentives for healthy lifestyles. To do this, we first attempt to provide general answers to three basic questions:

1. When is government intervention in health matters justified?
2. What "tools" can government use to carry out interventions?
3. Where should government aim its interventions?

The chapter concludes with six guidelines that can be used to develop government initiatives to promote more healthful lifestyles.

Focus on Lifestyle

To make writing this chapter a manageable task, we have elected to limit the focus to government's role in providing incentives to promote healthful lifestyles. The term "lifestyle" has come to be closely associated with health promotion initiatives and cuts across both the internal and the external environments of the individual. LaLonde[3] described the term in the following manner:

The expression "lifestyle" is related to the way people live in the social and historical context that is peculiar to them, but it is also related to the orientation given to their life, what is commonly called "philosophy of life." Lifestyles are initially imposed on us in our early years and from then on, we tend not to question our lifestyles unless we are prodded to do so. Moreover, lifestyles exist in harmony with the organized social milieu and with the physical milieu that have helped shape them. This latter aspect of the human condition results in lifestyles being partially ascribed for a given generation.

The lifestyle aspect of health promotion was selected because the question of whether and, if so, how the government should intervene to promote modification of lifestyles to improve the health of the population is surfacing with increasing frequency in health policy debates. The basic reason this has become topical is the widespread belief, based on epidemiological analyses conducted by researchers such as McKeown,[4,5] that the greatest potential for substantial improvements in the health status of the population lies in decreasing the incidence of self-destructive habits and increasing positive health practices. Haggerty, a physician, and Fuchs, an economist, provide succinct summaries of the lifestyle argument. Haggerty states:

One's lifestyle, including patterns of eating, exercise, drinking, coping with stress, and use of tobacco and drugs, together with environmental hazards, are the major known modifiable causes of illnesses in America today. Medical care, on which we spend so much has, in comparison, only a weak effect on health . . . . Education to alter personal lifestyle and illness behavior has quite naturally been advocated with increasing frequency as an "idea whose time has come."[6]

Fuchs concluded in his book, *Who Shall Live:*

The greatest current potential for improving the health of the American people is to be found in what they do and do not do to and for themselves. Individual decisions about diet, exercise and smoking are of critical importance, and collective decisions affecting pollution and other aspects of the environment are also relevent.[7]

Criteria for Government Intervention

When can government intervention to promote the health of the public be justified? The question must be faced squarely, since government actions designed to enhance some aspects of lifestyle and to curtail others may erode the individual's free choice — a basic societal value.[8]

It can be argued that the major function of our government is to protect the rights of the individual and the free market system for private enterprise. The nation's democratic tradition and economic system guarantee the right of private persons to exercise free choice with respect to all major life activities. They also allow private enterprise the right to produce and market goods and services in accordance with their own self-interest. In theory, individuals are free to pursue pleasure, and businesses are free to pursue profit, generally unencumbered by government interference. Programs to promote health must be conceived and carried out within a system of government based on the individualistic ethic, characterized by free choice within the limits of the law. That health promotion activities aimed at lifestyle do seek to change people's behavior is clear; when it is appropriate for government to step in and directly attempt to alter individual lifestyles is unclear.

Much of the uncertainty regarding the appropriateness of government action to influence people's values and lifestyles can be traced to confusion concerning the source of the intervention. Criteria for intervention shift as the party initiating the action changes. For discussion purposes, two types of health interveners can be specified: 1) private sector health providers and organizations, and 2) public sector (federal, state, and local government) health bureaucracies. Table 13-1 summarizes the two different sets of criteria for intervention.

Inspection of the criteria indicates that each list is grounded on a different set of premises. The first four private sector criteria are based on traditional medical-ethical grounds regarding doctor-patient relationships.[9] The fifth is the rationale for most public health efforts to prevent and control epidemics and to

Table 13-1. Criteria for health interventions by private and public sectors.

Private sector intervention may be warranted when . . .	Public sector intervention *may be* warranted to alleviate a market failure when a particular good or service meets one or more of four public finance criteria . . .	If the proposed intervention substantially satisfies one or more of the public finance criteria, then intervention *can be* justified if the . . .
1. Persons present themselves (or others for whom they are responsible) for care and the potential benefit of the action is thought to exceed the attendant risk.	1. It exhibits significant externalities (i.e., when there is discrepancy between private and public costs and benefits).	6. Functional impact on the population (in terms of quality, quantity, or productivity of life) is serious and prevalent; *and*
2. Persons indicate the desire to change health-related behavior but are unable to do so on their own.	2. It exhibits characteristics of public goods (for example, joint or non-rival consumption).	7. Cost-benefit or cost-effectiveness analyses suggest a favorable outcome.
3. Persons, as a result of age or handicap, are not able to care for themselves.	3. It is produced under monopoly conditions.	
4. Persons receive communications that reinforce potentially hazardous behavior.	4. When other market imperfections arise that provide a justification for public intervention (for example, when consumers lack the knowledge needed to make an informed decision).	
5. Ill effects of condition of (or actions taken by) one party present a health risk to others.	5. When it is a "merit good" (i.e., sociopolitical) decision that a given good or service is a "right."	

221

protect the public from environmental hazards. On the other hand, the first four public sector criteria are based on public finance grounds for government intervention. Public finance criteria are based on the premises that the market-place is the most efficient means of allocating resources and that government interference in the market system is warranted only when market failures occur.[10, 11, 12] The fifth criterion serves as a rationale for government's moving into areas that strict market-oriented economists consider "off limits" or at least questionable.[13]

There are several areas where intervention can be justified easily by both the private and the public sector criteria. Mandatory immunization for many vaccine-preventable diseases, such as smallpox, represents a situation that fits private sector criterion Number 5 (ill effects of actions taken by one party presents health risk to others) and public sector criterion Number 1 (exhibits significant externalities) because of its highly contagious nature and severity, as well as being covered by Number 2 (joint consumption). The government, however, is being pressured to enter, or has already become involved in, many other health areas which are not readily covered by the traditional public finance criteria. Much of the debate concerning national health insurance, for example, turns on the value of the "merit good" or right-to-health-care argument. Under these circumstances, advocates must attempt to justify action on the shakier grounds of "merit good." Consequently, in order to resolve controversy concerning whether or not a government action should be initiated, cost-benefit or cost-effectiveness analyses may be conducted, and data on the seriousness and prevalence of the condition are frequently cited. However, we contend that cost-benefit and functional impact analyses should serve as a secondary screen (to assist in the more efficient allocation of scarce public resources) *after* determining that government intervention is justified on public finance grounds.

We would suggest that health promotion activities which are entirely appropriate endeavors for the private sector may be improper for government. It is also proper for private sector health professionals to advocate public measures to boost their respective programs. But when the question arises whether government should expand further its health role, it should first determine whether the proposed program can be justified by public finance or merit good criteria, and, if it can, the government should then proceed to estimate the degree of functional impairment associated with the condition and the cost-effectiveness of measures taken to alleviate the problem.

Tools for Government Intervention

Though they will be dealt with in separate sections of this chapter, the question of when government intervention is justified dictates, to some extent, the tools government can use to intervene. The relationship between the two

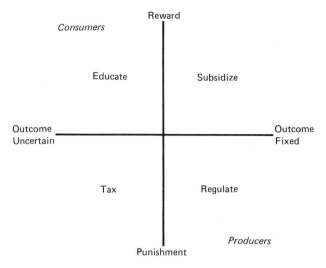

Figure 13-1. Incentives the public sector can use to promote health.

issues is obvious, since the readiness to use one or more tools the government has at its disposal to influence behavior is dependent upon having met the aforementioned criteria. Figure 13-1 shows the array of incentives the public sector can use to carry out health program initiatives.

By definition, an incentive is "something inciting to action or effort, as the fear of punishment or the expectation of reward."[14] The incentives, or tools, government may use to promote health can be divided into four basic categories:

1. *Education.* Communication to provide persons or organizations with the knowledge and motivation necessary to make an informed choice, taking into account health risks and benefits.
2. *Subsidization.* Actions taken to provide persons or organizations with tangible rewards for engaging in an activity judged to be healthful.
3. *Taxation.* Actions taken to provide persons or organizations with financial "punishment" for engaging in an activity judged to be health-aversive.
4. *Regulation.* Legislation designed to compel or force persons or organizations to engage in activity judged to be healthful or to refrain from activity judged to be health-aversive.

Each of the four basic categories of incentives can be implemented in myriad formats and combinations, depending on the target group (either producers or consumers) and on the source of the intervention (federal, state, or local government). Prior to focusing on specific formats, the key attributes of the incentive strategies are briefly mentioned. As Figure 13-1 suggests, the four incentive types vary on two fundamental dimensions: 1) reward versus punishment, and 2) outcome fixed versus outcome uncertain. Education and, particularly, subsidization incentives, on the one hand, versus taxation and regulation, on the other, represent the carrot and the stick. Accordingly, there is generally less resistance to education and subsidization, since no one's ox is gored outright (though, in the case of subsidization, some oxen may get supplemental feedings). Another distinguishing characteristic, namely the degree to which the outcome is predictable, separates education and taxation from subsidization and regulation. At the one extreme, use of education leaves the ultimate decision, and hence the outcome, in the hands of the informed consumer or producer. At the other extreme, regulation with stringent enforcement greatly increases the degree of certainty that behavior will be in the desired direction.

The point is that there is no single incentive type unequivocally superior to the others. Each has its respective strengths and weaknesses. For example, health education has been heavily criticized (sometimes justifiably, sometimes misdirectedly) for failing to produce the desired results. This is largely due to its "outcome uncertain" characteristic. But to the extent that fostering individual responsibility for one's own health is desirable, the "outcome uncertain" characteristic is also a major strength of the educational approach. Similarly, the regulatory approach which relies on centralized planning and enforcement may provide a direct and immediate solution, since, as Ball[15] states:

. . . goals and requirements can be written into law and into regulations giving the appearance, at least, of having solved the problem.

C.L. Schultze,[16] a top economic adviser, however, criticizes over-reliance on the regulatory approach, saying:

In a society which relies on private enterprise and market incentives to carry out most productive activity, there is a critical choice to be made beyond the question of whether or not to intervene. Should intervention be carried out principally by grafting a specific command-and-control module onto the private enterprise incentive-oriented system, usually in the form of a regulatory apparatus, or should it be undertaken by modifying the informational flow, institutional structure, or incentive pattern of that private system? Neither approach is universally appropriate to every situation. But our political system almost always chooses the command-and-control response and seldom tries the other alternatives.

The authors of this chapter agree with the position taken by Schultze. Government should attempt to be more creative in using their carrots —

educational approaches and subsidizations — to modify the incentive structure for producers and distributors and the habits of consumers in directions considered to be healthful and market-perfecting. Approaches relying more on internal than on external control may take more time and have a higher index of uncertainty. They may, however, be more likely to lead to patterns of production and consumption that are internalized over the long run, rather than being adopted grudgingly through short-term coercion.*

Based on the preceding discussion, it follows that a comprehensive effort to promote health should consider using a balanced mixture of all four incentive types, to influence both producers and consumers, and centralized (federal) and decentralized (state and local) governments' initiatives and incentive systems.

Targets of Interventions

Having considered when government intervention may be justified and what tools it can use, we are ready to consider the third question: Where should government aim its intervention?

Figure 13-2 is an eclectic model depicting the major actors and forces operating in the social environment to influence individual consumer decisions that, in the aggregate, characterize one's lifestyle. The two most potent factors influencing lifestyle are the family and the school or workplace.[18,19] The school and the workplace are the locations where most time is spent, where the greatest functional activity occurs, and where the closest social contacts exist. The family in which a child grows up makes a primary contribution to shaping his or her values, attitudes, and beliefs, while the schools the child attends have an increasingly strong impact on lifestyle as the child ages. This impact results from the models offered by teachers — non-family adults the child observes at close range — and by schoolmates — the circle from which most "best" friends come. The family life of the adult sustains and influences health-relevant aspects of lifestyle. Its influence is particularly strong during the child-rearing stage, when parents are concerned about the importance of setting a good example for children to follow. The workplace exerts a major influence on adult lifestyle as he/she spends approximately eight hours per day there. At work, the formal and informal systems combine to proscribe or prescribe specific behaviors, such as smoking and drinking, and there people interact closely with other persons similar to themselves in age, socioeconomic status, and lifestyle.[20]

---

*Kelman[17] asserts that, of the three different strategies most often used to modify behavior — coercion, imitation, and internalization — the latter is most effective in achieving long-term change, since it allows new patterns of thinking and acting to be integrated voluntarily into one's way of thinking and living.

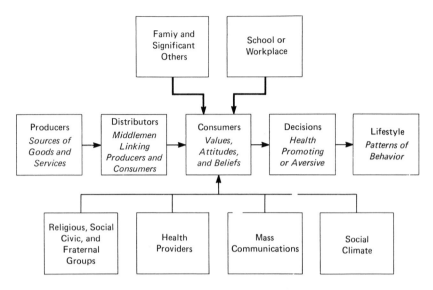

Figure 13-2. Actors and forces operating in the social environment of the consumer that influence lifestyle.

Several additional factors directly influence consumer values, attitudes, knowledge, and beliefs, and ultimately help determine lifestyle. First, an individual actively participates in *groups* (religious, social, civic, service, or fraternal), which can influence lifestyle and health status. Fuchs[7] provides an example of the impact of group membership on health by comparing health status indicators for the states of Nevada and Utah. The death rates for Nevada are 40-50% higher than those for Utah for most age groups. The major factor believed responsible for the better health enjoyed by Utah residents is their lifestyle. Ninety percent of the population in Utah is Mormon, and members of the Mormon church generally have a conservative lifestyle and a stable family life, and neither use tobacco nor drink alcohol or coffee. Residents of Nevada, in contrast, generally subscribe to a more "hard living" way of life, characterized by relatively high consumption of alcohol and tobacco,a less stable family life, and greater social mobility.

Health providers with whom an individual first comes into contact can influence lifestyle. Physicians often see patients at "teachable" moments and make recommendations that concern lifestyle issues (for example, smoking, obesity, drinking, and exercise). Though health professionals have great potential for influencing lifestyle, their current impact is limited: first, because people do not spend a great deal of time with their physicians (the average American sees a physician for 10-15 minutes per visit four or so times per year for an active complaint,[21] which leaves little time for general health counseling on fundamental aspects of lifestyle), and second, because physicians often feel the time spent on health counseling is wasted. Since many patients don't want to hear about their "bad habits,"behavior is hard to change even when a person wants to, and to do the task correctly would take a great deal of time (for which there is no ready source of payment). Health professionals could, however, exert more influence on health habits if they were to begin practicing "wellness" medicine as advocated by Ardel[22], "health hazard appraisal" as suggested by Robbins,[23] or the lifetime health monitoring approach outlined by Breslow and Sommers.[24]

Messages people receive through *mass media* represents a third set of forces which influence lifestyle. The newspapers and magazines people read, the radio programs they hear, and the television and movies they view reflect popular culture and thereby reinforce patterns of thought and living in countless subtle ways. For example, the most striking reaction one of this chapter's authors had to a rebroadcast of an Edward R. Murrow interview was Mr. Murrow's chainsmoking. The smoking habit once prevalent among television personalities did more to "date" the program than did anything else. Advertising has become increasingly effective at influencing consumers' decisions, by careful market segmentation linking a given product with a certain self-concept, mood, or lifestyle highly regarded by particular subsets of the audience.

Messages received from the mass media reflect the general *social climate,* a fourth broad category of forces shaping lifestyle. We sometimes forget that thought fashions exert a powerful influence on behavior. For example, Robert H. Ebert, M.D., former Dean of Harvard Medical School, recently wrote in the preface to a book on trends in physician career choice:

Dr. Funkenstein's book should be prescribed reading for all those who wish to influence the career choices of medical students . . . . Most medical school faculty . . . have a childlike faith in their ability to influence physicians in training by changing the curriculum and/or modifying the so-called educational environment . . . . [but] career choices seem to be related more to the general social atmosphere of the time than to anything that happens in college or medical school.[25]

Funkeinstein's book shows that, in the fifties, when popular interest and faith in science and technology were at their zenith, medical students elected to embark on bioscientific careers. When "thought fashion" changed during the sixties, however, and emphasis shifted to activism and social responsibility, career choice followed suit, and interest in biosocial medical careers became much more prominent. This is one illustration of the point that people's habits and values do change in response to variations in the social milieu. It is now apparent (witness the boom in running) that popular interest in physical fitness and health is on the upswing. Lester Breslow, M.D., one of the nation's leaders in prevention, states that "it's important to develop a positive [health promotion] strategy at this time to take advantage of a trend already in place."[26]

The preceding paragraphs describing Figure 13-2 are intended to highlight the field theory concept developed by the social psychologist Kurt Lewin.[27] Lewin theorized that the behavior of a given person at a particular moment in time represents the net impact of multiple positive and negative forces the person is striving for or trying to avoid. In a similar manner, the lifestyle adopted by any one person during a certain phase of life represents the net impact of many actors and forces influencing that person.

Before concluding this chapter, it might be helpful to discuss two techniques which can help improve outcomes of health promotion interventions aimed at producers and consumers, respectively. The first technique, "technological bypass,"[6] applies to producers. Technological bypasses, or "managerial solutions," are methods for shortcutting or reducing the need to change hazardous behavior or persons without actively involving them. Examples of technological bypasses are auto air bags, automatically locking seat belts, and "safe" cigarettes. Since complete elimination of all auto accidents and cigarette smoking is impossible, there is a genuine need to explore the potential for technological bypasses, for these and other problems, that are both acceptable to the public and profitable to the producer. But however true it may be that "man would rather rely on healers than attempt the more difficult task of living wisely"[28] or rely on inventors to protect himself from his own self-destructive behavior, science is unlikely to produce a "silver bullet" either to cure all our ills or to prevent all injury. Therefore, technological bypasses warrant serious consideration, and any of the four tools can be used to foster their adoption. Under most circumstances, however, use of technological bypasses in conjunction with other complementary programs of education, subsidization, regulation, and taxation will be desirable.

The second technique, marketing, applies to consumers and may be useful in developing sound health promotion interventions. A brief description of marketing is to:

1. Find out what consumers want.
2. Plan and develop a product or service to satisfy those wants.
3. Determine the best way to price, promote, and distribute that product or service.[29]

Though some persons, academicians especially, may bridle at the mention of the term "marketing," Kenneth Runyon[30] a leader in the field, states that "successful market is and always has been based on the behavioral sciences." The field of marketing is utterly pragmatic, a virtue sometimes in short supply in academic circles. Because modern marketing techniques are grounded in the disciplines of sociology, psychology, and social psychology, and rely on scientific methods to conduct market research, it cannot be taught cookbook fashion or be described adequately in a few paragraphs. Nevertheless, if marketing concepts are understood, and if marketing skills are applied to the development of health promotion strategies, then the chances of success will be greatly increased.

The marketing concept is consumer-oriented — built around the needs of the consumer, as opposed to selling a product. Using the marketing concept, one first finds out what the consumer wants and then produces the good or service that satisfies that need. The desired good or service is then delivered according to a marketing plan — a formal method for setting quantifiable objectives, developing strategies for reaching these objectives, and evaluating the extent to which the objectives are realized. A basic selling strategy involves "market segmentation" and can be described in the following manner:

Market segmentation is a customer-oriented philosophy. We first identify customers' needs in a submarket. Then we design a product and/or a marketing program to reach that submarket (segment) and satisfy those needs. Stated another way, in market segmentation we are employing a "rifle" approach (separate programs, pinpointed targets) in our marketing activities, as contrasted with the "shotgun" approach (one program, broad target).[31]

By tailoring programs to pinpoint at-risk groups, government can be more effective and make better use of scarce resources. Specific benefits of market segmentation include:

1. Designing programs that actually match customer behavior.
2. Determining what promotional appeals will be most effective.
3. Choosing advertising media more intelligently and determining how to better allocate the budget among the various media.
4. Setting the timing of the promotional efforts so they are heaviest during those times when response is likely to be at its peak.[32]

Conclusion

If government seeks to promote healthful lifestyles, then, to maximize effectiveness, it must aim simultaneous, synchronized interventions at the multiple factors making the most powerful contribution to shaping the lifestyle adopted by certain types of individuals. In light of the above, we offer the following guidelines for developing health promotion interventions, the aim of which is to influence health risks related to lifestyle:

1. Aim to influence behaviors that epidemiological analysis shows will lead to the greatest improvement in reducing premature disability and death in the population by identifying high-risk groups characterizable according to descriptive variables such as age, sex, socioeconomic status, and residence.

2. Study the high-risk groups to determine the trends in adopting and continuing the behavior and under what conditions the behavior pattern is formed and sustained.

3. Analyze the contribution producers and distributors make to promote or to retard the behavior, and determine if "technological bypasses" or "managerial" solutions are feasible.

4. Analyze the contribution that family structure and social environment within the school and workplace make to promote or retard the behavior.

5. Analyze the contribution health providers, mass communications, and social groups make to promote or retard the behavior.

6. Develop a marketing strategy which uses multiple tools and promotional techniques to work simultaneously with the key actors and forces that shape the behavior of well-defined segments within any given high-risk group.

REFERENCES

1. John E. Fogarty International Center and The American College of Preventive Medicine, *Preventive Medicine USA: Health Promotion and Consumer Health Education.* New York: Prodist, 1976.

2. McDermott, W., "Demography, Culture and Economics and the Evolutionary Stages of Medicine," in *Human Ecology and Public Health,* Kilbourne, E.D. and Wilson, G.S. (Eds.). London: Collier and MacMillan, 1969, pp. 7–28.

3. LaLonde, M., "Notes for an Address by the Honourable Marc LaLonde to the WOMCA 7th World Congress on Family Medicine." Canada: Health and Welfare Department, October 1976.

4. McKeown, T. and Lowe, C.R., *An Introduction to Social Medicine.* Philadelphia: F.A. Davis, 1967.

5. McKeown, T., *The Modern Rise of Population.* New York: Academic Press, 1976.

6. Haggerty, R.J., "Changing Lifestyles to Improve Health," *Preventive Medicine* 6: 276–289, 1977.

7. Fuchs, V.R., *Who Shall Live? Health, Economics and Social Choice.* New York: Basic Books, 1974.

8. Wikler, D.I., "Persuasion and Coercion for Health: Ethical Issues in Government Efforts to Change Life-Styles," *Milbank Memorial Fund Quarterly: Health and Society* 56. *3*:303–338, Summer 1978.

9. Bauer, K.G., "Averting the Self-Inflicted Nemisis (Sins) from Dangerous Driving, Smoking and Drinking," in *Consumer Incentives for Health Care,* Mushkin, S.J. (Ed.). New York: Prodist, 1974.

10. Blumstein, J.F. and Zubkoff, M., "Perspectives on Government Policy in the Health Sector," *Milbank Memorial Fund Quarterly: Health and Society,* Summer 1973, pp. 395–432.

11. Zubkoff, M. and Blumstein, J.F., "The Medical Marketplace: Health Policy Formulation in Consideration of Economic Structure," in *Proceedings: National Commission on Medical Care 1976-1977.* Chicago: American Medical Association, 1978, pp. 73–116.

12. Blumstein, J.F. and Zubkoff, M., "On Formulating National Health Policy," *Journal of Health Policy, Politics and Law*, in press.

13. Musgrave, R.A., "Provision for Social Goods in the Market System," *Public Finance* **26**, 1971; and Dunlop, D. and Zubkoff, M., "Consumer Behavior in Preventive Health Services," *Consumer Incentives for Health Care,* Mushkin, S.J. (Ed.). New York: Prodist, 1974.

14. *American Heritage Dictionary of the English Language.* New York: American Heritage, 1973.

15. Ball, R.M., "Background of Regulation in Health Care," in *Controls on Health Care* Washington, D.C.: National Academy of Sciences, 1974, pp. 3–22.

16. Schultze, C.L., *The Public Use of Private Interest.* New York: Harpers, May 1977, pp. 43–62.

17. Kelman, H.C., "Compliance, Identification and Internalization: Three Processes of Attitude Change," *J. Conflict Resolution* 2 *1*:51–60, March 1968.

18. Goode, W.J., *The Family.* Englewood Cliffs, New Jersey: Prentice-Hall, 1964.

19. Etzioni, A., *Modern Organizations.* Englewood Cliffs, New Jersey: Prentice-Hall, 1964.

20. Homans, G.C., *The Human Group.* New York: Harcourt, Brace & World, 1950.

21. *The National Ambulatory Medical Care Survey: 1973 Summary.* Washington, D.C.: DHEW. DHEW Publication No. (HRA) 76-1772, October 1975.

22. Ardell, D., *High Level Wellness: An Alternative to Doctors, Drugs, and Disease.* Emmaus, Pennsylvania: Rodale Press, 1977.

23. *Health Hazard Apprialsal: Seventh Annual Meeting of the Prospective Medicine and Health Hazard Appraisal of the Methodist Hospital Graduate Medical Center,* Robbins, L.D. (Ed.), 1970.

24. Breslow, L.R. and Somers, A.R., "The Lifetime Health-Monitoring Program," *New England Journal of Medicine* **296**, *11*:601–608, March 17, 1977.

25. Funkenstein, D.H., *Medical Students, Medical Schools and Society during Five Eras: Factors Affecting the Career Choice of Physicians 1958-1976.* Cambridge: Ballinger, 1978.

26. *The Nation's Health: Official Newspaper of the American Public Health Association*, August 1978, p. 6.

27. Lewin, K., *Resolving Social Conflicts.* New York: Harper & Brothers, 1948.

28. Dubos, R., *The Mirage of Health.* New York, Doubleday, 1959.

29. Stanton, W.J., *Fundamentals of Marketing, Fifth Edition.* New York: McGraw-Hill, 1978.

30. Runyon, K., *Consumer Behavior and the Practice of Marketing.* Columbus, Ohio: Charles E. Merrill, 1977.

31. *Ibid.*

32. Stanton, *op. cit.*

Insurance Issues

14

Health Promotion Strategies for Unionized Workers

Joann Grozuczak

United Mine Workers Health and Retirement Funds

Underlying the health promotion model is the premise "that good health and well-being is a goal within the reach of every individual."[1] Further, it has been suggested that social and political groups, by encouraging healthy lifestyles among their members, will build the foundation upon which the goal of good health can be achieved.

The health promotion model stresses the role of the individual in determining the quality of his or her health. Indeed, it is true that a healthy lifestyle is largely a matter of individual choice, and that the individual who flaunts the concept of healthy lifestyle cannot expect to maintain good health. And, of course, the more information and support society provides to foster individual health behavior, the more likely it is that the individual will change his or her perspective. The efforts of social groups to make this transformation are unquestionably well spent.

However, those groups must assume a much more difficult role if the health promotion concept is to succeed. While it may be true that an individual cannot achieve good health if his behavior does not foster it, no system of education and incentives can promise that, in American society, a healthy lifestyle will assure good health.

Society cannot demand that the individual bear the full burden of disease prevention. The promotion of healthy lifestyles is but one piece of what America's social, economic, and political institutions can do to work toward the prevention of chronic disease. There is much more in the realm of preventive health care that groups might accomplish, but it is far beyond the control of any one individual. Individuals, for example, make choices not to inhale cigarette smoke, but have no control over the toxic substances in the air they breathe; individuals can plan the healthiest of diets and still, unknowingly, consume carcinogenic pesticides and additives which nursing mothers may pass on to their infants.[2] And it is unrealistic to tell a coal miner, asbestos worker, or cotton mill hand to exercise to build up his circulatory and respiratory capacity, while also asking him to work in an environment that will very likely cripple those same functions.[3]

To ignore this in the health promotion scheme is to seal its doom. No matter how attractive the incentives may be, no matter how effectively peer groups are used, the health promotion model will fail if it makes false promises. And the lure of good health through individual behavior is little more than that unless the health promotion model includes an equal commitment to the prevention of the serious environmental health problems that threaten American society, and which are far beyond the control of any single member, whatever his or her behavior and attitudes may be.

Of all social groups which might take up the critical challenge of commitment and action in environmental health, the labor movement offers perhaps the best hope. Three compelling factors converge to dictate a strong labor role in this area: first, the concept of collective action on behalf of individuals who, alone, have little control over their environment is traditional and fundamental to the labor movement; second, it is in the workplace that substantial environmental threats originate and directly harm the workers who produce them; and third, the physical well-being of its members has historically been an important goal of the labor movement.

Labor unions evolved in western civilization to fill a need: to endow workers, collectively, with power that they could not possess as individuals The American labor movement, in particular, has remained intent upon the use of collective action to ensure that the basic needs of its individual members for appropriate wages, acceptable working conditions, and some measure of job security are met. From its earliest days, this single-minded goal has steered the course of American labor. In 1864, the Cigar Makers' International Union of America, one of the nation's first major unions and the training ground for the founders of the AFL, keynoted its constitution with the following statement of beliefs:

Labor is the creator of all wealth, and as such the laborer is at least entitled to a remuneration sufficient to enable himself and family to enjoy all those rights and privileges necessary to make him capable of enjoying, appreciating, defending and perpetuating the blessings of modern civilization. Past experience teaches us that labor has so far been unable to arrest the encroachments of capital, neither has it been able to obtain justice from lawmaking power. This is due to a lack of practical organization and unity of action. "In union there is strength." Organization and united action are the only means by which the laboring classes can gain any advantage for themselves.

The preamble of the Cigar Makers' 180th constitution further established the guidelines for effective collective action: "By organization we are able to assist each other in cases of strikes and lock-outs . . . and through organization only the workers, as a class, are able to gain legislative advantage."[4] Thus, over the last hundred years, unions have pursued their members' interests through the vehicles of collective bargaining and legislative pressure. When grappling with the issue of environmental health in the workplace, these traditional techniques would serve labor well.

The protection of the health of its members has long been a prime aspiration of American labor. Labor's expression of this concern, however, has had an uneven history, as unions have channelled both their bargaining and their political efforts into two health-related areas: medical insurance and job safety. Although labor's gains in both of these initiatives have been monumental, one must pause to examine the consequences and ask if labor's historical perspective on workers' health may not require broadening.

Labor and Health: The Traditional Perspective

The notion that individuals should be protected against the financial destruction of catastrophic illness, and the acceptance by the public of industrial unionism were products of the same era. Out of the Great Depression came the Wagner Act, which offered labor the basic legislative safeguards necessary for effective organizing and bargaining; and it was in the 1930's, too, that the founding discussions of New Deal social policy included the first glimmers of recognition that government should bear responsibility for the health of its citizens.

Although government never assumed that responsibility, the popularity of the health insurance concept grew in the post-Depression years, almost parallel with the rise of the American labor movement; it is thus not surprising that medical insurance grew to become an important collective bargaining goal. The first major employer-financed collectively bargained health plan, the United Mine Workers Health and Welfare Fund, was established to provide medical benefits to miners and their families in 1946. Since that time, nearly every major unionized industry has come to provide costly, comprehensive medical benefits for its workers. And, very clearly, the pattern of steadily increasing medical benefits that has characterized collective bargaining in major industries over the course of the last 25 years has occurred at the expense of other gains. In 1975, $2.73 billion was spent by American industries for medical benefits.[5] Between 1965 and 1974, dollars committed to health benefits through collective bargaining increased by 164%; wages, on the other hand, have increased in three major unionized industries – auto, rubber, and steel – by only 83%, 59%, and 85%, respectively, in the same period of time.[6] Labor, then, places sufficient importance on health care to allow a steadily greater portion of each collectively bargained dollar to be consumed by medical care costs.

One must wonder if some of this commitment is not misplaced. Following national patterns, there is, after all, no evidence to suggest that workers' health has improved in direct relationship with increases in medical benefits. And those benefits traditionally focus on conventional medical care, with its curative, technological, acute illness orientation. As the health promotion model suggests, there may be limits to what can be achieved by devoting further resources to medical technology and services. Having already achieved levels of medical insurance whose enhancement may produce dubious marginal gains, labor may now want to include prevention of illness as part of the bargain when it sits at the negotiating table.

Prevention of poor health, in and of itself, is not a totally alien concept to labor, but rather is one whose definition has been severely constrained, limited almost exclusively to the realm of job safety. The prevention of occupational injury – in contrast to the more complex issue of prevention of occupational disease – has been a historical concern of industry and government as well as of unions. The reasons are clear: when injuries occur on the job, they have immediate, overt consequences. The link between the injury and the workplace is obvious and its effect deleterious to both the worker and to the employer. Furthermore, problems of job safety have clear remedies – removal of the unsafe conditions.

As early as 1900, civic, industry, and labor groups recognized these factors and saw their lobbying efforts to establish state workers' compensation programs meet with success. In 1908, the first workers' compensation laws were passed, and, by 1920, all but six states maintained workers' compensation plans which paid injured workers up to 50% of their normal wages and covered injury-related medical costs for periods of up to three months.[7]

In concept, workers' compensation laws provided monetary compensation to individuals for lost working time, and compelled employers to internalize the costs of unsafe conditions inside their factory walls. The theoretical effect of workers' compensation is to distribute the social costs of occupational injury and, therefore, to provide an incentive for industry to maintain safe working conditions.

More than any other aspect of occupational health, the pursuit of industrial safety has met with some measure of success. Until the 1970's, however, legislative efforts to reform the workplace environment have accomplished little with regard to compensation for occupational diseases, and even less concerning their prevention. The rather simple system that charges the employer for the social costs of immediately hazardous working conditions and builds incentives for their elimination is not readily applicable to the more subtle process of occupational health maintenance.

Unlike safety hazards, the effect of health hazards may be slow, cumulative, irreversible, and complicated by non-occupational factors. While an unguarded blade in a circular saw may present a severe and immediate or "imminent" danger, it is often difficult to perceive the severity or imminent danger contained in a brief exposure to a potential carcinogen that can take years to cause a tumor or death. However, the probability of dying from cancer may be just as high as being injured by the saw.[8]

Indeed, occupational health hazards may figure into the morbidity and mortality statistics in this nation with startling impact.

Prevention of Disease in the Workplace

Recognition of the link between the industrial environment and each of the major, disabling chronic diseases is as critical to address as it is difficult to identify. Just as lifestyle can raise or lower an individual's risk of developing a chronic illness, broad environmental factors, originating with industry, may force devastating effects on society's efforts to prevent disease.

In the entire discussion of the link between environment and health, perhaps the most dramatic relationships occur between the work environment and carcinogenesis. The World Health Organization estimates that environmental agents, including, but not limited to, smoking and nutrition, cause 75–85% of the cancers which occur in industrialized populations. A substantial proportion of these agents can be traced to industrial chemicals or to other manufacturing substances.

These materials may be ingested or contracted through physical handling, but most are inhaled through polluted air. The likelihood of a toxic substance having a carcinogenic effect on an individual is heightened by two variables: the concentration of the substance inhaled or otherwise absorbed, and the duration of exposure to it. It is logical, then, that the worker who spends eight hours a day throughout a working life in a factory atmosphere laden with asbestos particles, benzidine, or vinyl chloride gas — all proven carcinogens — is at a great risk of developing some form of cancer.[9] To wit, 18% of all Americans die of cancer, compared to 50% of all asbestos workers.[10] A long-term rubber worker is almost 300 times as likely as the average American to develop lymphatic cancer.[11] Rare, exotic malignancies, such as mesothelioma and angiosarcoma of the liver, almost never seen among other groups, occur at alarming rates among asbestos and plastics processing workers, respectively. Coke-oven workers, copper and lead smelters, miners, textile workers, dye manufacturers, printers, dry cleaners, farmers, and insecticide sprayers are only a few occupational groups known to suffer inordinate cancer mortality as a result of constant exposure to toxic industrial substances.[12]

As if this small sample of grim statistics were not enough, it is important to note that the occupational diseases already identified probably represent the mere tip of an insidious, looming iceberg. The development of occupational diseases has been aptly termed an "epidemic in slow motion."[13] Scientists estimate that it takes 20–40 years for chemically-induced tumors to manifest themselves in the human body. The rash of sudden discoveries of occupationally-linked cancers fits into the early stages of an unfortunate time frame; the post-World War II spurt of industrialization, the growth of the plastics industry in the U.S. since 1939, and the ever-increasing development and use of hundreds of new chemicals in manufacturing each year over the past few decades have just begun to enter that 20–40-year period. Occupationally-linked tumors have probably just begun to appear. It is difficult to be optimistic about the future health of American factory workers.

The suspected carcinogenic effects of industrial substances are scant. Of the 13,000 known toxic industrial materials, only a handful have been subjected to animal studies, and even fewer to clinical trials. With the overwhelming number of potential industrial carcinogens before them, epidemiologists have only been able to study those chemicals which already appear to have had a harmful effect. Typically, they engage in research after an alarming cancer rate among some group of workers is discovered, often by their union – in short, after the damage has been done. Until the recent passage of the Toxic Substances Control Act, nothing was done to certify the safety of new or recent substances before they are put to use by industry.

The risk of cancer is not the only health threat to which labor must respond. Other chronic diseases have apparent environmental roots which trace back to the workplace. Heart disease is by far the most obvious lifestyle-linked condition, with its marked relationship to smoking, obesity, and cholesterol levels. However, these elements account for only 25% of heart disease risk, with 75% falling to as yet unidentified genetic and environmental causes.[14] It is strongly suspected that occupational stress correlates with heart disease. Moreover, the Coal Mine Workers Compensation Division of the Department of Labor recognizes heart disease as a complication of coal miners' pneumoconiosis.[15] Occupational factors, again, seem to contribute to the incidence of heart disease among American workers.

The example of coal mine workers' pneumoconiosis also serves to illustrate the link between the work environment and chronic respiratory conditions, such as emphysema and chronic bronchitis. Data suggest a dramatically high rate of respiratory disease among coal miners and former mine workers. Respiratory disease symptoms of persistent cough and dyspnea are reported among 10% of working miners and 24% of non-working miners, statistics approximately equal to the incidence of radiologic evidence of pneumoconiosis on mining populations.[16] The incidence of disabling respiratory disease among miners who worked at the mine face – the area of the mine where coal dust fills the air in the highest concentrations – is even more grim; X-ray evidence indicates that 22.3% of mine face workers and 33.3% of former mine face workers suffer from pneumoconiosis, with the incidence of the problem closely correlated with number of years in coal mining occupations.[17]

The Public Health Service estimates that 390,000 new cases of occupational disease occur annually and that occupational diseases cause over 100,000 deaths each year.[18] Alarming as this statistic is, it does not represent a final tally of the total threat of workplace health hazards.

The worker involved in the manufacture of a toxic substance is the classic "human guinea pig"; he or she is exposed to the substance for long hours day after day, year after year, in high concentrations and in various stages, from raw material to refined product. To belabor this inhuman analogy one step further, the workers' situation is not unlike the laboratory experiment in which the test animal is exposed to potential carcinogens in high doses during a compressed amount of time. In the experiment, the disease rate in the laboratory animal suggests the toxicity of the substance – albeit in an exaggerated manner – for humans; in the factory or minesite, the incidence of disease among highly exposed workers suggests a capacity of the finished product, or the waste produced in its manufacture, to damage the health of the community at large – again, in a more dispersed disease pattern. Recent research lends support to the contention that the risks of industrially-induced diseases are not confined to workers alone. Among the families of New Jersey asbestos workers, scientists have found abnormal X-ray results compatible with asbestosis – an occupational disease which cripples its victims' respiratory functions and is all too often followed by the appearance of lung cancer – at a rate of 38.4%.[19] Bladder and colon cancer rates among both males and females in chemical manufacturing centers significantly exceed national norms.[20] Perhaps most sinister of all, polyvinyl chloride, a plastics production substance which recently was found to cause liver cancers among the workers who manufacture it, is also linked with birth defects, premature births, and strikingly high cancer rates in the children of that worker population. Early findings suggest that this occurs not from direct exposure through working parents, but rather as a chromosomal, mutagenic effect, capable of passage from generation to generation.[21]

One cannot ignore, then, that industrial health hazards may have a wide-reaching effect, the potential damages of which cannot now be confidently assessed for workers or for their communities.

Occupational Health and the Health Promotion Model

In formulating its approach to the issue of occupational health, labor can both fall back on its own history and cull much that is new and useful from the health promotion model; the health promotion concept offers the union a set of goals which, once achieved, will shape political and economic institutions into a form compatible with, and supportive of, individuals' efforts to attain good health for themselves, their families, and their communities. To achieve them, labor can rely on the traditional mechanisms of collective bargaining and legislative intervention.

The health promotion model suggests that labor pursue three general purposes in its occupational health efforts:

1. To effectively use economic incentives to promote good health.
2. To strive to prevent health hazards, rather than react, with technology and monetary compensation to their results.
3. To recognize the importance of individuals' attitudes in determining the quality of their health.

Use of Economic Incentives. Collective bargaining is an economic activity, one which requires the parties involved to set a price on each item on the bargaining table, and to weigh the value of individual items against one another. As discussed previously, labor has placed a high value on worker health, but has not incorporated chronic disease prevention in its healthrelated bargaining goals. Indeed, the subject was so submerged that the NLRB did not even recognize occupational health as a mandatory subject for bargaining until 1966.[22]

There will be no preventive medicine gains at the negotiating table unless labor is willing to assess the value of occupational health highly when it bargains with industry. Occupational health must assume a high priority among other issues (such as wages, hours, and safety conditions). If the economics of collective bargaining dictate the attainment of occupational health assurances at the expense of other contract gains, labor must be able to shift its traditional economic values accordingly.

When translating the concept of occupational health into concrete bargaining goals, unions may pursue the following:[23]

1. A joint labor-management trust fund, based on employer contributions, to assess occupational health hazards.
2. Incorporation of OSHA and other relevant standards into bargained contracts.
3. Expedited arbitration proceedings over workplace health issues.
4. Unlimited union inspection rights.
5. Use and funding of impartial experts in disputes over workplace health issues.
6. Training of union health and safety stewards.
7. Periodic health screening examinations for employees.
8. Expanded use of health and safety committees.

Valuable as these measures are, however, they alone cannot alter industry's approach to occupational health. Whatever the incentives may be for unions to strive for a healthy workplace, they are not shared by industry. Thus, labor cannot rely solely on collective bargaining, but must turn also to major legislative intervention.

The American economic and political systems do not demand that industry bear the cost of the environment health hazards which it creates. In 1975, the average fine imposed by OSHA for a health and safety violation was $18 — clearly not sufficient to discourage, in itself, an unhealthy work environment. Furthermore, workers' compensation is rare in cases where an occupational link is suspected. Even in the case of asbestosis, which is one of the earliest identified and best documented occupational diseases, the economics of compensation dictated, to asbestos manufacturers, that the disease was cheaper than its prevention. Prior to the issuance of OSHA asbestos standards, the Johns-Manville asbestos company refused to make capital improvements to reduce the concentration of asbestos fiber in its New Jersey plant; it was estimated that those improvements would have cost $25 million in initial outlays and $5 million for annual operation, while the cost of disease in its workforce was only $900,000 — the company's yearly Workers' Compensation payment for asbestosis benefits at that time.[24] Only after years of dispute regarding the proper health standards in the asbestos industries had ended, and OSHA had promulgated final compromise standards, did the industry make any marked effort to improve its health conditions.

In this ultimate, positive outcome, the asbestos industry is a rare example, since asbestos is one of less than 20 substances for which OSHA has issued health standards. Because most industries and their resulting occupational diseases are now affected only by after-the-fact, workers' compensation legislation, it is critical for labor to work to use that tool to the fullest extent. For the moment, it is the best economic tool available for realigning occupational health incentives.

Labor's approach to industry's economic incentives must not be entirely punitive. To the extent that legislation protects industry and makes health condition improvements more attractive to the corporation, labor also gains. After all, the threat that an industry, and the jobs in it, will suffer due to costly environment improvement, is a grave one; and it is not always obvious that workers and government, when faced with a possible trade-off between health hazards and economic collapse, would opt for the latter. Whether or not it is justified, that possibility is raised by industry over and over again.[25]

Two legislative initiatives would serve in the interests of both occupational health and American industry, while remaining compatible with the overall goals of the labor movement. First, restrictive tariffs on imports, long promoted by labor to assure American workers' employment, should be applied to materials produced under unhealthy foreign working conditions. To fail to impose economic obstacles to such imports would cause both moral and economic dilemmas: if the market for a given manufactured good functions normally, the imposition of strict standards would upset an economic equilibrium in which the American-made product was priced lower than its substitutes, including foreign imports. With the added cost of environmental compliance placed on American manufacturers, importers not faced with the same regulations (i.e., most of industry outside Western Europe) would assume a competitive advantage, and capture the American market. They would thus be rewarded for their unhealthy conditions, American society would merely export its occupational diseases, and American workers would lose their jobs. Clearly, labor would wish to avoid this situation, and can do so through the familiar channel of lobbying to discourage imports — this time, with a focus on health as well as on economics.

A second legislative action which labor may want to support is a shifting of national priorities in the subsidization of industry. Governmental expenditures which encourage unhealthy lifestyles, with tobacco subsidies as a glaring example, should be abandoned and the same resources spent instead on grants to industries and independent researchers to develop substitutes for hazardous manufacturing processes and products.

The Preventive Approach. An effective worker's compensation program alone is not the answer to the occupational disease problem. Although it may alter industry's economic incentives and provide disease victims with minimal financial security, it will never repay the full social costs of occupational illness, nor will it assure that all feasible preventive measures are taken.

A preventive approach requires, first, the identification of occupational sources of disease. Prior to the passage of the Toxic Substances Control Act, the process of identification of hazardous materials was, at best, haphazard. Left to private industry and the limited capabilities of the National Institute of Occupational Safety and Health (NIOSH) only a handful of the estimated 13,000 known toxic substances had been tested for their health risks.

Funding for occupational health hazards research has been unquestionably inadequate. In 1976, NIOSH's budget included only $1.8 million for industrial cancer research, despite the fact that the cost to study a single substance exceeds $250,000. With these financial limitations and a staff of only 20 full-time researchers, NIOSH estimated that it could fully test and set standards for a maximum of 20 materials per year.[26] NIOSH is further charged with entering into conflicts of interest in some of its research, having often contracted the testing of toxic material to private research firms whose chief customers are the industries under investigation.[27]

In addition to a lack of data, a tendency to ignore existing information has hampered the prevention of occupational health hazards.

Industry has a dismal record in sharing its information regarding health hazards with relevant parties: workers, unions, government, and the scientific community. In the plastics industry, for example, evidence surfaced in the early 1960's to suggest an abnormal cancer risk among polyvinyl chloride processors; this data, however, was carefully suppressed, and its validity denied to anyone who inquired about it. Similarly, asbestos workers were not told of their high risk of lung disease from long-term employment in the asbestos industry until 1971, even though that information was available to the industry in the 1950's.[28]

OSHA, too, has fallen short in its responsibility to uncover and share relevant data. The tragic example of polyvinyl chloride again comes to mind. Italian animal studies performed in the late 1960's discovered a link between polyvinyl chloride and angiosarcoma of the liver. Based on that research, most of industrial Europe moved to regulate polyvinyl chloride exposure in the workplace. Although this information was publicly accessible, however, NIOSH chose either not to pursue the data or, possessing the information, not to act upon it.[29]

The past mistakes and ommissions in the task of identifying hazards and informing the public of them leave labor with a major role.

One hopes that the implementation of the Toxic Substances Control legislation will take place in a more systematic and comprehensive framework. Labor must monitor regulations as they are promulgated to assure that this commitment exists and must scrutinize their implementation to make sure it is met. Second, labor should strive to be sure that, in both the workplace and in government research facilities, information regarding health hazards is disseminated as soon as it becomes available.

Individual Attitudes Toward Occupational Health. Only when individuals are provided with adequate information and a suitable socioeconomic structure to foster a healthy environment can one finally speak of individual choice. But despite the overwhelming health risks which abound in the workplace, it is not clear that their elimination is high on the list of popular priorities. Fear for their livelihoods and unwillingness to break old habits prevent members of the public from spontaneously rising up against environmental health hazards. Labor's role as an influential peer group, here, is to change some widely held public attitudes.

First, workers must be assured that there is not a one-for-one trade-off between a healthy workplace and their jobs. Legislative action to subsidize healthy work conditions, and penalties for the use of unsafely produced imported substitutes, will provide vivid reassurances that government is substantively acting to prevent loss of jobs.

Labor can point to past experience to illustrate that industry's threat of collapse resulting from the cost of compliance with environmental regulations is often an idle one. The loudest warnings of this kind in recent years came from the plastics industry, which threatened that OSHA's polyvinyl chloride guidelines would paralyze the entire plastics industry and produce a loss of 2.2 million jobs[30] and annual sales of $65–90 billion.[31] A year after the issuance of those standards, however, all major plastics manufacturers are in compliance, and no economic downturn has been experienced by any of them. Their workers, ultimately, had gained a much healthier work environment with little additional cost.

A second attitudinal obstacle to a healthy environment is the unfortunate, but frequently-voiced, assertion that "next thing you know, they'll be telling us that *everything* causes cancer." Response to bans on artificial sweeteners imply a popular belief that scientists and government, in their efforts to identify environmental sources of disease, are public enemies, not valuable contributors to good health.

To counter this, labor must use its full force and influence. It must alter the belief that disease occurs randomly, that bad luck or God's will singularly control patterns of morbidity and mortality. It must convince its members that, to a significant measure, health is within society's control, and that responsibility for the prevention of ill health rests directly with its members.

It is at this point, then, that one can return to the individual aspect of the health promotion model. Having laid the political and economic foundations of a healthy environment, labor and other support groups must influence individuals to value that environment and to act decisively to maintain it in the face of contradictory goals. Appropriate incentives operating in industry, and a preventive approach guiding the government, the workplace, and, in large part, the community environment, will truly permit individual choice and individual responsibility for the quality of his or her health care.

REFERENCES

1. Mg, L.K.Y., Davis, D.L., and Manderscheid, R., "The Health Promotion Organization," *Public Health Reports* 93:446–455, September–October 1978.
2. Harris, S., Chapter 10 in this book.
3. Hunt, V., Chapter 9 in this book.
4. Litwack, L., *The American Labor Movement.* Englewood Cliffs, New Jersey: Prentice-Hall, p. 28.
5. Executive Office of the President, Council on Wage and Price Stability, *The Complex Puzzle of Rising Health Care Costs: Can the Private Sector Fit it Together?* Washington, D.C., 1976, p. 94.
6. *Ibid.*, p. 95.
7. Ashford, N., *Crisis in the Workplace: Occupational Disease and Injury.* Cambridge: M.I.T. Press, p. 398; and Hunt, V., *Work, Women and Health.* West Palm Beach: CRC Press, 1979.
8. Ashford, N., "Worker Health and Safety: An Area of Conflicts," *Monthly Labor Review* 98:5, September 1975.
9. Agran, L., "Getting Cancer on the Job," *Nation* 22:434, April 12, 1975.
10. *Ibid.*, p. 20; Davis, D. L. and Rall, D., Chapter 7 in this book.

11. Anderson, A., Jr., "The Hidden Plague," *New York Times Magazine,* October 27, 1974, p. 20.
12. De Coufle, P., Stanislawczyk, K., Houten, L., Bross, I.D.J., and Viandana, E., *A Retrospective Survey of Cancer in Relation to Occupation,* U.S. Department of Health, Education and Welfare (NIOSH), 1977, pp. 77–178.
13. Anderson, *op. cit.,* p. 20; and Davis, D.L., "Science and Regulatory Policy," *Science* **203,**4375:7, January 5, 1979.
14. Ashford, *op. cit.,* p. 492; and U.S. Environmental Protection Agency, National Cancer Institute, National Heart, Lung and Blood Institute, National Institute for Occupational Safety and Health, and National Institute of Environmental Health Sciences, *First Annual Report to Congress by the Task Force on Environmental Cancer and Heart and Lung Disease.* Washington, D.C.: Environmental Protection Agency, 1978.
15. U.S. Department of Labor, "Black Lung Medical Benefits," Notice to Beneficiaries, May 3, 1978.
16. Lambert, W.S., Doyle, H.V., Entershine, P.E., Henschel, A., and Kendrick, M.A., *Pneumoconiosis in Appalachian Bituminous Coal Miners.* Cincinatti, Ohio: U.S. DHEW, Public Health Service, Cincinatti, Ohio: 1969, p. 115.
17. *Ibid.,* p. 116.
18. Cited in Ashford, *op. cit.,* p. 93.
19. Mason, T.J.,and McKay, F.W., *Atlas of United States Cancer Mortality by County, 1950-1969.* Bethesda, Maryland: U.S. DHEW, Public Health Service, National Cancer Institute, p. 81.
20. *Ibid.,* p. 18.
21. Burnham, "New Peril Feared in Vinyl Chloride," *New York Times,* August 22, 1974, p. 13.
22. Ashford, *op. cit.,* p. 493.
23. California Labor Federation AFL-CIO and the Center for Labor Research, University of California, Berkeley, *"Report on the Proceedings of the Conference on Occupational Health and Safety,"* in Ashford, *op. cit.,* pp. 493–494.
24. Brodeur, P., *Expendable Americans.* New York: Viking Press, 1974.
25. *Ibid.*(The same problem, in a different industry, is also described in "B.F. Goodrich and Vinyl Chloride: A Study in Corporate Reaction," *Business and Society Review* **12,** *Winter 1974-1975.*
26. Hyatt, J.C., *"U.S. Inspection Unit Finds Itself Caught in Critical Crossfire,"* Wall Street Journal 54:1, August 20, 1974.
27. *Ibid.,* p. 1.
28. "B.F. Goodrich and Vinyl Chloride," p. 47.
29. Ibid., *p. 44.*
30. Brody, J. E., "Vinyl Chloride Exposure Limit Is Opposed by Plastics Industry," *New York Times,* June 26, 1974, p. 30.
31. Barry Kramer, "Vinyl Chloride Risks Were Known by Many before First Deaths," *Wall Street Journal* 54:1, October 2, 1974.

15

Neglected Issues in the National Health Insurance Debate

Representative George E. Brown, Jr.

United States Congress

Introduction: Improving the Health of the American People

The growing debate over National Health Insurance, and health care in general, neglects several major issues that are integrally related in determining the success of any National Health Insurance program. Because of this neglect, we do not have a rational framework which can explain why health care costs are increasing faster than any other major component in the cost of living index (food, housing, clothing, fuel, etc), with no commensurate increase in health or "wellness," as measured by lifespan, infant mortality, incidence of disease, or any other conventional measure of health.

There are two major interrelated reasons for this:

1. Our health care system emphasizes third party payment for medical treatment of disease and ill health, rather than individual and community responsibility for the prevention of ill health or the positive promotion of good health.
2. Our health care system emphasizes hospital care (the most expensive form of care), the most expensive technology, and the highest paid professionals available, rather than simpler home and community care, more appropriate (and less expensive) technologies, and a wide range of professionals and paraprofessionals available in the local community.

Given this situation, it becomes apparent that simply increasing the annual expenditure of billions of dollars for health care costs will never in and of itself improve the overall health status of the population. As the Canadians' experience with National Health Insurance has shown, no health care system, whatever its financing mechanism, can by itself achieve health.[1] The essential problems of health today stem from social, biological, environmental, and lifestyle factors, much more than they reflect inadequate facilities or curative services.[2] Wildavsky[3] reports that the medical system affects about 10% of human health, with the remaining 90% being determined by non-medical factors, such as individual lifestyle, social conditions, and the physical environment. Surprisingly, in both Canada and the U.S., over 90% of the health expenditures are on the treatment of illness, while less than 10% is spent on the prevention of illness and the maintenance of health.[4] In spite of these facts, the debate over health care in general, and the National Health Insurance in particular, has focused on medical care.

In order to make major improvements in the health of the American people, at costs which remain within reason, I suggest that we must:

1. Establish a system of paying for health care that emphasizes health promotion and disease prevention.
2. Utilize the full range of health care personnel and facilities more effectively, including not only hospitals and specialized physicians, but convalescent homes and hospitals, long-term nursing homes, home care, and the full range of paraprofessional and sub-professional health personnel.
3. Focus on the improvement of environmental factors which adversely affect health, including the home and workplace environments.
4. Focus on the simple lifestyle causes of poor health — poor nutrition, lack of exercise and sleep, overindulgence in liquor, tobacco, and drugs, and emotional and physical stress.
5. Focus on biological research that will reveal the answers to questions such as the causes of cancer and heart disease and the transmission of genetic disorders.

Unless we develop a health care program which includes these five points, we could spend untold billions of dollars for a new National Health Insurance Program which would do little to improve the health of the American people. There are many explanations of why these five points are not in the forefront of the discussion on health care system. The explanation which I find most compelling is the lack of short-term economic incentives for such programs, in contrast to the major vested interests and economic incentives involved in continuing the present approach to national health care, coupled with increasing deficiencies of current economic indicators as measures of national welfare.

Our economic system provides little, if any, incentive in the health area to encourage the concepts of personal responsibility, self-help, and long-term prevention of illness and disease. The costs of such activities may be large and immediate, while the benefits are indeterminant and remote. Every aspect of our personal lives is gradually being assigned a quantitative economic value, and our major national programs, ranging from environmental protection to public works projects, are increasingly being evaluated against economic criteria that were originally designed for entirely different purposes. The bias of economics, however, is on dollar flows and markets. Economics almost invariably overlook what are externalities to those marketplaces. Thus, the costs of benefits of environmental regulations, pollution control, good nutrition, preventive medicine programs, and the application of common sense are not measured in conventional economic terms. As such, they tend not to exist as serious components of economic discussions; and from this position, they literally disappear, obscured by the very real economic problems which are so central to public policy decisions.

Given this gradual evolution in the importance of economic criteria to public policy decision-making, it is little wonder that the current debate over National Health Insurance centers around such terms as "percent of the GNP," "increase in the cost of living index," or "contribution to the inflation rate." However, there is a great danger in this emphasis on economics criteria in the absence of data on non-market costs, such as the costs of environmental pollution, which pollution control programs prevent, or the costs of occupational diseases, which occupational health programs prevent. Former Congressman Paul Rogers, who had been known in the Congress as "Mr. Health," described the situation as follows:

The latest attack on the Nation's environmental and occupational programs, strangely enough, comes from the Council of Economic Advisors and the Council on Wage and Price Stability. The official inflation fighters have, it seems, singled out environmental and occupational health programs for their criticism. And yet in discussions with my staff, the President's top economic advisors admit that they really have no cost data on environmental and occupational disease. They said, "Well, we don't know really what the costs *are*. And since we don't know, we won't consider them." Furthermore, in what I think is rather a shocking assertion, they reject any responsibility to *gather* the data on the health care costs generated by environmental diseases.[5]

Besides diverting our attention away from the basic health issues, the economic arguments and the use of economic indicators, while important and of some value to decision-makers, can be genuinely misleading. The use of GNP (Gross National Product) as a measure of national welfare is an excellent example. The GNP is not a measure of progress, as many seem to believe, but is a measure of money flows. If the health of Americans gets worse, the amount of money spent on health increases. This, in turn, increases the GNP. If all other segments of our economy were constant, our GNP could still grow by simply having more sick people who have sufficient means (i.e., insurance) to pay for health services. This is, in fact, what has been happening in recent years.

Meanwhile, programs to prevent or reduce the causes of sickness, such as environmental protection programs, have come under attack because they are believed by many economists to reduce the GNP growth, causing inflation, and to generally divert capital into non-productive activities. There is, at present, simply no generally accepted way to quantify or calculate the benefits from preventing an injury or an illness. If we could allocate to a "plus" ledger the value of all of the *prevented* accidents and illnesses, and allocate to a "minus" ledger the value of all accidents and illnesses which actually occur, we would have an entirely different type of economic indicator. Unfortunately, there is little agreement on why accidents and illnesses don't happen, just as there is considerable disagreement on causes when accidents and illnesses do happen. And even when causes can be established with some certainty, a dollar value on costs or benefits is even harder to establish. As can be seen, our current economics are of questionable value in evaluating health promotion and disease prevention activities, not to mention non-market activities such as self-help programs.

The powerful motive force supporting the current health care system is based on it being highly profitable to a great many people involved in the health field, or, at the very least, on the present system not being unprofitable. The present, most prevalent, system of paying for health care today is through a system of third party insurance, where neither the physician nor the patient has a strong economic stake in controlling costs or even in preventing ill health. In fact, physicians are encouraged to increase costs. Only when we have developed a system which provides clear financial incentives toward the maintenance of health, instead of the treatment of sickness, can we expect health to improve and costs to decrease.

Despite all obstacles, much can be done to promote the five points described above, and to incorporate them into a national health program. Over time, our understanding of economics will change, and the value of promoting "wellness" will be appreciated. These five points will be necessary for the nation, regardless of the status of National Health Insurance.

Some elaboration of these points follow.

1. Establish a system of paying for health care that emphasizes health promotion and disease prevention. As stated above, we must replace the present system of paying for health care through a system of third party insurance, where there is no incentive to control costs. The system which appears to have the most promise in accomplishing this is an expanded national system of health maintenance organizations (HMO's), which would provide the consumer with a choice of competitive systems. HMO's have been shown to reduce hospitalization and other health care costs, and, in theory, if not always in practice, they provide a financial incentive for health promotion and disease prevention.[6]

Other methods exist that can provide a financial incentive for health promotion and disease prevention, such as the proposal to establish health promotion organizations (HPO's)[7]. Improvements are needed in the HMO approach, and new approaches, such as HPO's, need to be demonstrated in a realistic setting before we can be confident of their utility. Novel approaches should be explored to find the best institutional mechanism to meet the various health needs of the American people. Certainly, an extensive public education and awareness program which proclaims the virtues of disease and illness prevention is justified.

One thing appears certain, and that is that a National Health Insurance program, under the present third party insurance system, would dramatically increase health care costs. This is what happened when we went to Medicare and Medicaid, and it is what appears inevitable if we go to National Health Insurance under the present instititional arrangements.[8]

As Aaron Wildavsky[9] calls it, this is the "Law of Medical Money." which states that "medical costs rise to equal the sum of all private insurance and government subsidy."

The immediate role of the federal government should be to continue improving and implementing the various public laws that have been enacted to improve our Nation's capabilities in devising effective health promotion and disease prevention activities. All too often, while a major national debate is going on, as with National Health Insurance, sensible interim steps are not being carried out. Regardless of the eventual structure of a National Health Insurance Program, we will need the experience and information we gather from these interim steps.

2. Utilize the full range of health care personnel and facilities more effectively, including not only hospitals and specialized physicians, but convalescent homes and hospitals, long-term nursing homes, home care, and the full range of paraprofessional and sub-professional health personnel. This point seems obvious to a layperson, but needs to be made because it is frequently overlooked or disputed. Health insurance programs have only gradually begun to cover non-hospital or non-physician costs, and have yet to cover primary preventive medicine. Some arguments against broadening health care to non-professionals and non-medical facilities have centered on quality control and accountability. Ivan Illich,[10] in his book, *Medical Nemesis: The Expropriation of Health,* discusses the evolution of medical doctors and medicine into the modern-day equivalent of witch doctors and priests. Illich argues that modern medicine is overprofessionalized, and must be reversed "through a recovery of the will to self-care among the laity, and through the legal, political and institutional recognition of the right to care, which imposes limits upon the professional monopoly of physicians."

One need not agree with all or even most of Illich's thesis to recognize that he has identified a significant factor at the heart of the health care crisis in the U.S. Simply put, far too many people are unwilling to take responsibility for their own health, and far too many doctors are willing to assume a role that others can fulfill just as competently, and probably should for a variety of reasons. Rene Fox,[11] in her essay, "The Medicalization and Demedicalization of American

Society," also describes this phenomenon of the growth of responsibility, of doctors and medicine, which has occurred by a combination of chance and choice over the years.

While the concerns about using non-professionals or paraprofessionals and non-medical facilities for the treatment of illness have some validity, they are not compelling. We simply need to devise mechanisms to encourage these alternatives, and more fully use the entire range of resources available in the community. It would be better for all involved if we recognized this, and planned a health care system which accomplishes this goal.

3.   Focus on the improvement of environmental factors which adversely affect health, including home and workplace environments. This point has been increasingly stressed as our control of infectious diseases has improved. In August 1978, Congressman Paul Rogers, then Chairman of the Subcommittee on Health and the Environment of the Committee on Interstate and Foreign Commerce, and myself, then as Chairman of the Subcommittee on Environment and the Atmosphere of the Committee on Science and Technology, co-sponsored "The National Conference on the Environment and Health Care Costs,"[12] where this topic was the main concern.

There was a variety of diverse conclusions from this conference, but the following provides a summary:

The experts who participated in the Conference generally agreed that environmental protection and preventive health care are closely related. To assure public acceptance and effective consideration of that link, a specific, high-priority, ongoing program of research and development to include such factors as social, economic and perceptual considerations must be undertaken in a co-ordinated fashion. Some of the specific issues highlighted at the conference included the following:

1. More studies are needed to determine the effects of environmental factors on health. A high priority should be assigned to dose-response studies.
2. Efforts to improve knowledge of air pollution exposure need to be increased. These efforts could be directed at improved personal monitors and data quality control.
3. Policies directed at improving monetary quantification of disease and illness, with particular attention to the economics of prevention, need to be developed.
4. A reassessment of the status of preventive health professionals is needed.
5. Health improvement is presently possible if more attention is focused on personal factors involved in health. These factors include smoking, diet, exercise and preventive use of the health care system. This can be accomplished through health behavior modification, education and economic incentives. Important to any such effort, however, is the development of a coherent and credible data base through which the potential value of such personal health care factors may be reinforced.

Progress can be achieved, but it must be directed at specific objectives so that political, economic, social and scientific factors can be used to lower our health care costs while improving the environment in which we work and play.[13]

Various federal agencies are also emphasizing this topic in their research and regulatory enforcement programs, although there is still a long way to go in both areas.[14] Many perceive control of environmental health insults as not only the key to preserving wellness, but also as the most effective weapon in controlling health care costs, especially in the area of chronic disease.

In spite of this great concern, almost no work appears to have been done in integrating environmental protection programs with health programs. This need was articulately expressed in the January 1972 Presidential Message on "Environmental Pollution Effects on Health." In that message, then President Richard Nixon called for the enactment of several new laws, including the "Toxic Substances Control Act of 1971," the "Federal Environmental Pesticide Control Act of 1971," and the "Health Maintenance Organization Assistance Act of 1971," about which he said:

. . . together with proposals which were contained in my Health Message of February 18, 1971, and my Environmental Message of February 8, 1971 . . . [this will] provide the essential tools for dealing with the health effects of environmental pollution in the years ahead.[15]

The participants in the Conference that Paul Rogers and I organized in August of 1978 believed that something more than speeches, even Presidential Messages, was definitely needed. We have the laws we need largely on the books, and we have a verbal commitment from agency heads to consider environmental and occupational protection programs as preventive health programs. What we have lacked, however, is an organized and effective constituency for disease prevention and environmental health promotion.

Largely under the leadership of Paul Rogers, the "National Coalition for Disease Prevention and Environmental Health" was established in late 1978 to represent the common concerns of health services providers, health planners, voluntary health associations, health insurance companies, health and environmental scientists and researchers, environmental protection groups, labor unions, consumer groups, food and nutrition groups, and other organizations concerned with preventing the host of diseases caused by environmental factors. The "Principles" of this new coalition are worth repeating here:

1. Environmental factors and the general failure to implement adequate disease prevention measures are increasingly and more certainly linked to serious disease, injury and other health problems.

2. The social and economic costs of such disease, injury and other health problems are increasing to unacceptable proportions.
3. Sound preventive measures, including the enactment and enforcement of environmental health protections, can reduce human suffering, the costs of health care and other social and economic costs.
4. Protection and enhancement of the health of the American people and success in prevention of environmentally related disease and injury is dependent upon:

   a. a national recognition and emphasis on the social and economic benefits and necessities of disease prevention, including environmentally and occupationally related disease and injuries;
   b. the development and implementation of a comprehensive national policy of disease prevention, including environmental, occupational and consumer health protections;
   c. increased emphasis in Federal health research, training, public education, planning and services programs on disease prevention, including environmental, occupational and consumer protections;
   d. development and full implementation of environmental, occupational and consumer protection programs which are based upon consumer health protection needs (and adoption of the concept of the internalization of pollution costs by the polluter); and
   e. a realignment of economic and other incentives which presently inhibit disease prevention efforts or discourage the achievement of environmental health as a priority.

4.   Focus on the simple lifestyle causes of poor health — poor nutrition, lack of exercise and sleep, overindulgence in liquor, tobacco, and drugs, and emotional and physical stress. There are a host of proponents of this point. The best known research demonstrating the relationship between personal habits and personal health was done under the direction of Lester Breslow.[16]   Others are more outspoken, such as John Knowles,[17] who says:

Prevention of disease means forsaking the bad habits which many people enjoy — overeating, too much drinking, taking pills, staying up at night, engaging in promiscuous sex, driving too fast, and smoking cigarettes — or, put another way, it means doing things which require special effort — exercising regularly, going to the dentist, practicing contraception, ensuring harmonious family life, submitting to screening examinations.

There seems to be little question that an effective disease prevention and health promotion strategy must focus on the responsibility of individuals to take care of themselves. However, the tendency to "blame the victims" of diseases needs to be avoided. There is a fine line between what one can do of one's own free will, and what one cannot do. Society should take some responsibility for its members, and show compassion and understanding of individual failings. In addition, there are frequently circumstances (indoor smoking is one example) where only society can protect its members from one another.

5. Focus on biological research that will reveal the answers to questions such as the causes of cancer and heart disease and the transmission of genetic disorders. The rapid and dramatic increases in funding for biomedical and other types of research have probably come to an end. The present research budget however, if maintained, is still quite substantial and significant.

In the past, a disproportionate effort was put into looking for the "magic bullet," or the "cure for cancer." Today, the federal research programs are being broadened to include a greater emphasis on *causes* of diseases such as cancer and heart disease, to aid in the disease prevention programs of the federal government.

Efforts in epidemiology, which can show patterns of disease and alert us to unsuspected influences on our health, must be strengthened. Many areas of this research are operating on a very small scale, compared to traditional programs of treating diseases of individuals. The causative and preventive research programs need considerably more support. They can bring a growing awareness of health promotion, and disease prevention which will improve and make all of our health programs more effective.

Perhaps the most effective statement about the importance of this type of research was contained in the report prepared for the National Institute of Environmental Health Sciences, entitled "Human Health and the Environment — Some Research Needs."

In spite of astronomical and growing costs of medical diagnosis and treatment, an increase in investments in these areas will not yield significant improvements in average longevity, productivity or quality of life. Prevention of illness, disability and premature death will yield the greatest benefit to society and identification, evaluation and subsequent modification of the role of environmental factors in causing illness and premature death promise major payoffs in the prevention and control of disease.[18]

Conclusion

The National Health Insurance debate is obscuring several other important issues which are integrally related to health and to the makeup of our national health care programs. Primarily, we need to shift our flows from the treatment of illness to the maintenance of wellness. We must increase efforts to provide a healthy environment free from poisons in the air we breathe and the water we drink, and from toxic chemicals and radiation that attacks us from every side.

Every neighborhood and community must have a program of positive health care — a program operating through the schools, the churches, and civic organizations of all kinds — which emphasizes the individual's own responsibility for achieving good health through good living.

Every neighborhood and community must have an adequate infrastructure of health care institutions of all types, including adequate provision for home health care by a full range of health care personnel.

The present is a time for creating a new understanding of our nation's health problems — a time for examining our simplistic assumptions that mere access to hospitals and physician care would solve our health problems, and a time for understanding that individual human health and well-being is the result of a complex interrelationship of genetic heritage, lifestyle, environment, and access to a wide range of prevention and treatment facilities and personnel.

REFERENCES

1. Lalonde, M., *A New Perspective on the Health of Canadians: A Working Document.* Ottawa: Government of Canada, 1974; and Andreopoulos, (Ed.), *National Health Insurance: Can We Learn From Canada?* New York: John Wiley & Sons, 1975.
2. Andreopoulos, *op. cit.*, p. 262.
3. Wildavsky, A., "Doing Better and Feeling Worse: The Political Pathology of Health Policy," in Knowles, J.H. (Ed.), *Doing Better and Feeling Worse: Health in the United States.* New York: W.W. Norton & Co., 1977, p. 105.
4. Andreopoulos, *op. cit.*, p. 262.
5. *Proceedings of the National Conference on the Environment and Health Care Costs,* August 15, 1978, sponsored by Reps. George E. Brown, Jr., and Paul G. Rogers. Washington, D.C.: U.S. Government Printing Office, 1978, p. 3.
6. *Forward Plan for Health, FY '78-'82.* Washington, D.C.: U.S. Department of Health, Education, and Welfare, August 1976, p. 50; Saward, E., "Institutional Organization Incentives and Challenge," in Knowles, J.H. (Ed.), *Doing Better and Feeling Worse: Health in the United States.* New York: W.W. Norton & Co., 1977, pp. 201-202; and Sidel, V.W. and Sidel, R., *A Healthy State: An International Perspective on the Crisis in United States Medical Care.* New York: Pantheon, 1978, pp. 276-279.
7. Ng, L.K.Y., Davis, D.L., and Manderscheid, R.W., "The Health Promotion Organization: A Practical Intervention Designed to Promote Health Living," *Public Health Reports* 93:5, September–October 1978.
8. Davis, K., *National Health Insurance: Benefits, Costs and Consequences.* Washington, D.C.: The Brookings Institute, 1975, p. 4; and Klarman, H.E., "The Financing of Health Care," in Knowles, J.H. (Ed.), *Doing Better and Feeling Worse: Health in the United States.* New York: W.W. Norton & Co., 1977, pp. 215-234.
9. Wildavsky, *op. cit.*, p. 109.
10. Illich, I., *Medical Nemesis: The Expropriation of Health.* New York: Pantheon, 1976, p. 35.
11. Fox, R., "The Medicalization and Demedicalization of American Society," in Knowles, J.H. (Ed.), *Doing Better and Feeling Worse: Health in the United States.* New York: W.W. Norton & Co., 1977, pp. 9-22.

12. *Proceedings of the National Conference on the Environment and Health Care Costs*, *op. cit.*

13. *Ibid.*, p. ix.

14. U.S. Environmental Protection Agency, National Cancer Institute, National Heart, Lung and Blood Institute, and National Institute of Environmental Health Sciences, *First Annual Report to Congress of the Task Force on Environmental Cancer, Heart and Lung Disease.* Washington, D.C.: U.S. Environmental Protection Agency, 1978; and Interagency Regulatory Liaison Group, *Preventive Health and the Environmental Sciences: Research and Training for FY 1980 and Beyond.* Washington, D.C.: IRLG, 1978.

15. Nixon, R.M., "Environmental Pollution Effects on Health: Message from the President of the United States," House of Representatives, Document No. 92–241, February 1, 1972.

16. Belloc, N.B. and Breslow, L., "Relationship of Physical Health Status and Health Practices," *Preventive Medicine* 1:409–421, August 1972.

17. Knowles, J.H. (Ed.), *Doing Better and Feeling Worse: Health in the United States.* New York: W.W. Norton & Co., 1977, "Introduction," p. 59.

18. *Proceedings of the National Conference on the Environment and Health Care Costs*, *op. cit.*, p. 70.

16

Health Promotion and Health Insurance

Mathew Greenwald

Director of Social Research
American Council of Life Insurance
And
Health Insurance Institute

There is a new realism in the U.S. concerning strategies to improve the health of the population. In part, this realism has been fostered by indications that the massive investment our society has made in health care over the past quarter-century has not led to increased longevity or better health.[1] The proportion of total consumption expenditures on medical care went from 4.6% in 1950 to 9.5% in 1976.[2] Yet, in that period, many of the major causes of disablement and death in America, such as stroke and coronary heart disease, have declined only slightly, while many cancer rates have increased. There is evidence that a small decline in heart disease mortality is due to changes in smoking habits and preventive care, rather than to spending on medical care. The U.S. ranks fifteenth in the world in infant mortality; and the U.S. ranks lower in average longevity among developed nations than it did 50 years ago.

There appears to be a growing public disenchantment with doctors and hospitals. This may be related to the rising cost for services and it may also be related to the rate of deaths due to accidents resulting from medical procedures' complications. Over the past 20 years, this death rate has more than doubled.[3] The acceleration of malpractice suits may be an indication of this. Also, the public may be more questioning of biomedical research. A new relationship between the public and health care institutions is developing, with many people looking for new approaches to the allopathic medicine that dominates the health care system.

During the past quarter-century, there has been a great increase in the realization that lifestyle and environment factors influence morbidity and mortality patterns. Aaron B. Wildavsky[4] has estimated that the medical system affects only 10% of the health of the population, while 90% is determined by factors the system has little or no control over, such as lifestyle, social conditions, inherited traits, and the physical environment. It seems clear that, although efforts at improving the health care system, biomedical research, and related efforts will continue, a major thrust must be developed to encourage healthier lifestyles for Americans. The challenge before us, therefore, is to determine what the various institutions with a legitimate involvement in health can do to foster healthier lifestyles.

Two points must be emphasized here. First, no institution can or should deal with the entire problem of lifestyle change. Only by acting in a coordinated fashion can the various institutions hope to be effective. Second, institutions must confine themselves to roles which the population believes to be appropriate. For example, primary schools can have a key impact on children, but should not attempt to deal with the self-care habits of parents. Employers can play a positive role in improving the health of their employees, but there are some health-related areas where privacy and ethical considerations should prohibit them from involvement. Automobile insurers can play a role when automobile accidents — the leading cause of death among those aged 1–35 — are concerned, but they have little legitimacy in areas such as nutrition. For the food industry, of course, the reverse is true. By reviewing the two main challenges that some proponents of health promotion have put to the health insurance business, and then proposing appropriate methods by which I believe the health insurance business can encourage health promoting behaviors, their appropriate role can be examined.

The first challenge to the health insurance business relates to the basic design of health insurance policies. Drs. Lawrence K.Y. Ng, Devra Lee Davis, and Ronald W. Manderscheid[5] have written: "the patterns of institutions contribute . . . to current health problems. For example, the health care system provides economic incentives for sickness rather than health." John H. Knowles[6] has referred to health insurance as "disease insurance." These statements refer directly to the payment of claims only for the treatment of illness, and to the exclusion of coverage for regular medical screening, check-ups, and health education. Ng et al. and others believe that if health insurance covered regular screening, preventive medicine, and health education, the overall health of the population would be improved and more healthful lifestyles would be developed. Although I believe some screening and check-up strategies can be useful, I do not believe that health insurance policies should cover these services (although a few health insurance policies do provide these coverages).

There is evidence that many frequently used screening procedures have no impact on health status or medical expenses. Charles Phelps,[7] after an extensive review of the literature, stated: "direct tests of whether additional preventive treatment is cost-saving appear to show no effect. Whether or not health is improved is still untested in many dimensions, but preliminary data are again not wholly encouraging." The costs of screening cannot be overlooked, despite concern for health. Phelps concluded: "It now seems at least plausible that the hidden consequences of some of such tests make their monetary and psychic costs far outweigh their benefits."[8] The costs Phelps referred to were both monetary and the psychological problems that can result from the "false positive" test results that some screenings produce. However, as David Mechanic[9] has pointed out, medical care is finite, and any system of medical care includes an explicit or implicit rationing system. A rapid expansion of screening utilization will have an impact on other parts of the system, and an assessment of this impact deserves consideration.

The results of health education programs have been mixed. Some efforts appear to have been effective, but for many there are inadequate data available to make an evaluation. For some programs, a negative effect has been discovered. A well-designed experimental high school drug education program, which used a control group, found that the education effort increased knowledge of the drugs, but decreased fear of them. Those that attended the educational program exhibited increased use of alcohol and drugs.[10] An Alcohol Safety Action Project in Nassau County, New York found that those people convicted of driving while intoxicated who were assigned to an education-rehabilitation program had *more subsequent* accidents than those who went through the usual court procedures.[11] In sum, education efforts cannot be considered a panacea. More study needs to be done to determine how they can be utilized more effectively.

Insurance in general, and health insurance specifically, is designed to be a mechanism for sheltering individuals from unpredictable occurrences that would have a major, adverse economic impact. The benefits of dealing with risk through insurance are clear, and that the great majority of the public have purchased differing types of insurance coverage is testimony to this. Because insurance is so widespread, and is considered a necessity by most people — even legally mandated, in some cases — it is tempting to design it to meet more goals, even those not sought by the purchaser. But there are dangers in extending insurance, health insurance specifically, to cover predictable, non-risk situations such as health screening and health education. Because health insurance is basically a cost-sharing device, including health screening would force all insured to pay for screening and educational services that some may not use. There are, indeed, ethical considerations here that are made much more serious by the lack of evidence that these screening and educational services are effective. There is also some uncertainty about how many *additional* people would actually use such services, once covered, or follow through in ways the screenings or educational programs indicate. A survey commissioned for the Pacific Mutual Life Insurance Company[12] indicates that, in 1978, four-fifths of the public had had their blood pressure checked during the previous year. In a Health Insurance Institute Survey,[13] half the public reported that they typically get an annual medical checkup. Another third said that it was somewhat typical for them to get a regular check-up.

Shifting the financial responsibility for these services from the individuals to the insurance institution may not greatly increase utilization, but could have two adverse affects: 1) when people "freely" decide to use preventive medical services, and pay for them directly, they could be more likely to take the results seriously than if the services were purchased for them through insurance coverage; and 2) intrinsic to coverage for screening and education may be the subtle message that health is *not* the individuals' responsibility. As Knowles[14] and many others have argued, it is important for individuals to assume greater responsibility for their own health. But a medical insurance-government system which takes responsibility for many health-related decisions, and responsibility for the cost of those decisions, could reinforce a view that the responsibility for an individual's health lies with the institution.

A major problem of incorporating coverage of medical screening and education in health insurance policies is the subtle income class transfer of funds that would occur. If these services result in health cost savings in the short term, this transfer would not take place.[15] But there is no evidence that even long-term savings are realized. We know that middle and upper income groups are more likely to use the medical and non-medical services provided to them and are more likely to have their own doctors. Therefore, it should be expected that middle and upper income groups would be more likely to use screening and education services covered by health insurance. But because all income groups would be contributing equally to the cost of the participants' utilization of these services, lower income people would be subsidizing the services provided for higher income groups. Some policy designs might mitigate this effect, but it would be difficult to neutralize it.

Two developments appear necessary before consideration of screening, check-ups, and health education. First, more research needs to be done to develop better methods and to evaluate their effectiveness. When suitable methods are found and are proven effective, they should be encouraged and, in some cases, mandated. This can be done through school programs and job-related programs supplementary to health insurance plans. In some cases, health insurance companies could effectively administer these programs, but the distinction between these services and the basic principles of insurance must be clearly understood.

The second challenge to the health insurance business relates to the use of the risk classification system to encourage healthful activities and to provide incentives for health. Two methods have been proposed: 1) charging lower rates for health (and life) insurance to those who have positive health habits; and 2) giving premium reductions to those who improve their standing on certain indices of health, such as weight and blood pressure. Albert J. Struckard, Professor of Psychology at the University of Pennsylvania, has stated that the greatest potential for health behavior change by industry may be through the use of incentives represented by making reductions in health insurance premiums for individuals who make positive health behavior changes.

This idea has merit if utilized with care. Insurance policies should, and do, charge people according to their relative risk of suffering the consequences against which they are being insured. For example, older people, with a relatively higher risk of dying, should, and do, pay more for life insurance than do younger people, who, other factors being equal, have a lower risk of dying. Life and health insurance companies do require some applicants to undergo medical testing and do charge lower premiums to healthier people than to others. A number of life insurance companies offer substantial discounts, up to around 15%, to non-smokers (the insured who stop smoking after being insured can become eligible for these programs).

There are, however, a number of problems in expanding this concept. The most often stated goal of health promotion proponents is the population's adherence to Breslow and Belloc's[16] seven rules of good health: three meals a day, breakfast every day, moderate exercise, seven or eight hours sleep a night, no smoking, moderate weight, and little or no alcohol use. With some of the items, such as smoking and drinking, the relationship to health is conclusive. For many others (for example, eating breakfast), conclusive linkage to health is not available.[17] It is difficult to charge higher rates based on such weak evidence to people who do not follow such lifestyle practices. Additionally, there are problems with violation of privacy while collecting information concerning these behaviors, and it is very difficult to monitor continuation of these positive lifestyles. For example, there is no way of determining if an insured typically eats three meals a day or sleeps seven or eight hours a night.

Another concern in this area is the danger of "legislating lifestyles." Last fall, Oral Roberts University was charged with discrimination against fat people in their admissions policy. An asbestos company has announced a policy of not hiring those who smoke. A major chemical company, Monsanto, has made plans to keep track of the health of their 50,000 employees. To Harry Schwartz,[18] writing in the *Wall Street Journal*, the logic of linking lifestyles too closely to health care costs could have negative implications. He states: "If lung cancer comes from smoking, and heart disease from being obese, why should the rest of us help pay for the medical treatment required when the "health criminals" get their just desserts? Why shouldn't these irresponsible scoundrels be forced to pay for the damage their dissolute conduct caused themselves?" Exerting pressure on individuals to adopt healthier lifestyles can improve the health of the population, but unintended negative consequences must be guarded against, especially when the data are not conclusive concerning the positive impact of the behavior being promoted. Health insurance policies *can* provide incentives for healthy behaviors, but this would mean that people who do not exhibit healthy behavior could, especially in the short term, pay more for coverage, since insurance is a cost-sharing mechanism. At a time when health care costs are going up, this additional expense would be a much resented burden.

In sum, providing incentives for positive lifestyles through discounts in health (and life) insurance has merit if used carefully. In areas where there is a clear linkage between behavior and health, such as smoking and excessive drinking, premium incentives and disincentives are already in place. In other areas, which are hard or impossible to monitor and where the linkage to health is still not conclusive, it does not appear fair to provide a discount (and thereby charge more to those who follow other lifestyles).

When discounts are given, such as in the no-smoking case, the financial discount itself cannot be expected to motivate people to stop smoking. Even a few hundred dollars a year cannot change deeply ingrained behavior. But the symbolic nature of the discount is important. The message that smoking leads to higher health care costs is made, and the fact that smoking leads to illness is reinforced.

A health insurance policy design strategy which I believe would contribute to the public's sense of responsibility for their own health, provide efficient incentives for healthier lifestyles, and lead to more appropriate utilization of the health care system could be proposed. This policy design is the raising of health insurance deductibles and the raising of co-insurance levels. In past years, there has been a tendency to lower deductibles and co-insurance. Now, over eight in ten people pay deductible amounts of $100 or less, and most people pay 20% or less in co-insurance once the deductible is covered.[19] Even with this comprehensive coverage, many unions are seeking first dollar protection, and the public favors lower deductibles and less co-insurance.

Covering most or all health care costs with premiums and having the public go to little out-of-pocket expense when they utilize the system does not save individuals' money. Indeed, it unquestionably leads to over-utilization of the health care system, and thus tends to raise health insurance premiums. This type of comprehensive insurance protection also shelters the insured from direct financial responsibility for his or her self-health care. In any health insurance system, all pay in, and those who get sick make claims. Thus, the well subsidize the sick, and properly so. But with higher deductibles and more co-insurance, this subsidy would be reduced. Premiums would go down for all, and users of the health care system would pay somewhat more. This is a direct financial incentive for good health. This system is an easier one to manage than using the risk classification system to provide discounts to those who exhibit healthy lifestyles. There are no privacy problems with collecting the information, there is no need to monitor the insured to see if the healthy lifestyles are being maintained, and there need be no concern that the lifestyle may not *really* be related to better health.

Causing people to pay more of the cost of their health insurance directly would also reinforce the notion that health is the individual's responsibility. Today, I fear, the system of people going to doctors and hospitals when they are not feeling right, and having health insurance pay the cost, encourages the view that institutions have the major part of that responsibility. Higher deductibles and more co-insurance could also lead to more informed and careful use of the health care system, which will contribute to more efficient provision of health care services generally. (No one, of course, should be deprived of needed medical care, and health insurance policy design should not discourage needed utilization.) With the knowledge that some health insurance plans encourage overutilization, it seems useful to design health insurance plans that encourage more self-reliance.

The main criticism of higher deductibles and co-insurance is that it discourages needed utilization of medical care. Scitovsky's[20] study of the Palo Alto Clinic indicated that the initiation of a co-insurance factor of 25% for doctors' services led to a 24% reduction in visits to doctors in one year. A solution to this problem, as Herbert Klarman[21] indicates, is to relate out-of-pocket expense to income group. Thus, higher deductibles could be set for middle and upper income groups than for lower income groups. After a specified limit, differing by income, the policy would pay 100% of costs. Thus, for example, a person earning $30,000 a year may have a deductible of $250, clearly affordable, while a person earning $10,000 would have a $100 deductible. No one would be faced with overwhelming bills, while premiums would be lower for all. A study in Saskatchewan, Canada[22] found that the deterrent effect of higher deductibles on health care utilization wore off after a few years.

REFERENCES

1. Kisch, A., "The Health Care System and Health," *Inquiry* 11, 4:272, December 1974.
2. "Source Book of Health Insurance Data 1977–1978," Health Insurance Institute, p. 51.
3. Kristen, M., Arnold, C., and Wynder, E., "Health Economics and Preventive Care," *Science* 195:457–462.
4. Wildavsky, A., "Doing Better and Feeling Worse: The Political Pathology of Health Policy," *Daedalus* 106, 1:105–123, Winter 1977.
5. Ng. L.K.Y., Davis, D.L., and Manderscheid, R., "The Health Promotion Organization: A Practical Intervention Designed to Promote Healthy Living," *Public Health Reports* 93:448, September–October 1978.
6. Knowles, J.H., "The Responsibility of the Individual," *Daedalus* 106, 1:66, Winter 1977.
7. Phelps, C., "Illness Prevention and Medical Insurance," *The Journal of Human Resources* 13:204, Supplement, 1978.
8. *Ibid.*, p. 204.
9. Mechanic, D., "Rationing Medical Care," *Center Magazine*, September–October 1978, p. 22.
10. Stuart, R. "Teaching Facts about Drugs: Pushing or Preventing," *Journal of Educational Psychology* 66:189–201, 1974.
11. Preusser, D., Ulmer, R., and Adams, J., "Driver Record Evaluation of a Drinking Driver Rehabilitation Effort," *Journal of Safety Research* 8:98–105, 1976.

12. "Health Maintenance," Pacific Mutual Life Insurance Company, November 1978, p. 38
13. "Health and Health Insurance: The Public's View," Health Insurance Institute, 1979.
14. Knowles, J. *op. cit.*, pp. 57–80.
15. Short-term savings are necessary because most health insurance is provided through the group mechanism. Because of job mobility and retirement, long-term savings frequently would not have an impact on the group health care costs.
16. Belloc, N. and Breslow, L., "Relationship of Physical Health Status and Health Practices," *Preventive Medicine* 1, *3*:409–421, August 1972.
17. Thomas, L., "On Magic in Medicine," *Human Nature* 2, *1*:65–67, January 1979.
18. Schwartz, H., "Why Should We Pay for Medical Criminals?" *Wall Street Journal*, October 5, 1978, p. 24.
19. "Source Book of Health Insurance Data," *op. cit.*, p. 9.
20. Scitovsky, A. and Snyder, N., "Effect of Coinsurance on Use of Physician Services," *Social Security Bulletin* 35, *6*:3–19, June 1972.
21. Klarman, H., "The Financing of Health Care," *Daedulus* 106, *1*:226, Winter 1977.
22. *Ibid.*, p. 226.

17

The Role of the Insurance Industry in Health Education

Clarence Pearson

Health and Safety Education
Metropolitan Life Insurance

Although the U.S. is one of the most powerful nations on earth, rich in resources and committed to providing universal education, it has long suffered an unacceptably high infant mortality rate, a high incidence of disability due to degenerative disease among the aged, and a high incidence of vision and dental defects in comparison with those of other countries.

Against this, there is increasing evidence that many disabilities could be prevented or controlled if Americans would change their lifestyles and improve the environment in which they live – changes which would, incidentally, enhance their individual and collective well-being and increase the simple joy of living.

There is growing evidence that people *can* be motivated to make such changes by means of appropriate educational campaigns. For example, the recent adult education television series, "Feeling Good," produced by CTW and broadcast on PBS stations, enjoyed unexpected success. According to researchers at the National Opinion Research Center, ". . . 'Feeling Good' did have a significant impact on several different measures of health knowledge, attitudes, and behaviors in a sample of low-income women." And the Response Analysis Corporation reported: "The series, overall, had a measurable impact on viewer behavior and cognition in health areas both less critical and more deeply value-related."

As has happened in the past, a battle against illness may be about to happen again, perhaps on a grander scale. This is a time of great consequence in health education, a time of experimentation and testing – in part, because the needs are changing. Until recently, famine and contagious disease threatened human society. These two scourges killed tens of millions. But in the middle of the nineteenth century – another time of great importance for health education – society marshalled its scientific resources and embarked on a rigorous campaign to overcome these natural enemies. The campaign succeeded, but only in the industrially advanced nations of the world, where there existed the will and the wealth to commit to the struggle. There, economic growth and agricultural progress combined to help eradicate famine; infectious diseases were controlled through the efforts of public health physicians and sanitarians, who had discovered the benefits of purifying water and milk, disposing of sewage, and keeping food clean, and who are able to educate the people and their leaders in the necessity of doing so. The results were dramatic: today, except for isolated outbreaks, life-threatening communicable diseases have almost disappeared from the list of common causes of death in this country. Since 1900, the average life expectancy of Americans has risen from 47 to 72.5 years. Interestingly, however, it has risen very little in the past 25 years, in comparison to the earlier dramatic improvement.

Today, physicians and health educators are faced with new challenges: diseases caused not by the ancient enemies, famine and contagion, but by changes in our lifestyles and economies. According to the American Heart Association, the common causes of death and disability today are heart disease, cancer, and stroke. These illnesses are caused, at least in part, by our increasingly sedentary way of life, our poor eating habits, changes in our general environment, and occupational health exposures.

Ironically, the very success of public health and medical practice increasing the life span has compounded the problems associated with such diseases. Chronic and degenerative diseases are now involved in more than half of all the death in the U.S. As more Americans live longer, the incidence will rise.

Other elements complicate the problem. Since the turn of the century, we have changed from a predominantly rural to a predominantly urban country. Over 70% of all Americans now live in cities or urban complexes; about 80% live on less than 6% of the land. Such density may lead to health problems demanding new approaches to health education.

Many rural areas lack physicians, hospitals, and other sources of health care. As cities grow, the difficulties of providing adequate health care are compounded — especially for the poor, the under-educated, and the aged. They, like ethnic and minority groups, often need better and cheaper access to the health care system, thus presenting a dual challenge to health educators: motivating the people to adopt desirable personal health practices, and developing their ability to make effective use of the services available.

Times are changing, and the rate of change is accelerating. Although famine and communicable disease are largely under control, we now have an annual death toll from automobiles of some 48,000. Dental and vision defects that could be prevented affect individuals of all ages. Drug addiction, air pollution, crowded and substandard housing, and emotional disorders linked to high-tension urban living all affect the health and well-being of our citizens. Yet this need not be so if individuals and institutions can be educated to change their attitudes and their behavior.

The insurance industry recognized long ago that to change attitudes and behavior, people must be educated individually *and* collectively; that is, they must be educated not only to care for themselves, but also to think in terms of the community – in terms of their health citizenship, as it were. Each activity draws from and sustains the other. So, health education programs are being developed – in schools, homes, factories, and offices – and the formation of neighborhood groups is being encouraged, but in the best programs, the recipients are actively involved in the process.

As an example, Project Hi-Blood, funded by the Missouri Regional Medical Program, University of Missouri, attacks the problem of disability and death from strokes and cardiovascular disease secondary to hypertension in the inner-city, predominantly poor, black and white uneducated population, by demonstrating that hypertension can be controlled in the early stages. The project improves communication by utilizing indigenous people as Community Health Aides.

The challenge is enormous. Efforts to change any form of human behavior are usually met with resistance. Apathy, denial, and even hostility are common. Yet, health education can make a difference. The vigorous campaign to familiarize Americans with heart risk factors seems to have contributed to the recent drop in heart disease deaths. Although final results of the Stanford Heart Disease Prevention Program are not yet available, interim surveys have revealed success in expanding public knowledge. The program makes use of print, radio, and television, as well as direct intervention in the form of physical examinations and classroom instruction. According to Principal Investigator John D. Farquhar, M.D.: "It appears that, among other effects, the program increased the proportion from four to twenty percent of the people who believe saturated fats play a role in causing heart disease." Other equally striking effects have been noted. But there is still a need for more well-designed, better coordinated, and more widely available programs.

Too often, people equate "health education" with "health information." Health information is little more than facts, such facts as are available from physicians, radio and television, government agencies, and insurance companies. Simple awareness of the truth may lead to attitude change, but truly effective health education is a process that transcends such information conveying; it actually shapes attitudes and influences behavior. It attempts to motivate the recipient to accept the information, then to act on it. It is a complicated, long-term process.

Effective health education requires the active participation of the individual and his or her supporting institutions. It is the individual who eats and drinks too much, rests and exercises too little, drives carelessly, and ignores the signs that he or she should seek medical attention. And it is the individual, who, once in the health care system, forgets or ignores the physician's instructions. Scott K. Simonds, a member of the President's Committee on Health Education, has written: "The mass media can be effective in giving individuals correct knowledge, but personal contacts, especially those that reach individuals in small groups, help actualize the next step by providing the setting and stimulation for individuals to change old health practices or to adopt new ones. Believing that mass media alone can do the job . . . is a very unrealistic and simplistic approach in the eyes of the committee."

Although some health education programs have enjoyed success in the past, the insurance industry believes that it is time for renewed and intensified effort. We need look only at the ineffectiveness of automobile safety campaigns to understand the insurance industry's concern. The National Safety Council has reported that over $100,000,000 in cash and donated space and time is spent annually in this country in mass communications efforts to reduce traffic accidents, yet the incidence of traffic fatalities stands at an unacceptably high level. Campaigns to induce people to use seat belts are equally ineffective.

But programs must be continued. First, effective health education has the potential to ease the pressures of cost inflation and inappropriate use of medical care services, thus improving the environment in which health insurers must operate. Second, health education offers a very real potential for claims-cost containment over a period of time, by encouraging positive health behavior and thus reducing medical care expenditures. Third, if health education can be made a "marketable" benefit (that is, if it can be presented in such a way that people will attend to the message), it can generate the interest, support, and participation of the community in more effective health programs. Fourth, and most important, insurance companies recognize that effective health education can enhance a person's well-being.

At this time, the major areas in which more effective health education is needed are as described below.

Control of Communicable Disease

Health educators have already enjoyed considerable success in this area and will probably continue to do so. For example, when the Public Broadcasting Service (PBS) broadcast the special, "VD Blues," with Dick Cavett as host, on the morning after the broadcast, VD clinics in several major cities were flooded with clients; when questioned, they attributed their presence to having seen the show. Programs such as immunization, water purification, and disposal of human waste are generally accepted as ways of controlling communicable disease. Where they are not, it is usually because of ignorance rather than opposition. The education effort must continue.

Protection of the Environment

Insurance companies have long been aware of their responsibility — both as corporate citizens in their own communities and as insurers — in the attempt to control air and water pollution, noise pollution, radiation, and occupational hazards. They will continue their campaigns, through a variety of techniques, to meet that responsibility.

Attitude and Behavior Change

This area includes such obvious poor health practices as ignoring safety procedures, getting insufficient exercise, imbibing too much alcohol, eating the wrong foods, and smoking too much. Effecting change in this area has been one of the most difficult tasks faced by health educators. They have provided information, but the response has been disappointing. For example, a few years ago, PBS (then NET) broadcast a five-part series of television programs titled "Why You Smoke." It was unusual in that it not only provided information on health hazards from smoking, it involved the viewer directly by means of a paper-and-pencil test — a kind of smoker's "personality" profile. Yet an independent survey made one year after the broadcasts showed that only one person out of 20 who quit smoking after watching the shows was still not smoking.

Seeking Health and Following Advice

In this area, too, the American people have been given ample factual material. They know the signs of illness, but many do not respond and take appropriate action. Further, although some of those plagued with illness know how to manage it, they fail to follow the regimens prescribed. The opportunity exists to truly educate and motivate such patients.

Education Through Involvement

Individually and collectively, insurance carriers must not only provide information and guidance to individuals and groups, they must encourage them to develop their own education programs, to implement or acquire and manage their own health education facilities. When people who will be the ultimate users of material or facilities participate in their planning and development, they not only become more knowledgeable, they are more likely to acquire the motivation to take appropriate action. They also are often moved to disseminate the information to their neighbors.

Such are the dimensions of the challenge today – and tomorrow. This is a challenge which the insurance industry is confident it can meet. It has already committed enormous amounts of money, time, and energy to health education in the U.S., working alone and through a variety of organizations.

How Does the Industry Promote Health Education?

Basically, insurance companies are, as their name implies, insurers against loss. When loss occurs, the companies compensate the insured for the loss. But they also do more than that. They take appropriate actions to improve the delivery and financing of quality health care, and initiate programs aimed at containing health care costs, including programs designed to prevent disease and injury.

Through the Health Insurance Association of America (H.I.A.A.), the American Council of Life Insurance (A.C.L.I.), and other insurance trade organizations, insurance companies have pooled some of their intellectual and financial resources to achieve needed goals. For example, since 1970, the H.I.A.A. has had a committee to explore the subject of health education and determine possible ways in which the health insurance business might relate to program needs in this area. Also since 1970, the business has given wholehearted support to passage of the National Health Care Act, which would accomplish certain important objectives that have profound implications for stimulating health education activities.

The Health Insurance Institute, a division of the A.C.L.I., informs the public about financial protection against the costs of illness and disability. It provides information on health benefit plans to the print and electronic media and prepares educational materials for teachers, students, and community groups. Since 1959, it has published an annual "Source Book of Health Insurance Data."

About a third of the information developed for the media is concerned with personal health problems and how to deal with them – articles on such topics as preventive health care, mental stress, highway safety, cancer warning signals, nutrition, and immunization. Periodically, the institute published a new edition of a booklet entitled "Health Education Materials and the Organizations Which Offer Them."

In 1945, 148 life insurance companies in the U.S. and Canada combined to form the Life Insurance Medical Research Fund. By 1970, the fund had contributed over $26,000,000 to medical research and education.

In 1971, nearly 100 chief executive officers of the major life and health insurance companies held a conference on corporate social responsibility, and agreed to establish the Clearinghouse on Corporate Social Responsibility, a medium for the exchange of information in the area of social responsibility among life and health insurance companies. The Clearinghouse publishes a bimonthly bulletin, *Response*, which reports on the activities of its member companies.

The quality of life has long been a concern of the nation's insurance companies. As far back as the 1850's, companies such as New York Life and Manhattan Life were contributing funds for sanitary improvements, drains, and sewers. And, at the time of the Civil War, when the Sanitary Commission, precursor of the American Red Cross, was formed, life insurance companies contributed financial support.

It is interesting to note the similarities between the situation at the turn of the century and the situation today. The leading causes of disease and death at that time — tuberculosis and pneumonia — were being discovered. Many policyholders were immigrants or poorly educated native-born Americans who lived in unsanitary housing conditions. They knew little about protecting their health and often lacked the means to do so. Many states were creating public health departments to apply disease prevention measures such as environmental sanitation, enlightened infant care, and immunization. The insurance companies were assisting, too. Here are highlights of some of their supportive activities.

Aetna Life and Casualty. This firm has conducted a public information program on safe living for over 40 years, producing films, TV public service spots, and pamphlets on boating, bicycle safety, safe driving, and first aid. The company pioneered the development of the Aetna Drivotrainer, now used in more than 1000 schools and colleges. It supports development of curriculum materials, teacher training, and general administration.

Baltimore Life Insurance Company. Baltimore Life sponsors a publication, *Health Talk*, which is co-produced with Johns Hopkins Medical Institutions, and is distributed to policy-owners and the general public through field sales personnel. A significant portion of its advertising budget is allocated for health education.

Central States Health and Life Company of Omaha. This company has published a *Fitness Digest*, consisting of a series of articles on good health practices for widespread distribution to the general public.

Connecticut Mutual. Supporting mental health education programs, particularly for business and industry, Connecticut Mutual's contribution includes the distribution of booklets, the production of films, and the publication and distribution of the proceedings of the Institute of Living in Hartford, focusing on its lectures on psychiatry.

Equitable Life Assurance Society of the United States. Equitable conducts a wide range of employee education programs, including special programs for employees with emotional problems, sickle cell counseling, hypertension education and treatment, education in the Heimlich Maneuver (for those choking on food), life-support first aid counseling, Health Fair, group programs on smoking cessation, safety education, and accident prevention, physical fitness evaluation, and timely health information in health publications. It also publishes features on health in a policyholder publication, and has an informational program for group policyholders, covering all aspects of health care delivery and its costs, including promotion of involvement in health affairs.

Jefferson Standard Life Insurance Company. This firm has provided its facilities for the county medical association annual medical symposium involving national authorities for 28 years. The program is certified for graduate training credits for doctors. Also, the company holds various employee meetings on health education and publicizes in its employee magazine various community health programs (such as cancer detection).

John Hancock Life Insurance Company. John Hancock has a Health Clinic for employees and has long been involved in health maintenance. Recent additions include the Blood Pressure Detection and Monitoring Program, films on smoking, a diet workshop, education on nutrition, and CPR training for selective groups.

The Kemper Insurance Group. The first national award for the most outstanding occupational alcoholism program in the U.S. was given to the Kemper Insurance Group. It was presented in 1977 by the Association of Labor/Management Administrators and Consultants on Alcoholism (A.L.M.A.C.A.). Kemper employs two full-time counselors to help people with personal problems, alcoholism and drug abuse. The program began in 1964 and deals with immediate crisis situations, community referrals, follow-ups, etc.

The Liberty Corporation. Liberty is conducting a research project among employees, in cooperation with the University of South Carolina College of Health and Physical Education, designed to "scientifically examine the relationships between fitness, physical and psychological health, job satisfaction and productivity." The company is also engaged in advertising on health subjects, the publication of free health booklets tied to advertising, and a model speakers' bureau on health topics utilizing agents.

Liberty Mutual of Boston. This firm has had an ongoing health education program in effect for over 25 years. It works with policyholders in developing and implementing programs to improve health status of employees and families. This includes direct contacts with employees through health counseling, health maintenance exams, and the like, as well as outreach to families through health literature distribution. The subject matter includes all of the commonly encountered health problems and needs.

Life of Virginia. The company's program to detect hypertension, using an accurate new electronic instrument, has been recently emulated by other businesses in Virginia, which have established similar programs.

Metropolitan Life Insurance Company. Metropolitan launched its program of health and safety education in 1909. The program was a landmark in the history of health promotion by the insurance industry. During that year, the company distributed a booklet, *A War on Consumption*, which was published in 12 languages. This was followed by a continuing series of health and safety publications throughout the years. In the same year, Metropolitan established a visiting nurse service for its policy-holders. During its existence, more than 20 million policyholders received more than 100 million nursing visits. Metropolitan's advertisements in national magazines have conveyed health messages to millions of readers in the U.S. and Canada. Starting in the 1920's, they covered a wide range of topics. Another effective tool in health education has been the company's local health demonstrations. In 1916, for example, Metropolitan joined with the National Tuberculosis Association to demonstrate to the whole country how a community — in this instance, Framingham, Massachusetts — could bring tuberculosis under control. By 1923, the incidence of the disease had been cut by 68%. For 70 years, the company has conducted a health and safety education program through publications, films, TV, and radio, as well as demonstration projects, research, consultation, and cooperation with local, state, and national health organizations, both voluntary and governmental. More recently, it has shifted its focus to concentrate on two or three primary areas, using mass media campaigns to raise public awareness, while preparing fewer pamphlets and films. The first of these was a campaign on cardiopulmonary resuscitation, which began with an ad in the May 1975 *Reader's Digest*. The ad featured a wallet-size tear-out card with instructions on CPR. About 8,000,000 people removed the card, and Metropolitan filled requests for 2,300,000 more. A study showed that this was the highest scoring insurance ad in the history of the magazine. Successive campaigns have been on warning signs of a heart attack, emergency medical information, and (two) on childhood immunization. Each began with an ad in *Reader's Digest* and featured a detachable information card. Through this mass media approach, the company expects to continue to touch the lives of millions of families throughout the U.S. and Canada.

In the fall of 1977, the Clearinghouse on Corporate Social Responsibility conducted a survey of some 450 insurance companies to determine what their activities in these areas have been. Out of the 140 companies responding, most said that they conduct prevention and health education programs for their employees. These range from annual physical examinations, immunizations, personal counseling, smoking and drug abuse seminars, CPR courses, and columns on health education in their internal publications. Many of the companies also participate in a variety of community health education programs.

Of course, evaluation of public health efforts poses many problems. In those instances where it is attempted, it is often difficult to view the results with confidence. Perhaps the principal flaw in evaluation studies of the effectiveness of mass media educational campaigns is the absence of a control group. Nonetheless, campaigns to increase awareness of important health and safety information continue to elicit public interest and response in the form of requests for additional information — as noted above. Educational programs for groups, such as employees, for example, which offer information along with clinical testing and consultation, can evaluate effectiveness more specifically, in terms of control of high blood pressure, weight reduction, and other signs of compliance with personal counseling. A recent survey of insurance companies revealed many examples of such follow-up. Informal evaluations revealed a moderate rate of success.

The roster of insurance companies that have contributed directly to the promotion of health in the U.S. is long; their contributions of time and talent is immeasurable. And they are justly proud of their record. Yet they also play another, perhaps even more important, role — the support of health education in general. They have underwritten professional conferences and activities.

The Health Insurance Association of America strongly supported the enactment of P.L. 94-317, which was designed to achieve, through education, the significant improvement in personal behavior for the maintenance of health and prevention of disease. The association saw this as "a reasonable and responsible approach toward keeping people well, lowering health costs and reducing the number of work days lost through illness."

One of the most potentially significant contributions made by the insurance industry to the promotion of health in the U.S. — again as facilitator — has been its contribution of underwriting and manpower for the creation of the National Center for Health Education. The industry's involvement began in September 1971, when then President Richard M. Nixon established the President's Committee on Health Education. Of the 17 committee members, three were active in the insurance industry: Walter J. McNerney, Blue Cross Association; Charles A. Siegfried, Metropolitan Life Insurance Company; and J. Henry Smith, Equitable Life Assurance Society of the United States.

In its final report, the committee stated that "the needs, problems, and opportunities in health education are so great, so urgent, and so complex that progress will depend on a long-term, major commitment by both the public and private sectors." It recommended the establishment of two national focal points for the effort, one within the federal government, the other outside it. In response to the latter, the National Center for Health Education was established in San Francisco — and, again, the insurance industry contributed to its support.

Among those listed as contributors are Aetna Life and Casualty, Blue Cross and Blue Shield, Equitable Life Assurance Society of the United States, Health Insurance Association of America, Metropolitan Life Insurance Company, and Prudential Insurance Company of America. In the future, the center expects to function with the support of voluntary health agencies, professional societies, industry, labor, and philanthropy.

It is difficult to measure the success of the many varied health education programs underwritten and developed by the insurance industry over the past century, or, indeed, of any health education program. The individual human being is so complex, and the American population is so huge, it is not easy to "prove" that a given educational campaign "caused" an improvement in health, lowered a risk, or reduced a cost. Yet the history of the industry's involvement contains evidence of success that is reasonably valid. For example, in 1909, when Metropolitan launched its Welfare Division, its industrial policyholders had a life expectancy at birth of 46.3 years. By 1950, that figure had risen to 68.2 years. The mortality rate has declined almost continuously over that period, and reached a figure of 6.3 per 1000 policyholders in 1950 – about half the death rate in 1909.

Mortality from specific causes has declined strikingly: death caused by tuberculosis has been reduced 91%; from pneumonia and influenza, 87%; from the communicable diseases of childhood, 99%; and from accidents, more than 50%.

Data from studies of in-hospital patient education programs are easier to evaluate – and are equally encouraging. In North Brunswick, New Jersey, 100 congestive heart patients were assigned to experimental and control groups, with the former exposed to a broad range of educational activities. The educated group had one-third as many readmission days as the control group, and one-half the number of readmissions. They also followed their prescribed medical regimens more faithfully. Also, 47 patients in an experimental group who received pre-operation education before abdominal surgery at Massachusetts General Hospital were able to return home, on average, 2.7 days earlier than the 51 patients in the control group who were given minimal information and guidance. Again, it is difficult to read "cause" and "effect" into such results, yet there seems to be fairly substantial evidence that education in good health practices can affect attitudes and influence behavior. Education does make a difference.

Conclusion

For more than a century, life and health insurance companies have promoted health education for their policyholders and for the general public. They saw the need and responded to it. To do so, they utilized a variety of educational techniques and materials: pamphlets, films, advertising, and radio and television broadcasts. They mounted demonstration programs. They cooperated with government, voluntary agencies, and physicians. They stand proudly on their long and distinguished record.

Yet, as the President's Committee on Health Education concluded after taking 71 hours of testimony from almost 300 persons from 47 states and Puerto Rico, and meeting with directors of 22 neighborhood health centers: " . . . it is evident that the responsibility, the challenge, and the burden of meeting the widespread need, solving the problems and exploiting the opportunities must be shared by all concerned in both the public and private sectors of society . . . . at the same time, we must recognize that good health also is affected by broader opportunities for good jobs, a reduction in joblessness and its consequent poverty, more adequate housing, a higher level of education, and an upgrading of the physical environment."

The life insurance industry, well aware of its responsibility in that huge task, is committed to continuing the effort. In an attempt to achieve those goals it identified so long ago, it will continue to use tried-and-proven techniques, but also to adopt new ones. For example, in the *Blue Cross Association White Paper on Health Education* of August 1974, it was recommended that individual Blue Cross plans encourage health institutions to establish programs in health education and to support such efforts as reimbursable costs under insurance contracts. In 1977, the H.I.A.A. issued a Statement of Criteria for financing hospital-based patient education services by third party payers. The statement was hailed by many health educators and other interested persons as a significant breakthrough for achieving high-quality patient education.

The American Council of Life Insurance and the Health Insurance Association of America are studying several plans to broaden and intensify existing health education programs and establish new ones. One such program is designed to encourage the development of locally sponsored centers for public education, with technical guidance to be provided by the National Center for Health Education. Another plan would point up the critical importance of consumer and provider involvement in community health planning and provide practical opportunities for training of citizen participants in the National Planning and Resources Act programs throughout the country.

As observed in the opening of this chapter, the challenge is enormous, and the need urgent. In a variety of ways, the life and health insurance industry will continue to attempt to meet that need.

BIBLIOGRAPHY

American Life Insurance Association, *Contributions to the Nation's Health, Safety and Improved Environment by the Life Insurance Industry.* Washington, D.C.: American Life Insurance Industry, April 1973.

Metropolitan Life Insurance Company, *Brief History of Metropolitan Life's Health and Safety Activities – 1871-1971.* New York: Metropolitan Life, 1971; and *Catalog: Health and Safety Education Materials.* New York: Metropolitan Life, April 1978, p. 1.

Dublin, Louis I., *A Family of Thirty Million – The Story of the Metropolitan Life Insurance Company.* New York: Metropolitan Life, 1943.

Health Insurance Association of America, *Financing In-Hospital Patient Education: Proposed Criteria.* New York: Health Insurance Association of America, 1977.

Karson, Stanley G.,"An Historic Contribution,*" Response – A Clearinghouse on Corporate Social Responsibility.* VI,5: 2, September 1977.

National Center for Health Education, *Toward Health Improvement: A Design Proposal for a National Center for Health Education.* New York, 1975.

Report of the President's Committee on Health Education. *Health Services and Mental Health Administration.* Washington, D.C.: U.S. Department of Health, Education, and Welfare, 1973.

"Industry Body Approves Initiative in Health Education, Urban Affairs, Social Investments," *Response – A Clearinghouse on Corporate Social Responsibility.* VI, 4: 3, July 1977.

"Metropolitan Life Uses Magazine Ads to Educate Public on Health Matters," *Response – A Clearinghouse on Corporate Social Responsibility* VI, 5:6-7, September 1977.

"A Quote to Note – Speech Excerpt by R. Manning Brown, Jr., Chairman, New York Life Insurance Company," *Response – A Clearinghouse on Corporate Social Responsibility* VI, 6:13, November 1977.

Werlin, Stanley H. and Schauffler, Helen H., *A Survey of Consumer Health Education Programs.* Cambridge: Arthur D. Little, January 1976.

18

Coverage for Health Promotion and Disease Prevention

Duane R. Carlson

Blue Cross and Blue Shield Associations

It is a well known fact (and a matter of grave national concern) that for the past several years the total cost of health services has been rising steeply in Great Britain, Sweden, Canada, and the U.S. — under vastly differing systems of delivering and paying for these services. Thus, the means of seeking to modify the increases are also different, though not notably successful up to now. In the first three countries, where for some years government has been the principal source of payment for all health services, the chief method of seeking economy has been simply to cut down in one way or another on the services provided, shifting some of the burden from the government back to the population. In the U.S., where the bulk of the service is still provided by private rather than public sources, this method has been tried in a few states. These states have frozen their rates of payment for services rendered to poor people under the Medicaid program — a tactic that has had the effect of shifting the burden to the population, since it forces the providers to either limit their acceptance of Medicaid patients or to charge more for service to others. The federal administration also has been considering the imposition of ceilings on annual increases in total payments to hospitals from all sources, including the federal Medicare program that provides assistance for people over age 65, Blue Cross Plans, and other payers.

Most of those who oppose the effort to impose ceilings on payment to hospitals point to the reasons for increasing costs that are largely outside any substantial measure of control by hospitals. Briefly, these are as follows: the 15–18% per year inflation in the economy as a whole, which has increased the price of everything hospitals buy and has been particularly acute in the past two years in fuel oil and petrochemical products, of which hospitals are heavy users; increasing labor costs, especially loss of hospital exemption under the minimum wage and fair labor standards provisions of the National Labor Relations Act, which has resulted in steep wage increases and drives to organize unions of hospital workers; the burgeoning technology of medicine, with consequent pressure from physicians and the public for new equipment and the specialized, technically trained personnel to operate it; and the disposition of courts in many U.S. jurisdictions to hold hospitals and physicians responsible for negligence and actual malpractice and to award huge judgments, often out of all proportion to the harm or injury to the patient.

This is not to say that hospitals, Blue Cross and Blue Shield Plans, and others have been standing helplessly by watching costs go up, wringing their hands and not doing anything about it. Far from it. Opposed to the forces of inflation is any array of cost containment activities that is already making itself felt and seems certain to become increasingly effective. These may be grouped into six general classifications: management, planning, utilization review, reimbursement method, alternative delivery mechanisms, and new approaches to health.

Management

The biggest change in the management of health care institutions in recent years has been the rapid emergence and growth of institutional chains or multiple-unit management systems, mergers, shared services and joint enterprises, and similar systematic efforts to improve management economy by changing what has been, in effect, an industry characterized by small, independent units – unrelated, uncoordinated, and often duplicative and competitive – into networks of integrated facilities and services having the advantages and specialized resources of large-scale systems. Some idea of the extent of this movement was evident in a 1977 study that identified some 2000 of the nation's 7000 hospitals in multiple systems of some kind, and about twice that many in formal, shared service agreements.

In the years 1970-1974, there were 50% more mergers of hospital corporations in the U.S. than had been recorded in the previous 20 years, and, in many cities and small communities, hospitals were organizing consortia, or arrangements based on contracts, to conduct specified programs and activities together without disturbing individual institutional autonomy or management. Further, economies may be effected through administrative efforts such as joint purchasing, data processing, nursing education, and other functions. In some areas, Blue Cross Plans have taken the initiative in offering data processing, methods engineering, and other services to groups of member hospitals.

Utilization

The principal reason for hope that efforts to contain health care costs may stop short of such Draconian measures as sharply reduced payments or services is that an important cause of rising cost has been not any of the things mentioned as beyond the control of individual physicians and hospitals, but one that is largely within their power to curtail — excessive utilization of facilities and services. In the late 1950's, a Blue Cross Plan helped with the organization of the first hospital utilization review committees, and, a decade later, these committees were made mandatory conditions of participation for hospitals in the provision of services for Medicare patients.

However, none of these measures has been particularly effective in cutting down such excesses as the hospitalization of patients whose medical needs might readily have been met by out-patient or office services, over-use of hospital X-ray and laboratory services, unneeded medications, and the troublesome and always controversial problem of unnecessary surgery. One of the reasons for these practices, without much doubt, was that during most of those years when Blue Cross and Blue Shield Plans and health insurance offered by the major underwriters were enrolling millions of Americans, the Plans paid — in the main — for only inpatient hospital services; the bills for diagnostic work-up would be paid by Blue Cross Plans only if the patient was hospitalized.

This has long since ceased to be the case; for a number of years, Blue Cross Plans have paid more out-patient than in-patient claims (in total, Blue Cross Plans pay more than two out-patient claims for every in-patient one), but the convenient practice of ordering hospital admission and procedures, with somebody else paying the bills, has not been easy to control.

The advent of Professional Standards Review Organizations (PSRO's), mandated by the Congress in the Social Security Amendments of 1972, and brought on because utilization review by hospital staff committees wasn't working effectively and the Congress was determined to do something about rising Medicare and Medicaid costs, hasn't solved the problem by any means. Five years after the Act was passed, PSRO's are actually reviewing care in only a little more than half the jurisdictions, and even PSRO's best friends acknowledge that their potential promises more for improving the quality of care than for reducing its costs. But PSRO's represent a major cost containment effort by the government and the medical profession, working together, and the concept is not likely to be abandoned until there are clearer indications of how well it is working or not working.

Planning

Exactly the same thing can be said about another government program aimed at containing cost, the National Health Planning and Resources Development Act of 1974, which has established a network of Health Systems Agencies (HSA's) — about 200 of them in the U.S., generally corresponding to, but not precisely congruent with, the PSRO areas. Under the supervision of state agencies, the HSA's are responsible for seeing to it that health care services in their areas are "appropriate" to the needs for health care services of their populations — a broad assignment that is expected eventually to go to mandated regional integration of services of the kind envisioned in some of the more ambitious consortia, but which for the present is focused sharply on the problems of excessive hospital beds and duplication of expensive hospital equipment.

HSA's have unquestionably succeeded in forestalling many excessive install-ations, and the climate of austerity generated by the HSA's has probably dis-couraged some hospitals from even initiating the tedious process of trying to get approval. The most celebrated examples have been the proposals for computerized axial tomography, the so-called CAT scanners that cost anywhere from $300,000 to $700,000 and have become a symbol that the hospital is offering the very best, up-to-the-minute service, and, on the other hand, a challenge to the HSA to demonstrate that it is putting a stop to needless and expensive "keeping up with the Joneses."

Lawmakers and regulators haven't hesitated to put restraints on hospitals but have been notably shy about making any direct approach to doctors' practices or doctors' charges, so it is not clear just how this and other constraints on hospitals are going to be worked out. Meanwhile, HSA's, like PSRO's, constitute a major government effort to contain costs and rationalize the system. Nobody has seriously proposed it yet, but it may be inevitable that eventually the two agencies would be combined, a move that many have thought would make both more effective. Either way, both efforts are sure to be around for a long time.

Reimbursement

Since the early days of the Blue Cross organization, reimbursement of hospitals for services rendered to subscribers has been based on the cost of the services, and the reimbursement formulas have been worked out over years as needs have arisen for interpreting such factors as "free" care, bad debts, depreciation charges, and others. When Medicare and Medicaid came along in the 1960's, the cost-based formulas were well established and the practice was continued in these programs. But, as the cost of everything has risen steadily in these ten years, there has been increasing dissatisfaction with the method, which is widely believed to encourage excesses.

To avoid this tendency, there has been a strong movement in recent years toward switching from cost-based reimbursement to prospective reimbursement, in which the payer and the institution negotiate and agree in advance on rates to be paid for a specified period, at the end of which the institution may be penalized for expenditures in excess of the agreed rate, but may share in any savings. Many Blue Cross Plans are now reimbursing hospitals prospectively, and the Social Security Administration has been experimenting with Medicare payments on a prospective basis. Some hospitals understandably are not enchanted with the idea and point out that, when the method is changed, hospitals that have been efficiently and economically managed will suffer because there will be few, if any, opportunities to cut expenses without sacrificing service, whereas institutions that have been careless or extravagant can readily cut down and, in effect, benefit from past sins. Obviously, this would be true if historical cost were the only basis for establishing the prospective rate to begin with, but it can be assumed that negotiators would be sophisticated enough to examine management and financial practices in each case and arrive at rates that would still offer incentives for efficiency without rewarding poor performance. In any event, this is the direction in which payment practice is moving in both the private and the public sectors, and there is little likelihood that the "cost-plus" practices that some institutions have permitted in the past can be continued for long.

Alternative Systems

As was mentioned in describing the efforts to control utilization, Blue Cross Plans have been emphasizing out-patient services wherever possible, and government payers have created an elaborate system of controls aimed at ensuring that government beneficiaries get the services they need at the least expensive, not the most expensive, level of care. As a further means of achieving this objective, both government and Blue Cross Plans have been encouraging the organization and growth of Health Maintenance Organizations (HMO's) offering comprehensive physician, hospital, and other medical services, including preventive services, at an agreed annual rate. The prototype HMO is the Kaiser Permanente Health Plan, operating its own system with its own hospitals and clinics, in the Western states of the U.S., with a total enrollment now in the neighborhood of three million.

Kaiser experience over the years has demonstrated that, when all services are paid for, and when physicians who are partners in the enterprise have an incentive to seek the least expensive method of delivering the needed services, rates of hospital admissions and rates of surgery are consistently lower than they are in comparable population groups protected by Blue Cross and Blue Shield Plan coverage or insurance and seeking care in the traditional system. Many new HMO's have been organized in the past few years; Blue Cross and Blue Shield Plans alone have started, assisted, or are engaged in promoting and offering the services of 67 HMO's. Others have been organized by hospitals, groups of physicians, insurance companies, labor unions, and, in a few cases, industry. Their growth is rarely rapid, and over time it seems probable that HMO's will exist in enough communities so that a large share of the population will have the opportunity of choosing between this method and the traditional mode of delivery.

New Approaches

If all the activities that are thus underway in management, utilization review, planning, reimbursement, and delivery systems were to be continued aggressively, as seems likely to happen, there can't be much question that the rate of increase in costs will be retarded, and, in fact, there are data suggesting that this is already starting to happen. But there is a feeling also among some members of the health professional community, government officials, economists, and interested representatives of industry (which carries a large share of the cost in its contributions to the health insurance coverage of employees) that this isn't enough. We can keep on pouring more billions of dollars into the health care system, and in spite of all the efforts at cost containment, there will always be more spending as the population increases and the technology proliferates, unless at the same time we can also find other ways of improving the health of the population besides treating people who become sick or get hurt.

Despite all the scientific knowledge we continue to accumulate, despite the so-called technologic breakthroughs we achieve and the heroic measures we are prepared to apply and do apply, often with considerable success, the fact remains that millions of people do not get the coaching, care, support, information, and direction they need and must have if we expect to make measurable improvements in our nation's health. The minimum requirement for achieving this goal is that people must have the capability and the will to take greater responsibility for their own health. For some years now, we have been talking about the need for added emphasis on primary social medicine, preventive medicine, environmental medicine, and health education of the public. But while we talk, we keep right on concentrating our resources on specialized, high-technology medicine. Health status is known to be a compound of heredity, lifestyle, social and physical environment, and all kinds of emotional stimuli, as well as medical care; nevertheless, it can still be said that the medical system is going one way and the needs of society another. The directions are divergent — sometimes by 180 degrees — but when this misdirection obtrudes, we generally have turned our backs and considered readdressing it as someone else's job. Given what we know about just one set of issues — the relationships among poor nutrition, poverty, inadequate education and health — it is tragic that more has not been done.

Questions that need to be raised include these: Are we really using our formidable brains, hands, and money in the best way for maximum improvement in health status? What are we doing that we do not have to do or do not have to do so much? What should we be doing that we are not doing at all? How can we turn the system around so that its direction coincides, or at least does not collide, with society's health needs? How much of whatever it is that needs to be done is indeed our job, as professionals and organizations and institutions, and how much is someone else's? Who should be doing what?

The Blue Cross and Blue Shield organizations have much more than a passing interest in the cost considerations and implications of these concepts. These organizations are interested in holding down health care costs. That interest, goaded by private market as well as by governmental concerns, increases as health care bills rise. A healthier population means healthier Blue Cross and Blue Shield Plans, and we are interested in both parts of this equation. But over the years we have learned that we cannot get a healthier population, and hence healthier Blue Cross and Blue Shield Plans, simply by trying to help hospitals operate more efficiently (which we have done) or by encouraging and supporting regional planning of health care resources (which we also have done) or by paying for out-of-hospital health services, or promoting and supporting new organizational concepts such as health maintenance organizations. Our Plans have done all these things and will keep doing them, and more of them.

But more needs to be done. If we can discover how to design and manage constructive interventions in the social and environmental factors influencing health — how to inform, teach, and motivate people to take better care of themselves — then we will also find ways to support and pay for these activities. In fact, we have already begun to support and pay for such things as patient education services and psychological counseling in some of our Plans and groups. Some of these beginnings that are being made at achieving new, positive health strategies will be described here. Note, though, that this is no way an all-inclusive list but rather highlights certain developments we have learned about and are interested in. But first it should be pointed out that while health education is a key element in those new strategies, we need to recognize that providing information and educating, or actually motivating, are different things. Much of what we have seen labeled as "health education" is more accurately placed in the category of health information, randomly spewed forth without being part of a cohesive, pervasive program, and without any regard for measurement of its impact. Hampering the effectiveness of health information programs also are factors such as fragmentation, lack of any consistent integration and continuity, inadequate analysis of what consumers either need or want to learn, unimaginative or unnecessary technical presentation, and inadequate relation of information to the lifestyle, cultural background, economic, and educational level of the audience, environmental conditions, and existing services in the community.

Finally, it must be remembered always that, except under the most carefully controlled situations that are unsuited to most educational efforts except in limited population groups, results are extremely hard to measure. We know, for example, that people who have quit smoking or have changed their dietary or exercise habits as the result of intensive educational efforts of some kind are inclined to revert to their former habits of living and eating and exercising unless the educational thrust is sustained or reinforced over time. Even in controlled groups, such as employed or school populations, it is often difficult to make such observations regarding changes in behavior, and the results may be measured only imprecisely. Thus, for the most part, any broad-based educational or preventive programs that are undertaken by Blue Cross and Blue Shield Plans, educational institutions, industry, or others in a position to influence large population groups must be initiated largely on the basis of faith in the logic of education and prevention, and not as the result of precise cost-benefit analysis. Under the circumstances, it may be astonishing that so many groups have initiated so many programs in the last few years — and not that so few have done so little, as is more commonly supposed.

Schools, public health departments, Blue Cross and Blue Shield Plans, other health insurers, employers, and unions all have reasons to want to be well, and to keep well, and they have all made efforts in health education from time to time — sometimes elaborate and sustained efforts. It can be argued, too (and it is, on occasion) that public health departments are spending their entire effort on methods and programs having to do with sanitation, immunization, nutrition, prevention, and health education, and that the total of these activities does more to improve the health status of the population than everything that is done by doctors, hospitals, and nurses in the care of acute illness and injury. But nobody knows whether this is true or not, and the argument is witless anyway, because everybody understands that important things remain to be done in teaching and motivating people to take better care of themselves.

Hospital people insist that they do this. It is their proper and continuing job, they point out, to make certain doctors, nurses, and others are performing the educational functions that are components of patient care, as in instructing diabetic patients in their diet and medication requirements; teaching cardiac patients, colostomy patients, and others how to care for and live with their disabilities; etc. It's hard enough to see that these things are done, and done well, they argue, and then to get them into the budget somewhere so that somebody will pay for them. But some people will argue that to go beyond these tasks and consider health education for the whole community to be the responsibility of the hospital is impractical, because it doesn't make sense to divert any fraction of the hospital's always limited money, manpower, and facilities resources *away* from the essential tasks of saving lives and alleviating suffering, for the putative benefit of those who are not yet threatened or hurting, however much the total health economy might ultimately have to gain from such diversion.

There are forces, however, suggesting that the patient education functions of the hospital need to be improved and systemized, and that hospitals *should* be thinking seriously about the community education function, because this responsibility, which they have not assumed up to now, is likely to be thrust upon them before long. While it is true that some physicians, some nurses, some dietitians, and some training directors take their obligation to instruct patients seriously and fulfill it competently, there are unquestionably many more who are too busy with what they believe to be their more important duties to give the education obligation anything more than *pro forma* attention, and there are many who neglect it entirely. Thus, except in the most obvious cases, patients may suffer needlessly for want of any information, or because nobody has told them how important it is to follow instructions conscientiously, and nobody has bothered to find out whether they do or not. And this may happen even in the most obvious cases, where education is a known component of treatment, as in diabetes. A noted diabetes authority said recently that the number of diabetics who are treated in hospitals and then discharged with inadequate instruction in the proper care of their own conditions is appalling. He did not know, because there are few data on the subject, how much this inadequacy may contribute to the rate of readmission of such patients – but he was willing to estimate that the readmission rate could be drastically reduced if physicians were adequately prepared themselves, and were made responsible for seeing to it that nurses, dietitians, and others were properly prepared to train patients in their care during the period of hospitalization, and then to follow up systematicaly and make sure they were following instructions. Unquestionably, the same deficiency, and the same opportunity for improvement and avoidance of complication, exists for cardiac patients and for many others. In a less obvious example, consider the fracture patients who lose some function and suffer some disability simply because they were never instructed in the exercise necessary to restore full function following prolonged immobilization.

Patient education has been an important area of interest for the Blue Cross and Blue Shield organizations. It offers opportunities for reaching individuals at critical junctures in their lives, utilizing time in hospitals and physicians' offices to help them prevent further episodes of illness, to effectively handle chronic conditions, and to translate knowledge into effective action.

To further support such programs, the Board of Governors of the Blue Cross Association has passed a set of guidelines for programs in patient education. In summary, these guidelines, which were enacted because "it is appropriate that the Blue Cross organization encourage the development of cost-effective programs in patient education," state that:

1. The purpose and operational objectives of the program should be clearly stated and the techniques for meeting the objectives should be specified.
2. Patient education should be provided as an integral element of the total patient care process within a supportive organizational framework.
3. Necessary and appropriate health education should be developed and financed as a routine element of the care of each patient.

4. Educational methodologies should be directed to specific case types, and desired behavioral changes and the results of such interventions as to cost and quality of care should be documented.

Blue Cross Plans are also involved in experiments in the development of new benefits and utilizing claims data to develop occupational disease information with the federal government. Briefly, these include a project to study whether claims data can be used to help detect occupational diseases in certain industries and occupations; working with the National Cancer Institute to study various factors involved in providing cancer screening programs as a prepaid health care benefit, to determine whether early detection and treatment of cancer would lead to improved survival rates and lower treatment costs, and, if so, whether it would be economically feasible to offer the new benefit on a nationwide scale; and a project with the National Heart, Lung, and Blood institute to determine and develop the role of health insurance carriers in worksite-based hypertension education, screening, treatment, and follow-up services.

One of the most exciting programs aimed at educating and motivating individuals to achieve better lifestyles is the American Health Foundation's Health Maintenance Service Program. It offers an inexpensive primary prevention program for industry, which enables a firm to offer special benefits to its employees, and is aimed at better health for all. Some Blue Cross and Blue Shield Plans are doing pilot projects of the program with their own employees and may consider offering it to their subscriber groups.

This program, which may also prove to be an effective cost containment technique, involves a brief, simple medical screening, identification of high-risk personnel, and effective preventive interventions to reduce the risk factors for those identified as having more than one risk factor. It also can include a component of "administrative cost containment," including second opinion surgery, peer review of non-emergent hospital admissions and elective surgery, and medical review of excess absenteeism. The goals of the Health Maintenance Service are to reduce smoking, alcoholism, overweight, hypertension, and hyperlipidemia; the most effective methods are those that make use of allied health professionals in programs that give preventive medicine an outreach arm at the place of work and work with groups of employees who have been identified as high-risk.

Group therapy has proved to be most effective in smoking cessation clinics, and taking the screening, intervention, and educational programs to the workplace removes a major barrier to participation and compliance. Dr. Ernst L. Wynder, President of the American Health Foundation, has pointed out that going where the people are and where the action is involves having staff available to work with night shift employees. "We in preventive medicine have to be there at any time we are needed, just as we expect the therapeutic sector to respond," he says. "Preventive medicine must not just be preached, it must be practiced. Our kind of 'lifestyle medicine' can have a ripple effect from the individual to the workplace group, the family, and the whole community. Blue Cross Plans can help accomplish this, and if the private sector doesn't act, certainly the government will."

Also among the interesting positive health programs now underway is the Sun Valley Executive Health Institute, a program which combines a broad-gauge physical examination (including stress EKG and pulmonary capacity exam) with education and motivational techniques; it is designed to instill healthy lifestyles in its participants. Developed under the theories "human asset appraisal," the course has been utilized primarily by businessmen, with their wives also taking part. Held in Sun Valley and utilizing the facilities of Moritz Hospital and the Sun Valley recreational complex, the four-day course begins with a physical exam, and the rest of the time is spent in a succession of group programs, exercise periods, and individual consultations with a physician, a dietitian, an exercise specialist, and, on an optional basis, a physical therapist and a sex therapist. This extraordinary combination of education, motivation, group work, and individual consultation has thus far registered significant reductions in body weight, blood pressure readings, cholesterol levels, and other indices, as secured from follow-up exams. A "mini-version" of this course — to be provided in five consecutive two-and-a-half-hour evening sessions — is now being tested. Initial trials at Blue Cross of Idaho, for employess and spouses, have shown considerable promise.

Among many efforts initiated by Blue Cross and Blue Shield Plans, to emphasize the new, positive approach to health, is a statewide public education program undertaken by Blue Cross and Blue Shield of Rhode Island, designed to help Rhode Islanders recognize and treat one of our most serious health hazards — our lifestyles. Called "Change Your Mind About Your Body," the program includes a general education effort aimed at all Rhode Islanders, and specific efforts aimed at leaders of government, labor, business, and industry.

The Rhode Island program is designed to do two things: first, to help all Rhode Islanders recognize the serious health implications of careless lifestyles, and secondly, to guide them to the resources available in the community which can help make lifestyle change not only possible, but enjoyable. The communications effort is also being directed to Rhode Island government, labor, business, and industry, which continue to finance a large percentage of the health care bills for their employees and members. By promoting at-work screening programs, quit-smoking programs, exercise programs, weight control programs, and educational efforts on alcohol abuse and stress, it is felt that substantial inroads in the areas of health benefit costs and lost production time can be achieved.

A promising program under development in the Blue Cross and Blue Shield Plans is the Education and Screening for Employees (EASE) program of the North Carolina Plan. Developed with Dr. Siegfried Heyden, professor of community health at Duke University, it features workplace screening — in this case, an intensive screening specifically for smoking, obesity, hypertension, diabetes, and cancers of the prostate, cervix, breast, colon, bladder, and mouth. The screening is accompanied by educational activities and materials, and positive results of the EASE screening are checked and rechecked prior to referral of the patients to physicians.

Area physicians and industry management in North Carolina have responded positively to the benefits of the program, Plan officials have reported. The results of screening in the first large company in which Dr. Heyden conducted the EASE program — Cannon Mills — included the following:

In one year, 15,000 were educated and 10,000 were screened (conducted by one physician and nurse — about half-time — with support of two plant nurses and a secretary, the latter primarily involved in screening and follow-up). Conditions discovered included high blood pressure, 15% (a third previously undiscovered), most now under medical care with diet, low salt, and/or drugs; diabetes, 8 per 1000, with 75% under control with weight reduction (diet) and cancer, 20 cases in 10,000 exams (treatment cost approximately $2000: asymptomatic and no spread; this compares with an average expenditure of $20,000 if there is sign or symptom spread — if the patient survives the first year). Approximate costs of the program were $8.50 per male and $12.50 per female; the cost would be approximately $10-15 elsewhere.

Since Dr. Heyden has begun his work with the Plan, the EASE program has been conducted for Plan employees and is being done, on a pilot basis, for several thousand members of the Plan's largest group, the State of North Carolina employees.

Another program being studied by Blue Cross and Blue Shield Plans is the lifetime Health Monitoring Program developed by Lester Breslow, M.D., professor of public health at the University of California at Los Angeles and former president of the American Public Health Association. This is a lifetime schedule or series of packages of effective individual preventive procedures that can be incorporated into existing patterns of medical practice. The "packages of preventive services" are those which have been proved most effective for specific age and sex groups; for each of ten such groups, a set of distinct health goals, and the preventive services most likely to result in their attainment, are presented. Introducing the concept at a 1975 conference on preventive medicine at the National Institutes of Health, Dr. Breslow warned that "in deciding on incorporation of preventive medical procedures into personal health services, scientific skepticism is properly applicable not only toward many things that have been included in medicine for years but also toward what is new in preventive medicine. Because clinical trials may take years to complete and even then may not be definitive, it will be necessary to make decisions on the basis of prudent evaluation of what evidence exists." Walter J. McNerney, President of the Blue Cross and Blue Shield

Associations, said: "We may not be far from the time when some such benefits will be mandated in the federally funded programs, and some of the states may readily move in the same direction."

California was the site of another interesting group, the Institute for Humanistic Medicine in San Francisco. These people held the belief that medicine can be responsive to total human needs, comprehending the mind, body, will, and aspirations; that both the questions and answers about a person's health lie within the individual. What the Institute sought to teach physicians, nurses, and others in its training programs and publications can be summarized as follows: 1) the patient cannot be seen simply as his or her disease and the physician not simply as a technician — the healing power is in the patient; 2) every person achieves a unique interdependent relationship of body, mind, emotion, and spirit, and health is the dynamic integration of these; 3) the patient and the physician in the health relationship are colleagues; 4) illness may provide an opportunity for personal growth; and 5) illness must be seen in the context of the life span of the individual, not for 15 minutes or 2 months. The Institute — in its too brief history — conducted programs in a humanistic approach to medicine for physicians now in practice, as well as for medical students.

A somewhat related and interesting concept is on trial at the Wholistic Health Center project in Hinsdale, Illinois, where four years ago the Kellogg Foundation funded the model for a new kind of primary care embodying preventive medicine, health education, psychological and social counseling, and patient participation, as well as nursing and medical care. Essential components of the model are establishment of the out-patient service in a church facility, staffing by clergy trained in psychological counseling and by trained volunteers, in addition to physicians and nurses, and an initial planning conference in which patient, physician, counselor, and nurse together examine the patient's problems, agree on a course of treatment, and accept mutual responsibility for the outcome.

The Wholistic Health Center at Hinsdale Union Church, and its companion center at the United Methodist Church of nearby Woodridge, Illinois, have been supported by a $375,000 grant from the W.K. Kellogg Foundation, administered by the Department of Preventive Medicine and Community Health of the University of Illinois Medical School. In mid-1980 the original centers had become self-sustaining, and centers had been established in 11 communities in the metropolitan Chicago area, elsewhere in the midwest, and in Washington, D.C.

The method is obviously effective: In a recent survey of several hundred center patients, 85% of those for whom the plan of treatment included a change of living habits reported that they had followed the recommended course of action, at least in part. The few comparable studies that have been made in traditional settings suggest that 50% compliance is an unusually high score, and 0% is not uncommon. Center personnel are now engaged with the Department of Medicine at the University of Illinois in the design of further studies aimed at making specific comparisons of outcomes by diagnosis in larger groups of Wholistic Health Center patients and others.

Obviously, all these and the many other, similar new services are not going to be introduced and financed overnight. Progress moves slowly along an evolutionary path for a number of reasons. First, the health care field has been so thoroughly institutionalized for so many years that these new, non-institutional services are not readily accepted. Also, there is some difference of opinion about the value of these services within the professional and scientific communities. Technology has its ardent and influential defenders who are skeptical, if not hostile, to the concept that there are limits to what medicine can accomplish. Any consequential moves toward eliminating occupational and environmental hazards to health involve major expense and determined opposition for industries and communities.

Change, inevitably, can be accomplished only gradually. For years, we have been teaching people to depend on physicians and medical institutions for everything related to their health, and it is not easy now to turn them around and get them to accept a large share of the responsibility for their own health. The process is made more difficult by the overwhelming volume of advertising on television and in print that encourages people to use products and engage in activities that are basically inimical to health — junk food, cigarettes, etc.

Finally, for all its unquestioned importance, the New Directions concept remains somewhat amorphous and lacking in specific goals. Who is responsible for what? What groups encompass both the new and the traditional approaches? Doctors? Hospitals? Blue Cross and Blue Shield Plans? Public health departments? *Who*? Again, for what specific purposes? How far should health status extend? Does it include, for example, such unquestionably health-related conditions as anxiety and periodic depression? Do we need new institutions to project the new services? We do see the Carter administration addressing welfare, unemployment, housing, and other problems having an impact on health. These are encouraging signs, but the truth is that we simply don't know the answers to most of these questions.

Here is an opportunity for leadership. For Blue Cross and Blue Shield Plans, as well as for health institutions and professions, the time for addressing hospital services and medical care alone is passed. Increasingly, the emphasis is going to be on broad health services, of which hospitals and medical care will be important parts, but not the whole. The concept that has considered institutional and medical care and all the other activities related to health as separate entities is no longer defensible, nor is the sharp line we have drawn in the past between the sick and the well. The services, like the populations, must be seen as continuums.

"We are starting a new era," McNerney said in an annual report to Blue Cross Plans. "We are emerging from a preoccupation with illness to a parallel concern with health. We are growing from a self-image of a facilitative force to one of performing a broad, critically important role. While still dedicated to acutely ill patients, we are on the verge of daring to ask how they got ill, and to devote our resources more to root causes involving individual lifestyle and environmental issues, both physical and social. Involved here is a fascinating array of education and benefit programs, new linkages with industries, schools and other community institutions, as well as the individual subscribers. Our mission increasingly will be, in significant part, keeping people well. We are also on the threshold of assuming a bolder role in the delivery of both preventive and curative services."

Undoubtedly, diagnosis is easier than prescription. How to motivate people to change their habits and how to foster a more enlightened relationship between the human organism and its environment are complex and challenging questions. But now is the time to address the issues; there must be no delay. The social as well as the human cost of our current path is too much for us to bear.

Health Promotion: Action and Strategies

19

The Practice of
Health Promotion:
The Case of Obesity

Albert J. Stunkard, M.D.

Department of Psychiatry
University of Pennsylvania

Obesity is a particularly fit topic for a volume on the theory and practice of health promotion. Just about every reason why people are interested in health promotion applies to obesity. It is a condition resulting to an unusual degree from lifestyles and personal habits. Unlike other disorders linked to lifestyles, however, an enviable body of research defines this linkage. Obesity is a condition whose contribution to hypertension, adult onset diabetes, and the hyperlipidemias alone ranks it as a foremost cardiovascular risk factor — and half of all deaths in our country are cardiovascular deaths.

But obesity is of interest to health promotion for reasons far beyond its contribution to ill health or the extent of our understanding of its origins. Obesity is unique in the extent of the health promotional activities that have already been undertaken for its control. As we shall see, some of these activities have had equivocal and disappointing outcomes and the war is far from won. But the battle has been joined, the campaigns are underway, and the practice of health promotion can find valuable lessons from the case of obesity.

This chapter describes the impact of the social environment producing obesity and how this environment may be modified to aid in the control of obesity. It describes briefly the impact of unplanned and uncontrolled factors such as social class, and then, at greater length, extensive research on the behavioral control of obesity. Finally, we look at how the findings of this research may be utilized in future large-scale programs for the control of obesity.

The first evidence of how the large-scale social environment influences obesity was obtained by the Mid-Town Study, a comprehensive survey of the epidemiology of mental illness.[1] This study showed a striking association between socioeconomic status and the prevalence of obesity, particularly among women.[2] Figure

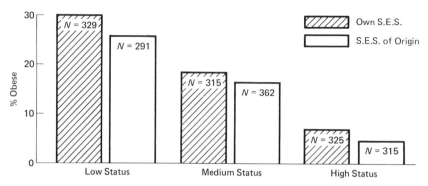

Figure 19-1. Obesity by socioeconomic status (Women).[22]

19-1 shows that 30% of lower class women were obese, compared to 16% among those of middle social class and 5% in the upper social class.

A notable feature of this study is that it permitted causal inferences about the influence of socioeconomic status. This was achieved by ascertaining not only the socioeconomic status of the respondents at the time of the study, but also the status of their parents when they were eight years old. Although a subject's obesity might influence his or her own social class, it is unlikely that this problem in his adult life could have influenced his parents' social class. Therefore, associations between social class of the respondents' parents and obesity can be viewed as causal. And these associations were almost as powerful as those between the respondents' own social class and their obesity. Since this original work, a number of other studies in various parts of the world have confirmed the strong relationship between social factors and obesity; social factors must be considered as among the most important, if not *the* most important, influence on the prevalence of obesity.[3]

The full implications of these findings for our understanding of obesity and for its control have yet to be realized. For they mean that whatever its genetic determinants and its biochemical pathways, obesity is, to an unusual degree, under social environmental control. And they suggest that a broad scale assault on obesity need not await further understanding of its biochemical determinants. Understanding of its social determinants may be sufficient. Such understanding has been greatly advanced by recent studies of the influence of the behavioral therapies.

The Influence of the Behavioral Therapies on Individuals and Small Groups

In the past, it has been fairly easy to assess the effectiveness of any out-patient treatment for obesity because the results of traditional treatments have been so uniformly poor and the treatments so obviously ineffective. Only 25% of persons entering conventional out-patient treatment for obesity lose more than 20 pounds, and 5% more than 40 pounds.[4]

Against this background, Stuart's report on "Behavioral Control of Overeating"[5] stands out. It describes the best results obtained to that time in the out-patient treatment of obesity, and it constitutes a landmark in our understanding of this disorder. Even the absence of a control group does not vitiate the significance of its findings. The 8 patients who remained in treatment out of an original 10 lost large amounts of weight: 3 lost more than 40 pounds and 6 more than 30 pounds.

A description of the essential elements of behavioral treatments for obesity is beyond the scope of this report, and the interested reader is referred to the extended descriptions of Mahoney and Mahoney,[6] and to the detailed manual by Ferguson.[7]

Soon after Stuart's landmark program, the first controlled outcome study of behavior modification of obesity reported an average weight loss of 10.5 pounds over a four-month period among moderately overweight women university students.[8] Subjects in a no-treatment control group gained 3.6 pounds, a significant difference ($p < 0.01$).

A no-treatment control group, such as that used by Harris, was quite acceptable in psychotherapy research in 1969. Yet it has serious disadvantages: refusing treatment to someone who has come seeking it is far from a neutral event. The resultant disappointment could well produce weight gains that would make the treatment condition appear to be more effective than it actually was. The problem calls for the use of a placebo control group to match the attention and interest received by patients in the active treatment program. An elaborate study by Wollersheim provided precisely such controls and opened up new vistas in research on psychological treatment.[9]

Wollersheim's elegant factorial design contained four experimental conditions: behavioral treatment, "non-specific therapy" based upon traditional psychiatric methods, "social pressure" modeled on lay weight control programs, and, finally, a no-treatment control group. Four therapists each treated one group of five patients in each of the three treatment conditions for ten sessions over a three-month period. Figure 19-2 shows that, at the end of treatment, and at eight-week follow-up, subjects in the behavioral ("focal") treatment condition had lost more weight than those in the no-treatment condition. In addition, they had lost significantly more weight than those in the two placebo control conditions, who had themselves lost significantly more weight than those in the no-treatment condition.

Wollersheim's study solved the problem of placebo controls, but in so doing, brought psychotherapy research face to face with a new problem: experimenter bias. Although the placebo therapy controlled for the patient's expectations of treatment, it did not control for the therapist's, and this is not a trivial matter.

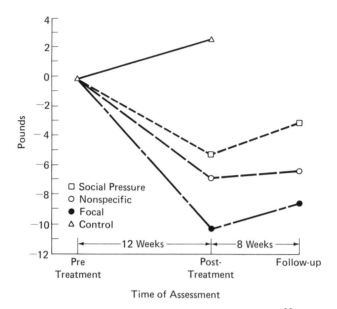

Figure 19-2. Comparisons of results of treatments.[23]

The double-blind experiment in psychopharmacology has shown how powerful this influence can be in the administration of drugs. It is surely more powerful in the more emotional case of the psychotherapies.

The problem of experimenter bias was approached in an ingenious manner in the study by Penick *et al,*[10] which was also one of the few to deal with severely (78%) overweight persons. Therapists were selected to treat the control group on the basis of their great skill in the treatment of obesity and their use of the entire conventional therapeutic armamentarium, including medication; behavior modification, on the other hand, was carried out by persons with no previous experience in treatment. In all, 15 patients were treated with behavior modification and 17 with conventional therapy. Both therapies were on a once-a-week basis for two hours over a period of three months.

The results of treatment favored the behavioral approach. Thus, weight losses of the control group were comparable to those in the medical literature; none lost 40 pounds and only 24% lost more than 20 pounds. By contrast, 13% of the behavior modification group lost more than 40 pounds and 53% lost more than 20 pounds.

The most important implication of the Penick study lies in its promise of greater applicability of the behavioral therapies. It showed that behavior modification, devised by a team with little experience in the modality (indeed, without any clinical experience), was more effective in the treatment of obesity than was the best alternative program that could be devised by a highly skilled research team. In fact, the inexperienced therapists achieved a two-fold increase in weight loss over conventional measures. Lesser increases in effectiveness have brought about major changes in the management of other disorders. The question arose: "How can the advantages of behavior modification be exploited most effectively?"

Application of Behavioral Measures to Large Groups

The first controlled effort to explore the application of behavioral measures to large groups was carried out with TOPS (Take Off Pounds Sensibly), a 30-year-old self-help group for obesity that enrolls over 300,000 members in 12,000 chapters in all parts of the U.S.[11] The study involved all 298 female members of 16 TOPS chapters situated in West Philadelphia and its adjacent suburbs.[12]

Four treatment conditions, each containing four matched TOPS chapters, were employed for a total of twelve weeks: behavior modification by psychiatrists, behavior modification by (lay) TOPS chapter leaders, nutrition education carried out by TOPS chapter leaders (who had received an amount of training in this area comparable to that provided the chapter leaders in behavioral modification), and, finally, continuation of the standard TOPS program. The most striking effects were upon attrition rate, a major problem in TOPS and, indeed, in all large-scale weight control programs. Figure 19-3 shows that the attrition rate in the two behavior modification conditions was lower during treatment, and significantly lower one year later. At follow-up, 38% and 41% of subjects had dropped out of the chapters which had received behavior modification, compared to 55% for the nutrition education and 67% for the standard TOPS programs. The difference between the behavioral treatment and other treatments was highly significant statistically.

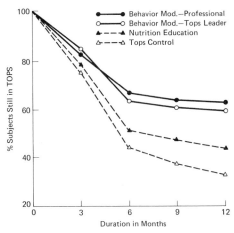

Figure 19-3. Comparison of attrition rates.[24]

Despite the bias against the results of behavior modification resulting from the differential attrition rates, behavior modification produced significantly greater weight loss than did the control conditions, both at the end of treatment and at one-year follow-up.

This program was a useful feasibility study. It taught us that behavior modification can be introduced into large populations through appropriate institutional auspices. TOPS, apparently, is not to be such an institution. It has made no effort to capitalize upon the program to which it made such an important contribution. Ironically, the chief beneficiaries are TOPS' main competitors, the commercial weight reduction organizations. They have already begun to develop strong behavioral components to their programs, which had traditionally been confined to inspirational lectures, nutrition education, and group pressure. It is estimated that 400,000 Americans are now exposed each week to behavioral measures for the control of obesity under commercial auspices. Controlled clinical trials of these programs are sorely needed. They represent one of the first approaches to the control of obesity that is sufficiently far-reaching to warrant description as a public health measure. Traditional public health efforts in the field of weight control have been conspicuous for their absence until quite recently. Three non-traditional programs, however, have been carried out in the very recent past and each has profound implications for health promotion.

The Stanford Heart Disease Prevention Program. The first of these studies was the Stanford Heart Disease Prevention Program, which consisted of a broad spectrum intervention to reduce coronary risk factors in three towns of 14,000 each.[13] A rigorous evaluation has added to the value of this highly innovative project.

The major intervention in the Stanford three-community study was an intensive and sophisticated media campaign, which contained, during each of two years, 50 television and 100 radio spots, three hours of television, and several hours of radio programming; columns, stories, and advertisements in the local weekly newspapers; posters and billboards; printed matter sent via direct mail; and other materials. The dominant characteristic of the media campaign was its organization as a total integrated information system based initially upon data gathered from preliminary surveys and later upon information collected during the course of the campaign. In one of the three towns, the media campaign was supplemented by a face-to-face instruction program directed at two-thirds of the participants identified as being in the top quartile of risk of coronary heart disease. One town received no campaign and served as a control.

Although coronary heart disease, rather than obesity alone, was the target of the campaign, and although much of the program was not specifically behavioral, this experiment is highly relevant to efforts to control obesity (or any condition which is based, at least in part, upon lifestyles and personal habits).

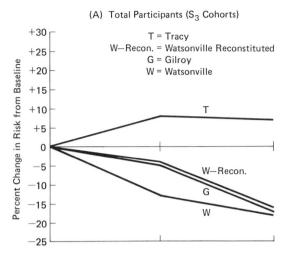

Figure 19-4. The reduction in risk factors among high-risk participants in the Stanford Heart Disease Prevention Program. Percentage change in baseline (0) in risk of coronary heart disease after one and two years of behaviorally-oriented health education programs in three communities. *T*, the control town, shows no change in risk factors. *G*, the "media only" town, shows a steady decrease in risk factors over the two years of the program, as does *W-RC* (subjects in Watsonville who did not receive face-to-face counseling), which shows a rapid decline during the first year and then no further change.

Its results were most encouraging. By the end of the second year of the campaign, the risk of coronary disease had decreased by 17% in the treatment communities, as measured by the Cornfield risk index, whereas it had increased by 6% in the control community. Even more striking are the results shown in Figure 19-4: a reduction in risk factors among high-risk participants of 30%. Such a reduction in coronary risk has been compared to an increase in life expectancy at age 45 of 5 years, a greater increase in life expectancy for middle-aged men than that achieved by all the medical advances that have occurred during the present century.

The Swedish "Diet and Exercise" Program. The second large-scale, non-traditional health promotion activity was the most broadly based program yet to be undertaken: the "Diet and Exercise" program of the Swedish National Board of Health and Welfare.[14] The origins of this effort go back to the mid-1960's, when leading Swedish nutritionists were asked to prepare a report for a governmental committee dealing with agricultural policy. The resulting report, with recommendations such as reductions in the proportion of fat in the diet to 35%, was disregarded by the governmental planners. However, the report did alert leading academics to the problems posed by the high animal fat and low vegetable content of the Swedish diet.

These problems of the Swedish diet were serious, although it should be noted that they were not much greater than those of other affluent Western societies. There had been some improvement in the Swedish diet since the turn of the century, largely in the increase in the particularly low level of intake of fruits and green vegetables. But in almost all other categories, the diet could be said to have become more unhealthy, with increasingly higher levels of caloric density and lower levels of nutrient density. For example, there had been a great increase in the consumption of fats and sugar, in high-fat dairy products such as cheese and cream, a shift in meat toward higher fat content, and a marked decrease in the consumption of bread and cereals. Because of these dietary changes, it was necessary to consume 2500 calories in order to meet daily requirements for several essential nutrients. Yet the concomitant reduction in physical activity during this period meant that no more than 20% of the *adult, male* population had caloric expenditures this high, and the figure was considerably lower for women.

This state of affairs led a leading Swedish nutritionist to describe an average family in the 1960's as follows: "The mother is obese, the father has started to get his first symptoms of coronary heart disease, the daughter has anemia, and the son has been given his first false teeth. All of them are generally fatigued, suffer from cold and are constipated."[15]

Background information on diet and exercise such as that described above was published in 1971, in a pamphlet with a circulation of 180,000 (for a country of 8 million), initiating the "Diet and Exercise" program. The program was composed of a number of special project groups:

The *project group "Institutions"* carried out studies of institutional food service programs and held conferences all over the country, at which dietary recommendations were made to those people responsible for employee restaurants, old age institutions, and nurseries. The group produced special information packages to be used in the training of the staffs of institutions and distributed posters with simple texts for further instruction of both staff and guests.

The *project group "Exercise"* worked with 200,000 leaders of the sports movement, aiding their activities and enlisting their help in promoting the dietary programs. The considerable publishing and public relations capabilities of the sports movement were thus obtained at no cost to the "Diet and Exercise" program.

The *project group "Diet and Expense"* had considerable success in developing and promoting reasonably priced and nutritionally well-balanced daily menus. This effort was particularly important in view of the widespread belief that nutritious food is too expensive for the average person to afford.

An *Advisory Committee on Industrial Questions* was formed some time after the original project groups, as a result of the unanticipated interest of industry in the original pamphlet that initiated the campaign. Much to the surprise of the staff, this pamphlet was voluntarily accepted by the food industry as its official guide for product development. Both the food industry and other commercial organizations gave considerable backing to the program as it developed.

Two project groups were notable for their relative lack of success. They were the groups devoted to *"Mass Media,"* which tried to establish liaison with these agencies, and *"Education,"* which tried to introduce improved nutritional education into the schools.

A major operational activity of "Diet and Exercise" was through concentration on special themes. One of the first, derived from research showing that Swedish breakfasts were poor from a nutritional point of view, was entitled "Start Your Day in a Better Way." Recipes for simple nutritious breakfasts were widely publicized, along with a program of calisthenics. Fifty percent of retail stores took part in the campaign by mounting attractive window displays showing appropriate breakfasts and by distributing large numbers of pamphlets produced by "Diet and Exercise." Newspaper coverage reached 95%.

Another thematic program, carried out in cooperation with the Bread Institute, was designed to increase the limited consumption of bread by 25%. The theme of this program was very widely publicized — "The National Social Welfare Board wants you to eat six to eight slices of bread every day." High visibility was achieved; 81% of the people reported having seen the slogan, and, several months later, the number who remembered it was as high as the number of those who remembered the colors of the Swedish flag. The injunction, "The National Social Welfare Board wants you to . . . " even became the starting point for bawdy jokes, an encouraging sign of observer recognition. And the program seems to have worked. Sales of bread increased by 5% — a major success by traditional marketing standards. Furthermore, this increase interrupted a trend of decreasing bread consumption of several years' duration and occurred in the face of an increase in the cost of bread and during a time when the consumption of pastries fell by 9%.

One of the major lessons of the "Diet and Exercise" program was that economic reasons required the utilization of established channels for the dissemination of information, making it difficult to target specific audiences with specific messages. The four major channels were schools, places of employment, large households, and local government. This constraint meant that liaison with local authorities and opinion leaders became critically important.

What have been the effects of this unprecedented nationwide health promotion program? Unfortunately, evaluation has not kept pace with intervention. The results are fragmentary, and, in some critical areas, absent. Although rather detailed plans for evaluation had been drawn up, and an extensive baseline survey of knowledge, attitudes, and behavior of individuals had been carried out, lack of funds has prevented follow-up surveys. A major lesson of the "Diet and Exercise" program, thus, is the need for assured funding for evaluation prior to embarking on intervention programs.

Three kinds of evaluation were considered: studies of the behavior of individuals, studies of the consumption of foods, and studies of health benefits (such as mortality and morbidity rates). As we have noted, the first type was not funded. Regarding impact of the program on health indices, a decrease in the rate of coronary heart disease was noted, but Swedish authorities believe that the effects of the program cannot be distinguished from secular trends affecting other affluent societies. There appeared to be an interruption in the rising prevalence of obesity in surveys taken in the Gothenburg area, and "Diet and Exercise" may have been responsible. Only in the area of food consumption was it possible to draw some conclusions, and even here the nationwide character of the campaign made it difficult to evalate that part of the impact which could be attributed to it.

In general, measures of food consumption reflected the goals of the campaign. Thus, there was a small but significant reduction in consumption of sugar and sugar products (such as soft drinks), and the aforementioned arrest and reversal of the decline in the consumption of bread (and cereals). The dairy industry developed a special low-fat (0.5%) milk and promoted it so successfully that it captured 25% of the market. Increasing consumption of cream and other milk products, however, meant that the total consumption of fat from dairy products remained at about the same level. Ironically, all of these efforts have been without effect upon the national agricultural policy, the starting point of the program.

Despite shortcomings, from which we can also learn, the Swedish "Diet and Exercise" program is a landmark in the mobilization of an entire nation in the interests of health promotion. We need to learn more about this program. To date, it has been reported largely in the Swedish literature, and then in no great detail.

The German Television Weight Reduction Program. The third large-scale nontraditional health promotion activity was a German exploration of the use of television in a program of weight control. It represented a cooperative effort of the second of two television channels of the German Federal Republic and the Max Planck Institute of Psychiatry in Munich. The program consisted of seven "packages," or sections. Each lasted one month and consisted of a major 45-minute show in prime time on one Sunday evening a month, together with 3-minute reminder shows on the other Sunday evenings. By virtue of its prestigious sponsors, the size of the population reached by the program was unprecedented for a health promotion program: 7.8 million people in a country of 60 million. The standard television rating system revealed that 35% of these viewers − 2.8 million − were overweight, of whom 1.8 million viewed more than one of the major shows and 140,000 viewed at least five.

The program contained most of the features of traditional behavioral programs, such as self-monitoring, stimulus control, methods of changing eating habits, and self-reinforcement, with contracting with stimulus control playing a major part.

In addition, considerable information was given regarding overweight and its hazards, nutrition, and counting calories. A total of 37 rules were carefully sequenced from simple principles and techniques to more complicated ones. Modeling played an important part in the program, carried out by ten obese persons, half men and half women, who demonstrated the various behavioral techniques and discussed their use and problems that arose in implementing them. They lost unrealistically large amounts of weight for a behavioral program, 37-54 pounds during 7 months, probably as a result of crash dieting and other "unbehavioral" behaviors.

The investigators made an effort to evaluate the cost-effectiveness of the television program by comparing it with two other conditions. One condition was their own extensively studied "bibliotherapy," a kind of correspondence course in weight reduction. The second condition was a combination of television plus bibliotherapy. The evaluation of these programs was a high point of this endeavor. It began a year before the television program in order to evaluate the bibliotherapy and no-treatment conditions without the possibility of contamination by the television program. For this purpose, an invitation was extended over the second television channel to viewers to participate in a free weight reduction program for 300 people. Interested persons were to send to the station a postcard noting their name, address, age, sex, height, and current weight. A total of 32,000 replies were received, from which two samples of 300 were drawn for the "bibliotherapy" and "no-treatment control" conditions. The following year, a similar appeal netted 100,000 replies, out of which two samples of 300 were again drawn, for study of the television alone and the television plus bibliotherapy conditions.

The first two groups were matched on age, sex, height, and weight, and these values were then used as the criteria for matching the second two conditions. The result was four unusually well-matched samples that averaged 41.8% overweight,* 40.4 years in age. Women constituted 63.9% of the subjects. It is worthy of note that matching upon these four variables resulted in very close matching on other variables studied, including marital status number of children and years of education.

Each of the four samples of 300 persons were then broken down into two sub-samples, one of 250 which received the standard treatment and one of 50 which was selected for more intensive study. Later analyses confirmed the wisdom of this precaution, for the intensive study was reactive in the "television

*Percentage overweight was calculated from the Broca Index (normal weight in kilograms = height in centimeters - 100). In accord with current practice in Germany, 20% was subtracted from the Broca-derived normal weight to yield the normal weight used in the study. These weights are less than those for comparable heights according to American height/ weight tables, meaning that the extent of overweight in this study was overestimated by American standards.

alone" condition — where subjects lost 11 pounds in the intensive study condition and only 5.5 pounds in the standard treatment condition ($p < 0.01$) — but not in the other three conditions.

Another check on the quality of the data provided valuable information about the validity of self-reported weights. One week before the end of the program, a 10% sample of participants was contacted and asked if they would agree to a home visit to discuss the program. No mention was made of weight in the inquiry. At the time of the visit the interviewer weighed the subject on scales brought to the house for this purpose. Measured weights were remarkably close to self-reported weights.

After this vast amount of effort, the results of the television treatment were disappointing. The values for the standard treatment conditions are summarized in Table 19-1. The most striking finding is the effectiveness of bibliotherapy alone — and its far greater effectiveness than television alone. Considerable confidence can be placed in the bibliotherapy results, since they are remarkably similar to those obtained in two previous studies carried out by this same research group. Television alone produced a weight loss (5.5 pounds) which was statistically significantly greater than that in the no-treatment condition (2.5 pounds). This difference of only 3 pounds, however, is not impressive, and the addition of television did not significantly increase the weight loss over that produced by bibliotherapy alone.

Why was this effect so limited? The most likely explanation is that the frequency of the television programs and the length of individual programs was not great enough to achieve significant impact. Face-to-face behavioral weight reduction programs traditionally utilize weekly meetings of at least an hour, and

Table 19-1. Values for standard treatment conditions.

Treatment	Dropout Rate (%)	Weight Loss (lb)	Success Rate (Feinstein 1960 Criterion, %)
Control	52	2.2	3
TV alone	54	5.5	5
Bibliotherapy alone	40	16.3	25
TV and bibliotherapy	38	18.7	32

$x = p < .01$
$xx = p < .001$

efforts that we have made to increase the length of this interval have resulted in a decrement in performance. Although the effectiveness of television in changing behavior has not been systematically studied, market research suggests that frequent, multiple impacts are necessary to change buying patterns even marginally. And the Stanford Three Community Study, which used such frequent, multiple impacts, exerted a cumulative effect which continued to grow for two full years.

Disappointing as have been its substantive effects, the Max Planck Institute study has been a valuable feasibility study and has laid the foundations for the evaluation of large-scale media efforts at changing health behaviors.

The Many Potential Influences of the Future

Leadership in broad-scale efforts to control obesity is passing to non-medical agencies. As we look to the future, there is every reason to believe that this trend will accelerate; the most promising new methods for controlling obesity seem to lie almost entirely outside the province of the medical profession. For obesity is, in very large part, a result of the way we live (our lifestyles) and the most effective means for controlling obesity today appear to lie in alterations in our lifestyles. Such an undertaking as altering the lifestyles of a nation is far beyond the capability of a profession such as medicine. It will require changes in those powerful social and economic forces which have given rise to these lifestyles and which sustain them.

Those forces are powerful indeed. Consider the impact upon our nutritional practices of the amount spent each year by the food industry in the U.S. to advertise its products — $1.2 billion.[16] Efforts by physicians to treat individual patients on a one-by-one basis pale by comparison. They might be likened to exhortations to a swimmer to persevere against a raging current. What are the possibilities of swimming *with* the current?

Changing the social and economic forces which maintain our lifestyles is by no means as overwhelming a task as it might at first appear. In the first place, relatively small changes in each of the institutions could, by their cumulative — and perhaps potentiating — effect, bring about considerably larger changes in the end product. Second, these forces are not simply blind, economic ones. They involve human beings in positions of responsibility that enable them to make choices between alternatives. Within their constraints, people choose what helps over what hurts. Finally, there is the possibility of generating powerful new social forces which can change existing patterns. Interest in personal health can be precisely this kind of force. The persuasive "Perspective on the Health of Canadians"[17] and the subsequent activities of the Long-range Planning Committee of the Canadian Department of Health and Welfare illustrate how many agencies might be mobilized in the interest of improved health and the prevention of disease. Consider first the contribution of industry (see Table 19-2).

Industry. The leadership in the control of obesity currently exercised by industry depends largely upon one type of activity: direct service to clients. But such direct service to clients is only one of five approaches which would seem ideally suited to industry efforts at research and development. The other four are development of new food products, delivery of food through restaurants and catering services, provision of opportunities for exercise through health clubs, health spas, and sporting goods manufacturers, and, finally, insurance incentives.

One of the most notable of the foods developed for weight reduction purposes was Metrecal, developed from the "Rockefeller Diet" of the mid-1950's. Metrecal was taken up by the public with an enthusiasm which astonished its pharmaceutical manufacturer, and it broke a variety of sales records before its poorly understood decline and fall. Diet foods have become increasingly popular since Metrecal, and low-calorie beverages are beginning to occupy an increasing part of the soft drink market. But the potential for development of new products for weight control seems virtually unlimited. Two promising new areas of research are the development of non-absorbable fats and non-nutritive sweeteners.

The third component of an integrated industry approach to weight reduction is comprised of the restaurant and food service industries. Despite the widespread concern with body weight on the part of vast numbers of persons who eat out, most find it awkward or impossible to secure satisfying low-calorie, non-atherogenic foods in restaurants. Even when restaurants serve low-calorie dishes, all too frequently the choice is limited and the selection uninspired. There is a great need for restaurants which serve an assortment of attractively prepared low-calorie dishes. This need could be met either by the establishment of specialty restaurants or, perhaps more promisingly, by modifying some of the items on the menus of traditional restaurants and by appropriate promotion of them. One pilot study has already produced encouraging results. A restaurant chain in Houston, Texas has begun to list the caloric content of a few items on its menu, selected for their limited fat and calories and prepared with polyunsaturated oils.[18] The initial response was an increase in consumption of these items sufficiently promising to induce the company to expand their number and to introduce a special menu to describe them.

The growth of large catering agencies which furnish complete food services for schools, businesses, and other institutions provides another important strategic opportunity for nutritional intervention. Large (and increasing) numbers

Table 19-2. Industry.

(Clinical) service delivery
Product development
Delivery systems-restaurants
Delivery systems-health clubs and spas
Insurance incentives

of people eat in facilities served by these agencies, and the nutritional education they receive in the process doubtless carries over to meals eaten elsewhere and to their future eating practices. Any improvement in the nutritional quality of the foods provided by these agencies would thus benefit vast numbers of people now and in the future. And such improvement need not await the uncertain outcome of efforts at building a market in the highly competitive restaurant business; it could flow directly from management decisions involving a small number of experts in the relevant disciplines. Indeed, the most successful of the "Diet and Exercise" efforts was that devoted to modifying the food served by large catering agencies.[19]

Health clubs and spas have already demonstrated their appeal to a large and growing market, even as free-standing enterprises. They might be more effective, and less costly, as part of an integrated network of weight reduction agencies which also included restaurants, food products for eating at home, and nutritional/behavioral programs of direct service to clients. Enlisting the sporting goods industry in such enterprises is an unexplored area of possibly great effectiveness.

The greatest potential for health behavior change by industry may lie in an almost totally unexplored agency — life and health insurance. Assessment of the risk of death and disability lies at the heart of the insurance industry and the industry has achieved remarkable accuracy in predicting such outcomes for population groups and in modifying predictions on the basis of changing health contingencies. It has not, however (with rare exceptions) attempted to alter these contingencies. In that direction may lie an unparalleled promise for the future. The insurance companies may well possess the most powerful incentives for health behavior change in our society today.

The Media. The results of the Stanford Heart Disease Prevention Program have documented the effectiveness of an integrated media campaign in changing unhealthy lifestyles in small populations. It has been followed by programs on at least two U.S. commercial television stations in which an attractive, mildly overweight newscaster has described and carried out a step-by-step description of a weight loss program over periods of 8-10 weeks. These programs demonstrated conclusively that commercial television can go far beyond its traditional health behavior functions of conveying information and, to some extent, attitudes, and can teach in an apparently persuasive manner health behavior skills such as weight control. Furthermore, by daily presentations and by the use of modeling, these efforts possess strengths that are not available to traditional clinical weight reduction programs. Unfortunately, these possibly quite effective programs were not evaluated. But we have learned from the large-scale German study described above how to carry out such an evaluation. The time is ripe for combined effort.

Education. Schools furnish a golden opportunity to provide nutritional education and practical experience with good nutrition. The current deterioration of food quality in American schools and the failure of the "Diet and Exercise" program to influence significantly the Swedish school system are particularly regrettable and suggest the importance of informing parents and school boards of the need for vigorous advocacy of a more adequate nutritional policy in the schools.

Failures of nutrition education do not, of course, stop at the elementary school level. The low state of nutrition education in schools of medicine must play a part in our nutritional problems, including obesity.

Government. The potential of government in the control of obesity is as yet almost totally unrealized. The taxing function could become a powerful tool for modifying health behavior: Just as improved health behavior might lead to lowered insurance premiums, so might it also lead to tax rebates. A second area where government could have a major impact is in the improvement of the nutrition of the vast number of government employees that it feeds every day, in and out of the military. Finally, the climax of a vigorous, integrated program of obesity control could be capped by the promotional activities of prominent government figures. Franklin Roosevelt had a great impact in transforming poliomyelitis from a feared plague to a national challenge. Here is a power which can be exercised with remarkably little cost to remarkably great effect.

Work site Treatment. A promising opportunity for changing health behavior is provided by the use of work sites for conducting medical service programs. "On the job training" has a long and honorable history in industry. On the job training for improved health behavior can be just as rewarding, to worker and employer alike. The potential of the work site as a locus for the provision of long-term health care has recently been demonstrated in a pilot project in an area related to obesity. Hypertension, like obesity, is rarely cured, but it does respond to effective and available treatment. A large percentage of hypertensive persons, however, receive treatment that is inadequate to control their blood pressure.[20] Thus, a survey of its members by the United Store Workers Union in New York City revealed that less than 50% of the hypertensives in conventional treatment had achieved satisfactory results. By contrast, a specially designed, union-sponsored work site program achieved long-term control of blood pressure in over 80% of hypertensives and radically reduced days of hospitalization for cardiovascular causes.[21] This chapter's author has recently completed a pilot study with this union, which showed that work site treatment for obesity was feasible and can be carried out by the workers themselves.

Voluntary Agencies. Some religions inculcate an enviable series of health behaviors in their members and offer assistance to others. The Smoking Cessation Clinics conducted by the Seventh Day Adventists are landmarks in such endeavors. Other health promotional activities could be carried out under other religious auspices; weight control would be a prime candidate.

Fraternal organizations often take a special interest in the health of others — the Shriners in crippled children and the Lions in those with visual impairment. An enlightened membership might decide to deal with its own health problems — obesity, for example — as well as those of its beneficiaries.

Recreational organizations have traditionally had a strong interest in health behavior. The gymnasiums of the Young Men's Christian Association are among the important health facilities of many American communities; they are now being increasingly utilized in the rehabilitation of patients following myocardial infarction. Obesity control would be a logical next target.

Voluntary health agencies, such as the Heart Associations in different countries, occupy a special position in the health care system. They have great promise for disseminating new information about weight control and new techniques for achieving it.

Youth groups have traditionally had a major concern for health. This concern can now be more effectively translated into action by use of the newer behavioral techniques.

Permutations and Combinations. This chapter has outlined what might be called single-factor approaches to the control of obesity. But future approaches are not likely to be limited to such inefficient, one-by-one forms of intervention. Combinations of different interventions seem particularly promising. Combining interventions may accomplish more than simply adding their effects; it may actually multiply them.

Summary

Systematic studies have shown that social forces exert a powerful influence upon the prevalence of human obesity. This susceptibility of obese persons to social forces has been utilized by behavior modifiers to construct programs of obesity control that are more effective than traditional ones. These programs have quite recently been successfully utilized with large population groups in the first approach to the control of obesity which is sufficiently broad to warrant description as a public health measure. But this is only a beginning. A variety of agencies and institutions stand at the threshold of major new capabilities of controlling obesity. Industry is the most developed. No less than five different potential agencies can be identified: clinical services, food product development, food delivery services, health clubs, and insurance incentives. But government, education, and numerous voluntary agencies are not far behind. Each could multiply its effectiveness by developing the enormous unused capabilities of the media for weight control. The prospects of work site health training programs are almost entirely unexplored. Development of the capabilities of any of these agencies will contribute significantly to the control of obesity. Combining their capabilities in integrated programs of weight control could bring as yet unimagined benefits.

Health promotional activities in the field of obesity have developed so rapidly in the very recent past that a comprehensive series of recommendations was one of the major products of the October 1977 Fogarty International Conference on Obesity. These recommendations follow.

Recommendations of the Fogarty International Conference on Obesity

The Public Sector *Education:* We recommend that the Federal Government encourage and coordinate public pronouncements on health behavior, including nutrition and exercises.

School experiences help to set the stage for later health practices, and therefore schools should be models for sound dietary and exercise patterns for a lifetime.

Regulation: We recommend extension of rules on labeling to emphasize caloric content of all packaged foods.

We recommend setting of standards to promote better nutrition as, for example, lowering the fat content of grades of meat and processed meat.

We recommend regulations requiring disclosure of caloric content of food in food advertising.

We recommend regulations encouraging the use of stairs instead of elevators in buildings, and facilities for walking and cycling instead of riding automobiles in communities.

Food service: We recommend that more options be provided for lower calorie and more nutritious selections in government-controlled food services.

Financial incentives: We recommend research to explore the feasibility of rewarding improved health behavior by means of tax rebates and lowered insurance premiums, the first carried out directly and the second encouraged by regulations.

The Private Sector We recommend that the food industry continue to develop more nutritious and lower calorie options (decreased energy density and/or decreased portion size) in processed food and that the price of these goods not add additional cost burden to the consumer.

We recommend that the food industry increase the information about calories and nutrients in processed foods.

We recommend that the restaurant and food service industries provide nutritional information about the foods they serve.

We recommend that both food catering services and institutions which feed their own employees provide options for lower calorie meals.

We recommend that life insurance and health insurance companies continue and expand their programs for public information and that they experiment with incentives for improved health behavior through variations in their rate structures.

We recommend that the communications industry explore the possibility of integration of health behavior messages throughout an entire network and that nutrition and exercise receive careful consideration as topics.

We recommend that the womens' magazines — a major source of information about obesity and its management — be enlisted in a more informed effort at reader education in this field.

We recommend that health clubs, sports clubs, and sporting goods manufacturers continue and expand their promotion of exercise and that they encourage also nutrition education.

We recommend that the medical services organized and/or sponsored by industry and labor unions provide also preventive services and that they evaluate these efforts.

Voluntary Agencies We recommend that the voluntary agencies continue and expand their traditional functions in the health area, including the promotion of better nutrition and exercise. We further recommend that they focus attention upon the health of their own members in addition to that of the groups which they have been organized to serve.

REFERENCES

1. Srole, L., Langner, T.S., Michael, S.T. *et al., Mental Health in the Metropolis: The Midtown Manhattan Study*. New York: McGraw-Hill, 1962.
2. Goldblatt, P.B., Moore, M.E., and Stunkard, A.J., "Social Factors in Obesity," *JAMA* 192:1039-1044, 1965.
3. Stunkard, A.J., "From Explanation to Action in Psychosomatic Medicine: The Case of Obesity," *Psychosomatic Medicine* 37:195-236, 1975.
4. Stunkard, A.J. and McLaren-Hume, M., "The Results of Treatment of Obesity: A Review of the Literature and Report of a Series," *Arch. Intern. Med.* 103:79-85, 1959.
5. Stuart, R.B., "Behavioral Control of Overeating," *Behav. Res. Ther.* 5:357-365, 1967.
6. Stunkard, A.J. and Mahoney, M., "Behavioral Treatment of the Eating Disorders," In *Handbook of Behavior Modification and Behavior Therapy*. Englewood Cliffs, New Jersey: Prentice-Hall, 1976, pp. 45-73.
7. Ferguson, J., *Learning to Eat, Leader Manual and Students Manual*. Palo Alto: Bull Publishing Company, 1975.
8. Harris, M.B., "Self-directed Program for Weight Control: A Pilot Study," *J. Abnorm. Psychol.* 74:263-270, 1969.
9. Wollersheim, J.R., "The Effectiveness of Group Therapy Based Upon Learning Principles in the Treatment of Overweight Women," *J. Abnorm. Psychol.* 76:462-474, 1970.
10. Penick, S.B., Filion, R.D.L., Fox, S., and Stunkard, A.J., "Behavior Modification in the Treatment of Obesity," *Psychosomatic Medicine* 33:49-55, 1971.

11. Stunkard, A.J., Levine, H., and Fox, S., "The Management of Obesity: Patient Self-help and Medical Treatment," *Arch. Intern. Med.* **125**:1367–1373, 1970; and Garb, J.R. and Stunkard, A.J., "A Further Assessment of the Effectiveness of TOPS in the Control of Obesity," *Arch Intern. Med.* **134**:716–720, 1974.

12. Levitz, L. and Stunkard, A.J., "A Therapeutic Coalition for Obesity: Behavior Modification and Patient Self-help," *Am. J. Psychiat.* **131**:423–427, 1974.

13. Farquhar, J.W., Maccoby, N.M., Wood, P.D., Alexander, J.K., Breitrose, H., Brown, B.W., Haskell, W.L., McAlister, A.L., Meyer, A.J., Nash, J.D., and Stern, M.P., "Community Education for Cardiovascular Health," *The Lancet*, June 4, 1977, pp. 1192–1195.

14. Isaksson, B., "Diet and Exercise. Assessment of the Swedish Program," in *Recent Advances in Obesity Research: II* J. Bray (Ed.) London, Newman Publishing, pp. 477–485.

15. *Ibid.*

16. McGovern, G., "Dietary Goals for the United States," *Report of the Select Committee on Nutrition and Human Needs of the United States Senate.* Washington, D.C.: U.S. Government Printing Office, 1977.

17. Lalonde, M., *A New Perspective on the Health of Canadians.* Ontario: Information Canada, 1974.

18. Scott, L. W., Foreyt, J., Manis, E., O'Malley, M.P. and Gotto, A. M., Jr. "A Low-Cholesterol Menu in a Steak Restaurant," *J. Am. Dietet. Assoc.* **74**: 54–56, 1979.

19. Isaksson, *op. cit.*

20. Wilber, J.A., "The Problem of Undetected and Untreated Hypertension in the Community," *Bull. N.Y. Acad. Med.* **49**:510–520, 1973.

21. Alderman, M.H. and Schoenbaum, E.E., "Detection and Treatment of Hypertension at the Work Site," *New Engl. J. Med.* **293**:65–68, 1975.

22. Stunkard, A. J. and Brownell, K. B. "Work Site Treatment for Obesity," Am. J. Psychiat. **137**: 252–253, 1980.

20

The North Karelia Project: Health Promotion in Action

Pekka Puska, M.D., Pol. Sc.

North Karelia Project
Epidemiological Research Unit
Central Public Health Lab.
Helsind, Finland

Principles of Comprehensive Community Programs for Control of Cardiovascular Diseases

Cardiovascular Diseases: A Public Health Problem. Cardiovascular diseases can be considered the main cause of mortality in the world. They are distributed all over the world. Some of these diseases are universal, although the prevalence rates vary in different regions. Some of these diseases occur only in certain geographical areas. In the developed countries, generally, approximately half of the deaths, nearly a third of the permanent invalidity, and a high proportion of the use of the basic health services are due to cardiovascular diseases.

It is already rather well known that the burden of coronary heart disease is not of equal size even in all developed countries. According to mortality statistics, the respective mortality rates of middle-aged males in Finland seem to be the highest. And, within Finland, it is the county of North Karelia in the East that occupies the worst position. This is confirmed by the results obtained from the World Health Organization (WHO) register study that also included non-fatal heart attacks. The annual incidence rate per 1000 males aged 20-64 seems to be roughly 1 in Sofia, 2 in Innsbruck, 3 in Warsaw, 4 in Prague, 5 in London, 6 in Helsinki, and 10 in North Karelia (which seems to be the highest known incidence rate in the world in this age group).

The high mortality and morbidity of cardiovascular diseases today are not connected only with the aging of the population. In many developed countries, some 40% of all the deaths in the middle-aged population are due to cardiovascular diseases, and about three-quarters of these are due to coronary heart disease. There are also good indications that this mortality among the middle-aged has, in many countries, considerably increased. The relevance of the problem for the middle-aged population is particularly evident in the most pathological areas: for instance, in the county of North Karelia in Eastern Finland, where approximately two-thirds of all the acute myocardial infarctions of males occur in the middle-aged group.

General Principles for Community Control of Cardiovascular Diseases. Considering the magnitude and nature of the problem, the facts that cardiovascular diseases are so common and that the preceding stages and risk factors involve a major proportion of the population, it is quite evident that we are dealing with a community problem. Accordingly, the aim should be the *control of these diseases in the whole community.* The attitude toward the problem should be similar to that toward controlling any epidemic in the community.

Because the cardiovascular diseases are connected with one another in many ways concerning their natural course or the needed control measures, it is sensible *to integrate the control activity in the community in a comprehensive way.* A comprehensive control program thus includes *primary prevention, treatment of the acute phase, rehabilitation,* and *evaluation and research.* Considering the community nature and the magnitude of the problem, it is natural to base the control program as part of *the existing service structure in the community;* that is, to direct and develop the existing services to meet the needs of the program. *The emphasis in the program should be in the primary prevention* of the disease, in which treatment in the clinical stage always has a limited role. Considering the high prevalence of the risk factors, primary prevention means an *activity practically directed to the whole population,* and not only to individuals who have clinically extreme findings. Because the task is essentially to influence people's behavior, and because we know that the development of these behaviors is in a complex way connected with the social structure of the community, the full support and involvement of the whole community is needed. This means a community action and a service structure supporting this; i.e., an activity which aims at establishing a healthy environment, healthy forms of health behavior, and comprehensive treatment of risk factors.

Community control of cardiovascular diseases implies that the scientific knowledge can be applied to help the population. Even if continuous basic biomedical research is of extreme importance in the control of cardiovascular diseases, the main steps at present depend on the progress in the field of application of the already existing knowledge for people's benefit. Final scientific proofs of the possibilities to prevent coronary heart disease may never be obtained from controlled trials, since large numbers of people and many years are needed, and many human and behavioral problems are encountered. Instead, carefully evaluated programs can gradually diminish the level of uncertainty and guide the progress in the society. The control of cardiovascular diseases should accordingly be *implemented in the form of a systematic and planned program, the contents of which are determined by sound review of the existing knowledge and by many local factors, and which is followed by appropriate evaluation*, upon which continuous decisions concerning the program can be made.

In the first stage, it is advisable to implement the control program in a *restricted area* ("pilot" area or "model" area) and under so thorough scientific evaluative research that the feasibility, the (favorable and unfavorable) effects, and the ratio of costs and benefits can be evaluated. When the activity later on is applied on a national level, the evaluation of the effects can, at best, be restricted only to the follow-up of the main indicators of the success of the program. This is important because later on, in the changing morbidity situation, an intensive, large-scale intervention and an extensive program can be unnecessary considering the ratio of costs and effects.

Implementation of the North Karelia Project

Start of the North Karelia Project. Faced with the exceptionally big problem of cardiovascular diseases (CVD) in North Karelia, the representatives of the local population in North Karelia signed a petition in 1971, asking for national assistance to reduce the high mortality and frequency of cardiovascular diseases. After the planning stage, the North Karelia project was launched, in 1972, to meet the urgent need of the local population. The project was to consist of a systematic, comprehensive community program to control cardiovascular diseases in the county of North Karelia — a mainly rural area with some 180,000 inhabitants — and its scientific evaluation.

Planning of the Program. In the planning stage, it was decided to start a comprehensive cardiovascular community program integrated with the service structure and the social organization of the community. The comprehensive intervention was planned to consist of both primary and secondary prevention.

The *main objective* of the program was defined to be decrease of the CVD morbidity and mortality among the North Karelia population, and especially the middle-aged male population. The epidemiological consideration of the available information from abroad and from Finland, as well as the situation in North Karelia, led to a heavy emphasis on primary prevention of the numerous disease attacks by a general reduction of the risk factors of smoking, serum cholesterol (i.e., change of diet), and high blood pressure among the population. The generally high level of these risk factors among the male population in the area has been shown. It can be mentioned that it is a matter of mainly rural people who carry out heavy exercise in their work and are rarely overweight. Because of the need to establish a comprehensive program, activities to promote secondary prevention had also to be considered.

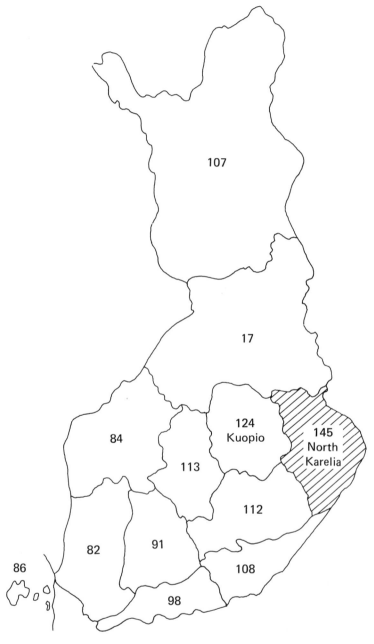

Figure 20-1. Age-standardized mortality from ischaemic heart diseases in Finnish counties in 1969 (100 = whole country).

After having set the main objectives of the program, the *intermediate objectives* were outlined: i.e., those factors through which it was likely to arrive at the main objectives. The basis was the epidemiological knowledge about the natural course of the disease (about the risk factors through which the occurrence or progress of the disease could be changed). At the same time, consideration was given to the prevalence of these factors in the target population. Considering the complex problems of the community intervention, it was decided to restrict the program to only a few factors of strategical importance. Those were chosen to be smoking, serum cholesterol (diet), and hypertension.

Accordingly, chosen as *intermediate objectives* were 1) reduction of smoking, serum cholesterol, and high blood pressures in the community (primary prevention), and 2) to promote early detection, treatment, and rehabilitation of heart disease patients. As a national pilot program under the national health authorities, the *national objective* was to test the feasibility and effect of this type of community control of CVD and to provide tested field methods for national use concerning CVD and related health problems.

When the intermediate objectives of the program had been outlined it was possible to start developing the contents of the program; i.e., the measures through which it would be possible to arrive at the intermediate objectives. The contents of this program were built up from practical *measures* or *services*, the nature of which were to depend on the local conditions.

Before planning the details of the program, background information of the problem in the community was collected, and a kind of "community diagnosis" was made. The aim of this was to obtain a comprehensive picture of the baseline situation for a deeper understanding of the problem and the strategical factors to be intervened upon. It was also to form the basis for continuous analysis of the changes in the community.

Important was *epidemiological knowledge* about the disease or diseases, the mortality and the morbidity, the distribution of this within different groups in the population, the factors possibly influencing the natural course of the disease, and the prevalence of these factors in the target population. It was also important to understand the typical features of the population and the area. It was essential to have good information on the forms of behavior related to the risk factors, on the ongoing process in the community concerning these behaviors and behavior complexes, and on the leadership and social interaction structure in the community. For the implementation of the program, the support of the population was essential: this is why it was attempted to find out how the population and its representatives saw the problem and how they felt about the possibilities to solve it. The same concerned the health personnel working in the area, because the program would be, to a great extent, dependent upon on their cooperation. Before implementing the program, it was also necessary to have information about the *resources* and the type of *service structure* existing in the community.

Finally, in the planning and implementation of the program much had to be built upon *previous development and outside expert opinion*. The elements in the control of coronary heart disease have been developed within the cardiovascular program of the WHO during the last few years. Concerning primary prevention of coronary heart disease, especially important are the recommendations of the expert working groups in Rome (1972), Innsbruck (1973), and Berlin /GDR (1976). The elements of a comprehensive community program of CDV have since been further outlined by the WHO Expert Group in Koli (1976).

Concerning the mass nature of the cardiovascular program and the fact that the problem is closely related to the behavior and lifestyles in the community, the program could be built only as part of the service structure and the social organization of the community. The services had to fit into the social and cultural situation of the individuals, the groups, and the whole community. In order to involve the whole community, a general "community action" was found necessary in mobilizing the community resources, and this was to be supported by a systematic service structure. In order to reach the whole population, the basic services were planned to be delivered in a systematic and "routine" way, often integrated in all the services.

The following were the main elements of the intervention: services to change the *environment* were planned (many of them, unfortunately, were not available for a local health program); general *information and health education* to the public was to make the population aware of the problem and the methods to solve it (which usually implied the participation of the population itself); and, in a key position, were *individual services*, to be developed and created so that the need of the program could be included in every possible case in a systematic way. Because primary prevention was so essential, it was found to be of special importance to deliver these services for the population in a simple and routine way, in the daily living conditions of the population, and in a way socially and economically acceptable to the population. An important element of the program was *training and further education* of the personnel, especially health personnel, participating in the program. This training was to cover both the general principles of the program and the practical tasks that each personnel group was supposed to do within the program. Within the program, *information services* were developed to help to manage and direct the activities from the single field worker to the leaders of the program. This implied different kinds of forms, from the practical patient files to special disease registers (etc.).

Evaluation of the Program. Evaluation was planned as an integral part of the program. The tools for the evaluation were the information services by which the development of the program could be followed and the indicators of the objectives measured. The evaluation of the program and its information services can, in principle, be divided into two parts: internal and external.

Every practical subprogram had to include such information services, which helped to arrange the services within the program and to enable the individual worker to follow the impact of his work. This *internal evaluation* consisted of files, patient cards, etc. This type of information could, of course, mainly not be used in the scientific external evaluation of the program, due to bad standardization and often inadequate coverage. However, these information services have had a most central role in the operation of the program.

The *external evaluation* was carried out at the research center of the project attached to the University of Kuopio. This kind of evaluation and *evaluative research* were especially important for the program because they assessed the *feasibility and effect* of the program, the *costs*, and the *process* that actually had taken place.

The evaluation of the feasibility of the program was to reveal to what extent it had been possible to implement the practical activities that had been planned. The necessary information was obtained from the description of the activities and from various statistics on the activities. In the assessment of the *effect* of the program, the achievement of the main and intermediate objectives were followed during the program period. Because the observed changes could have been due to other development than that caused by the program, it was necessary to follow the indicators of the objectives in the same way in another reference community, as similar as possible to the program community.

The assessment of the *costs* of the program was to enable one to get a picture of the ratio between costs and effects in the program or the efficiency of the program. Careful assessment of the costs involved in the program should give information not only about the costs of the total program but also about the relative costs involved in various subprograms. By detailed and comprehensive information, it was aimed to get a careful picture what kind of *process* in the target community really led to the achievement or non-achievement of the objectives. It is especially important in a scientific evaluative research to reveal not only the intended effects but also the possible unintended effects, both positive and negative. Examples of negative unintended effects could be side-effects caused by increased medication, decrease of income in some population groups (for example, producers), and increase of stress due to anti-smoking health education.

The methods for the evaluation and the information system for monitoring the changes in the community included in the project for the *main objectives*, a *myocardial infarction and stroke register* and *mortality and hospital data*, and, for the *intermediate objectives, random sample surveys* covering risk factors and other information. A comprehensive survey was carried out in the program community and in the matched reference community at the beginning and at the end of the five-year program period (baseline survey, terminal survey). In addition, a lot of other information was collected to follow changes in the program area (especially so-called follow-up surveys, done by mail twice a year to different random samples of the middle-aged population).

Implementation of the Program. Subprograms were established to work toward ameliorating each of the three risk factors for coronary disease on a community-wide basis.

Smoking: A county-wide campaign to reduce and, where possible, to eliminate cigarette smoking in the population was launched in 1972. Laws were passed banning smoking in all public vehicles and public buildings. This was supplemented by anti-smoking posters in public places, lectures in schools, and anti-smoking advertisements in newspapers, on radio, and on television. Special efforts were made to reduce the incidence of smoking among health personnel, teachers, and those individuals identified by screening programs as at high risk for developing CVD or in whom disease was already present. Group therapy sessions for confirmed smokers were also established.

Diet: This program sought primarily to reduce to total fat consumption in the regular diet of the people of North Karelia, where dairy products, sausages, industry, low-fat (and then non-fat) milk was introduced and became the staple dietary product. Margarine was substituted for butter and even the ubiquitous sausage was modified to include 25% mushrooms to lower the fat content. Use of vegetable oil was encouraged. The consumption of fresh vegetables, seldom seen in the standard diet of the North Karelians, was encouraged even to the point of having families establish vegetable plots. In addition, high-risk individuals with hypercholesterolemia not normalized by dietary change were placed on lipid-lowering agents.

Hypertension: A county-wide screening program to detect individuals with elevated arterial blood pressure was undertaken. Those with hypertension were registered in the special register and usually placed on anti-hypertensive therapy, followed by public health nurses operating out of special dispensaries.

Other programs: Special efforts were made to identify individuals with clinically evident coronary heart disease and, if they were not already under a physician's care, to initiate treatment. Coronary care units were either established or improved in the main hospitals of the county; these were supplemented by improved ambulance and mobile coronary care transportation. In addition, community programs to teach cardiopulmonary resuscitation were established. A rehabilitation program was also started for the medical follow-up of patients who had suffered acute myocardial infarction. This included organized group activity for secondary prevention and rehabilitation. In addition, a separate, intensified service was established for primarily the middle-aged male population found to be at high risk for CVD.

It is to be emphasized that all of these programs were organized on a community basis with wide public participation. The aim was to establish a county-wide framework for the necessary basic services to reach everybody in the community in need of the service in question, and to support that with a major community action.

Most of the programs began in 1972, with intense public education through the news media and community meetings. By 1973, most of the individual services (screening programs, hypertension, clinics, hospital and out-patient services for patients with CVD and rehabilitation programs) had been established: efforts to introduce environmental changes were also well underway. By 1976, efforts were being made to continue the community effort to reduce CVD risk after the project period ended in 1977. This involved the training of lay people as "agents" on CVD control to continue educational efforts and to maintain local community services.

Management of the Program. The program had been implemented as an integrated activity in the existing service structure and social organization of the county, with the administrative body the Department of Social and Health Affairs of the county. Thus, the Chief of the Department had been responsible for the final decisions. In addition to the "normal" staff of the department (the county medical officer and two county public health nurses), extra persons were employed because of the project (a health education secretary, a nutritional secretary, an office secretary, and two clerical persons). In addition, the director of the project, who was in charge of the general planning and coordination, and other research investigators, were in continuous contact about the intervention with the staff of the department.

The running of the program was continuously discussed at the steering committee of the project, which was an advisory body of the department. The steering committee was comprised of the above-mentioned officials plus some other key persons of the community. The program was divided into practical subprograms. Every subprogram had a responsible person to annually make the proposal for the next two years' plan and, twice a year, the practical plan for the next half year. The principal investigator was to make the final proposal of the whole program for the steering committee.

Based on these plans, the people of the project have run the practical program. To a great extent, it has been done by official orders to the health centers (which are responsible for the basic health services in the area) and supported by educational meetings and courses for the health personnel arranged by the department. Direct contacts have been taken to various institutions in the community: other sectors of county administration, voluntary organizations, food producers, etc. Suitable health education material has been produced by the project to be distributed through various channels in the community.

Practical Contents of the Intervention. TV has not been available, because there are no local TV possibilities. Local radio programs have frequently been used.

The project has had continuous personal contacts with the few reporters of the local radio and some official contacts with the management in Helsinki to get the formal support. The reporters are constantly given news about the project for the local news transmission. Extra programs about practical aspects and activities of the project are made jointly with the reporters and the project staff. The types of programs has been interviews, lectures, courses, question/answer (for example, a smoking cessation course, a nutritional lecture series).

All the county newspapers have actively published articles, news, and other texts on the risk factors and the activities of the project. Most of the texts are prepared by the journalist in cooperation with the project. There has been a text concerning the theme approximately every second day throughout the years of the intervention.

The project has prepared a set of leaflets on the prevention of heart disease. The texts have been prepared jointly with the staff of the project, national experts, and local people. The leaflets have been printed in the local printing companies owned by the local newspapers. The leaflets have been distributed personally in connection with the created services in the area.

Several posters have been prepared by the project and printed locally. The posters are designed and used to support the activities in the field.

Jointly with the county school department, various campaigns have been carried out at the local schools. Usually, the material for a specific activity has been prepared by the project, and sent to all the schools in the area by the project with the administrative orders of the school department about the contents of the activity.

Various kinds of health education gathering have constantly been arranged in the area. Many voluntary organizations are interested in the topic, and experts on the project are continuously asked to lecture. More systematic occasions have been arranged, especially by the local heart associations and the local housewives' associations ("Martha Associations"), which operate in every local community. They both have an administration on the county level, which are in continuous personal contact with the project. The heart associations organize meetings for small local communities, usually with a doctor addressing the people. The Martha Associations organize meetings for local housewives, especially with nutritional information.

The health personnel are mainly employed by the health centers or the hospitals. Training courses or meetings are organized by the county health administration as official training for the personnel. The project plans the contents of the training based on the practical tasks of the various personnel groups in the subprograms of the project. The members of staff of the project give themselves a major part of the teaching. In addition, the project prepares written texts, guidelines, memorandums, feedback of the activities, etc., which are sent to the personnel. The county health department and the project encourages practical and systematic local training at the health center level.

Through the respective county departments, the project participates in the regular training courses of other personnel groups, teaching them the background of the activities and their practical tasks in the program. Leaders and counselors of the voluntary organizations have been trained for the purpose of their tasks in the subprograms. Journalists and reporters have been trained, as well, through courses, meetings, and personal contacts.

Different types of community leaders are taught by the county health department and the project. In the first instance, a practical list of approximately 1200 key persons, including labor leaders and leaders of various civic organizations, was used for mailing leaflets and the bulletin of the project. Community councils were contacted by the project. At a later phase, a systematic program for training voluntary lay people as "agents" of CVD control has been carried out jointly by the project and the county heart association, giving them practical tasks in their own neighborhoods.

A systematic organization of basic public health services is a major component of the intervention. Especially the health services (especially health center activity), but also other services, have been carefully analyzed by the staff of the project. Based on this and on the objectives of the program, the practical subprograms have been developed. The subprograms include detailed instructions about what tasks should be carried out by various normal basic services in order to meet the needs of the CVD control program. The implementation of these activities has been realized by official instructions of the county health administration and the administration of the health centers and by the above-mentioned training activity. Some health center activities have been partly run or assisted by voluntary organizations (myocardial infarction rehabilitation groups by local heart associations). To instruct, ensure, and check the activities at the local communities, the staff of the county health department and the project make regular visits to the local communities to have meetings with the community leaders and the leading workers of the health center. At these meetings, the situation of the subprograms in the respective communities are analyzed. Through this mechanism, the activities have been integrated in the administrative five-year planning system of the health centers.

In addition to the official public services, several other organizations give to the population services supporting the project. The Martha Associations organize counseling of the housewives in the preparing of food. The nutritionists of the project, together with the staff of the Martha county organization, have prepared detailed "packages" for a nutritional counseling to instruct the housewives to prepare healthy types of dishes. Institutes for the education of the adult population have, on the request of the project, included several courses to the population on various health education topics.

Gradually, new, specific, and deeper services have been introduced in the area to support the basic activities in the subprograms. These have been prepared and tested by the project and introduced gradually through the most feasible channels. They include anti-smoking groups, nutritional groups, and special activities for the drop-outs of the hypertension program.

Environmental changes have been mainly restricted to the possibilities within the national legislation (i.e., to the decisions that can be made locally). The project has, however, in some cases, contributed to national decisions supporting a desired activity in North Karelia.

On the recommendation of the county health administration and the project, the local community administrations have contacted health centers, schools, voluntary organizations, restaurants, and offices to ask them to prohibit or restrict smoking in their facilities. To facilitate this, signs ("DO NOT SMOKE HERE — we participate in the North Karelia project") have been distributed by the project through mail (to all public addresses) and through other channels in great amounts. The project has contacted public transportation organizations, which, jointly with the project, have introduced non-smoking in public vehicles.

Great proportions of the total fat consumed in the area come from the dairy products. In the area, there is one great dairy (serving most of the area) and a smaller dairy (in the Northern part). There has been close personal contact between the staff of the project and the management of each dairy to find low-fat products that are advantageous for the dairy and to promote their consumption. Accordingly, new products have been introduced and special campaigns carried out.

A lot of fatty sausage is consumed in the area. Contact between the staff of the project and the managerial persons of the sausage company, some of whom participated as patients in the rehabilitation groups of the project, has led to two types of low-fat sausage being developed and introduced, and joint campaigns have been carried out.

Vegetables are expensive and not easily obtainable in the shops of the area. Accordingly, the project has asked all the counseling organizations in the area to carry out practical campaigns to get people to grow vegetables themselves in the spring and later on to harvest, store, prepare, and use them. This is supported by general information.

The project has contacted the shops to promote the possibilities of the population's obtaining the recommended food. The county health administration has asked all health inspectors in the county to collect structured information on the marketing and advertising of tobacco products. They are asked, through their normal shop visits, to draw the shopkeepers' attention to the attempts to reduce smoking and to change the dietary habits.

The services used to guide and manage the activities of the project are called "information services." Hypertensive patients (in the register) and myocardial infarction patients (in the rehabilitation groups) each have a special card giving information both to the patient and to different health workers. Various patient files have been influenced by the project by training and official orders to include the practical information needed by the workers to get feedback about their work in the subprograms of the project. Every hypertensive is registered and followed up annually. The project runs a central register, but copies of the record form are at the health centers. The project gives continuous feedback to the health centers and the personnel from the computerized central register, in the form of reports and memorandums.

The project runs a centralized and computerized myocardial infarction and stroke register based on the standardized data collected by special nurses at the health centers and the hospitals. The project gives continuous feedback about the register concerning the amount and type of disease attacks and factors associated with them to the health centers and their personnel.

To monitor the changes in some of the key indicators of the intermediate objectives of the program, a postal survey is made by the project twice a year, every time for a different random sample of the 25–59-year-old population (N = 2500). By these trends (smoking and nutritional habits, blood pressure measurements, and the use of anti-hypertensive drugs, for instance), the whole population is followed. The trends and other results concerning the area and are continuously related to the personnel. The population is also informed.

Other available information is collected by the staff of the project and distributed to personnel in the field for the benefit of the guidance of the activities. The health centers make annual reports to the county and to national administration. These reports include some key elements of the CVD control program and are used in the continuous planning of the program.

Experiences

Interim Results. During the first four-and-a-half years (1972–1976), the feasibility of the program was good in the area with rather scarce medical resources. The cooperation of the local population, community leaders, and health personnel has been experienced in many ways; participation rates to the surveys have averaged 90%. There is no question that a major community action has been accomplished.

So far, no final results from the evaluation (most data from the reference area) are available, but a lot of information is already at hand about the changes in the program area, and clear changes were noticed during the program period in the indicators of the intemediate objectives in the community.

An interim evaluation of changes in the community during the first four-and-a-half years indicates that smoking among males was reduced from 54% to 43%. Smoking remained at a level of 12% among females. The decrease of smoking among males was observed both in rural and urban area, in different socioeconomic groups, and especially among individuals at high cardiovascular risk. Approximately 38% of the smokers who attended a smoking cessation group had remained non-smokers six months later. The preliminary five-year "terminal" data confirm the above-mentioned reduction in the percentage of male smokers in the area. It showed reduction also in the reference area, although not of the same magnitude.

Considerable dietary changes have been observed: the percentage of males who consume low-fat milk increased from 17% to 50% and that of users of butter on bread decreased from 86% to 69%. The percentage of males who reported to use at least 10 grams of fat on bread reduced from 60% to 38%. The serum cholesterol was measured for more than half of the middle-aged males in the community. The preliminary results concerning the five-year changes in the serum cholesterol level indicate among males an average reduction of 10 milligrams in the area, compared with no change in the reference area.

Since the beginning of the program, blood pressure measurements gradually increased so that they covered practically the whole population. The number of registered hypertensives increased so that, at the end of 1976, nearly 17,000 hypertensives were registered, which approaches 9% of the total population. Out of these subjects, more than half became aware of their condition only during the program. The frequency of the control visits of those with known

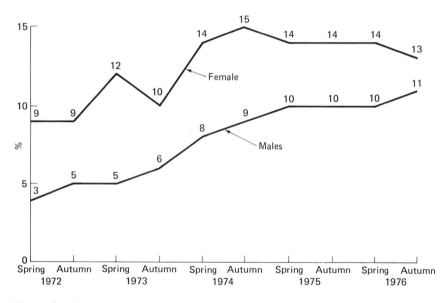

Figure 20-2. Percentage of persons under anti-hypertensive drug treatment amonth the 25-59 year-old population in North Karelia.

hypertension increased so that it led within the first years to an adequate situation for practically every known hypertensive.

An interim study showed also that adherence to the follow-up and to the treatment were good. During the first year, only 1% of the registered missed their annual follow-up visit. The adherence to the treatment was then 94%.

After four-and-a-half years of the intervention, the proportion of the middle-aged population under anti-hypertensive drug treatment increased among the males from 3 to 11 and among the females from 9 to 13 (Figure 20-2). According to the register, the percentage of normotensive subjects increased during the first year from 12 to 28, and at the fourth follow-up to 38. The mean change in blood pressure during the first year was a 15 mm Hg reduction in the systolic and a 6 mm Hg reduction in the diastolic blood pressure for those patients who had had this follow-up. It must be noticed that 65% of these hypertensives were already under drug treatment at the time of the registration.

Preliminary data from the five-year terminal survey indicate that the proportion of elevated diastolic blood pressure values ($> = 95$ mm Hg) in the whole community reduced among males by 25% and among females by 45%. They showed practically no improvement in the reference area.

According to the myocardial infarction register that has been operating in the area throughout the period following WHO criteria, the annual incidence rate of acute myocardial infarction among middle-aged (30-64) males was 13.8 per 1000 in 1972, remained stable during the following years, and was 13.9 in 1975, but started to reduce after that and was 10.9 in 1977 (Table 20-1). A preliminary observation has also been made that there is a change from the more severe "definite" cases toward the less severe (so-called "possible") cases.

In the respective annual incidence rate of strokes, a drop has been seen from the third year onwards: from 2.6 per 1000 in 1972 to 1.8 in 1975, among males, and from 2.1 to 1.3 among females (aged 30-64). The low level has been maintained in the continuation.

Table 20-1. Annual incidence rates of acute myocardial infarction among the population aged 30-64 during 1972-1977 in North Karelia, according to the register (preliminary data).

		Annual Incidence Rate per 1000 Persons				
	1972	1973	1974	1975	1976	1977
Males	13.8	14.3	13.7	13.9	11.6	10.9
Females	2.6	2.7	3.1	2.8	2.6	2.4

Table 20-2. Annual total mortality rates among males and females aged 30-64 during 1972-1977 in North Karelia. (preliminary data).

	1972	Annual Mortality Rate per 1000 Persons				
		1973	1974	1975	1976	1977
Males	11.9	12.5	12.4	12.5	11.6	10.6
Females	4.6	4.3	3.8	3.8	3.6	4.0

Table 20-2 shows how the reduction in the cardiovascular accidents is also reflected in a reduction of the total mortality rates of both males and females in the area.

Other Experiences. The good feasibility and full support for the program in the community has been mentioned earlier. Also a great national interest has been observed, which, of course, could make the use of the reference area more difficult.

The project has been financed by funds of the Finnish government (funds from both scientific and health service sources). The annual budget of the project organization has been only approximately $250,000. The cost of the activities in the community is much greater, and, as stated, is a target of the evaluation. It can be noticed, however, that the program has been implemented in the health services practically without any extra resources for the program. There are also indications that most of the activities have been accomplished by a more effective and systematic use of resources, and that the share of total resources used for CVD control might not have much increased.

In order to acquire information about the opinions of the activities among the local health personnel and the decision-makers, a special survey was made in the area and in the reference area. These groups were asked how sufficient they felt the various CVD control measures to be in their own health centers. There was a clear difference between the counties: The North Karelian subjects were more satisfied with the CVD control activities in their own health centers than were their counterparts from the reference area with their services. This was the case for all the aspects included. The North Karelian subjects were especially more satisfied with the hypertension control and the heart disease patients rehabilitation as well as with CVD control in general. Health personnel more often expressed satisfaction with the CVD control activities than did decision-makers, who often demanded still more sufficient activities.

With this kind of intensified activity within the given resources, there is always a danger that other fields of health care will become neglected. Thus, in the study, the subjects were asked about the sufficiency of other activities in their health care centers. There were no marked differences between the counties

Table 20-3. Opinions of health personnel and local decision-makers about the sufficiency of the health center activities in North Karelia (NK) and the reference county (Ref.).

Activity	Consider the activity to be sufficient in the local health center:					
	Physicians		Public Health Nurses		Decision-makers	
	NK (%)	Ref. (%)	NK (%)	Ref. (%)	NK (%)	Ref. (%)
CVD control						
CVD control in general	52	18	49	7	20	7
Anti-smoking	45	30	34	19	28	18
Nutritional education	35	13	31	18	24	10
Hypertension control	79	42	90	47	45	31
Heart disease patients' rehabilitation	52	13	44	9	21	8
Health examinations	59	35	49	23	28	22
Other health activities						
Physicians' appointments	47	42	48	42	43	38
Child and maternity counseling	73	75	91	80	88	77
School health	61	63	77	78	65	65
Domestic care	24	23	35	34	23	24
Occupational health	34	28	34	24	34	31
Function of the health center as a whole	43	42	38	39	42	40

in this respect — these other services in North Karelia were considered to be at least as often sufficient as in the reference county. Among health personnel in North Karelia, the satisfaction with the CVD control activities was higher than the satisfaction with the function of the health center in general, while the situation was the reverse in the reference area (Table 20-3).

Conclusion

Cardiovascular diseases constitute a major health problem in most of the world, and in the developed countries the improvement of the health situation of the populations is heavily dependent upon the success in the control of these diseases. Accordingly, health services should strive at the control of cardiovascular diseases in the community. Because the diseases, their precursors, and their risk factors are so common, the control programs should be directed to the entire population in a comprehensive way.

Because of the nature of the diseases, the potential progress in their control lies on primary prevention, which is based on general reduction of the known risk factors. The programs should be planned in a systematic way — including a hierarchy of objectives and a collection of comprehensive background information of the problem and the community. The program should be implemented in a systematic way and integrated with the existing service structure and the social organization of the community. An appropriate information system is necessary to guide the program and to evaluate its results. The evaluation should aim at assessing the feasibility, effects, and costs of the program and at obtaining a reliable picture of the overall changes in the community.

The exceptionally pathological situation in the county of North Karelia in Eastern Finland led to a strong local demand for control of cardiovascular diseases in the area. After a careful planning stage, the North Karelia project was launched to carry out a systematic community program based on the principles stated above. The comprehensive community program was started in the area in 1972, under the Finnish health authorities, and assisted by the WHO, to form a pilot program for the national planning.

The main objective of the program was a decrease in the mortality and morbidity of acute myocardial infarction in the population, and especially in the middle-aged population, which has relatively the highest risk. The implementation of the program took place in a systematic way and integrated with the social organization and the health services of the area, and with strong community participations. The project included a scientific evaluation of a five-year period of the program.

The experiences gained so far have shown that the comprehensive program was feasible and was strongly supported by the population. The available information indicates that there are clear changes in the indicators of the intermediate objectives toward the wanted direction: smoking has reduced, dietary habits have changed, and hypertension control has greatly improved in the community. There is also some preliminary information about favorable changes in the mortality and morbidity, although it is very early for such conclusions. The program in North Karelia will continue, and follow-up and risk indicators are organized to assess the long-term changes.

Based on the positive experiences gained so far, many of the methods used in the project have already been planned for the national control of cardiovascular diseases through respective national plans. It is felt that community-based and systematic programs integrated with the existing services and with built-in evaluation are needed for the control of cardiovascular diseases, as well as many other great health problems of our times.

21

Incentives for Health Through Educational and Medical Services*

Emily H. Mudd, Ph.D.

Helen O. Dickens, M.D.

Celso-Ramon Garcia, M.D.

Karl Rickels, M.D.

Ellen W. Freeman, Ph.D.

George R. Huggins, M.D.

Jacqueline J. Logan

Department of Obstetrics/Gynecology
Department of Psychiatry
University of Pennsylvania

Introduction

A long-overlooked area for developing incentives for health is that of the provision of educational and medical services for teenagers. In the health services program conducted for high school students by the Medical School and Hospital of the University of Pennsylvania, three incentives for personal involvement in health care were identified:

1. Educational discussion groups to promote sharing of ideas among peers and among professionals and patients.

*This project was made possible, in part, through grants from The Lebensburger Foundation and the Foundation for Educational and Social Development. The authors acknowledge with appreciation the participation of Pearl Jimperson, nurse adolescent educator, and the assistance and cooperation of the entire clinic staff of the Family Planning Service, all of who functioned with tact and caring.

2. Medical services offered with concern for educational and emotional guidance and support.
3. Opportunities for continuing contact with a health program through frequent appointments and individualized counseling services related to sexuality and health care.

The aim of these incentives is to develop sound principles of self-management among young people who are building the foundations of their future behavior patterns and formulating their attitudes about their own roles in the promotion and preservation of health.

The Problem

In the nuclear family structure of our society today, an adolescent may have no clear concept of his or her relationship to health care services. On one hand, teenagers are viewed as children who depend on parental guidance and consent. On the other hand, they may be biologically capable of establishing families themselves.

In 1976 and 1977, one-fifth of all U.S. births were to teenagers. Females age 17 and younger constitute the only age group in the U.S. for which the birth rate has not declined. Between 1970 and 1974, births to 14-year-old females increased from 6.6 to 7.2 per 1000 births; for 15-year-old females, it rose from 14.7 to 19.2; and, for 16-year-olds it decreased to 37/7 per 1000.[1]

The Pilot Program

Personnel in the department of Obstetrics and Gynecology in the school of Medicine of the University of Pennsylvania have been concerned for a number of years with adolescent health care.[2] Three years ago, a health education and medical service program for never-pregnant high school students was initiated in cooperation with several city high schools. The program has two distinct components:

1. Through cooperation with schools, it strives to reach students through presentations and discussions in school classrooms (before pregnancy occurs).
2. It offers continuing consultative and supportive services without fee to students who request contraceptives. It also responds to students who request medical or counseling services, and, if necessary, provides referral without fee.

The program includes a series of six instruction and discussion sessions offered in classes in three high schools. These sessions stress attitudes and personal relationships as part of health care. Topics include menstruation and pregnancy, venereal disease, family planning, and social and sexual attitudes. Classes are led by members of the hospital team, who are assisted by classroom teachers. This team also works in the hospital Family Planning Service and interviews and counsels students who later apply for medical services. At the end of each classroom series, any student may request contraceptives or other gynecological services during school hours or on Saturdays at the Hospital Family Planning Service Examinations, counseling, and contraceptives are given without charge or parental consent. Anonymity is respected. Continued student contact is explicitly sought by scheduling a follow-up visit in six weeks, followed by visits every three months, or as prescribed, for a minimum period of two years.

The Pilot Study

Areas for further program development have been explored. All students who enrolled in this Family Planning Program were followed for the duration of their enrollment. The data allow comparisons of the demographic and emotional factors of girls who continued contraceptive use with girls who discontinued the program or who had unplanned pregnancies after enrollment in the program. This investigation is an initial step in the process of exploring how teenagers experience their sexuality and the kinds of health services they need and use.

All students in the study of never-pregnant girls were unmarried and were attending high school. Parental consent was not required for contraceptive treatment. The importance of this issue in teenage programs is reflected by the fact that nearly half of the group (46%) stated that their parents did not know about their contraceptive use. Most students (88%) chose oral contraceptives; 4% chose the IUD; 2% chose foam; and one student selected the diaphragm (6% did not elect to use contraceptives because they stated they were not sexually active). Ten students who were pregnant by the time of their initial visits were referred to obstetrical services and were not enrolled in the contraceptive program.

Results

Continuing Contraceptors. During 1973-1975, 161 students enrolled in the Family Planning Service, and 94 students could have continued for two years. Of those 94 students, 63% continued the contraceptive program for one year without pregnancy; 34% continued the program for two years without pregnancy.

The continuation rate of approximately 63% of students in the program through one year may be compared to continuation rates of 34-80% reported by U.S. family planning programs designed to serve all women of reproductive age.[3] Teen clinic reports show an even broader range of continuation rates for participation than do programs serving all women of reproductive ages. One teen clinic program reported a low continuation rate of 23% after one year[4] while another reported a 97.5% rate of continuation.[5]

Occurrence of Pregnancy. Sixteen unplanned pregnancies occurred among 161 students enrolled in the program: an incidence of 10% of the total program. In addition, there were 5 planned pregnancies which occurred after a year or more of contraceptive use.

Social and Demographic Characteristics. The small group who had unplanned pregnancies were compared with those who continued contraceptive use. The social and demographic data indicated only one significant difference: older girls (16-18 at time of pregnancy) were more likely to have unplanned pregnancies than younger girls (14-15 at time of pregnancy). A possible explanation could be that older girls experience more regular sexual activity.

No other comparisons showed significant differences. It was found that younger girls (14-15 at enrollment) were as likely to continue in the program as were older girls (16-18 at enrollment). Parental knowledge of contraceptive use did not differ between girls who continued contraceptive use and girls who became pregnant. Whether the student lived in a single-parent household headed by the mother or in a two-parent household did not affect statistics. Nearly all students indicated their relationships with their parents were "happy" or "average."

Emotional Assessments. We have begun investigation of attitudional, personality, and emotional factors involved in the election and discontinuation of contraceptives. The aim is to identify predictors of effective/ineffective contraceptive use and to develop services which best meet the health needs of these teenagers. Preliminary findings have appeared:

1. Those teenagers who continued in the program and those who discontinued did not differ on the nine symptom distress dimensions assessed by the SCL-90, a self-report inventory developed to extend the Hopkins Symptom Checklist.[6]
2. Teenagers who became pregnant while in the program differed from the others in only one of the nine SCL-90 dimensions assessed — somatization, a dimension which includes such symptoms as weakness in parts of the body, pains in the heart or the chest, faintness or dizziness, and/or headaches. This finding may partly reflect difficulties encountered by these females with their chosen contraceptive methods.
3. Teens did not differ significantly from adults in dimensions of emotional psychopathology (i.e., somatization, anxiety, and depression), but did differ significantly from adults in areas assessing interpersonal relationships and social adjustment. The teenagers showed higher scores, indicating more difficulty in these areas.

Conclusions

The findings from this study of contraceptive use by a program emphasizing education and emotional support indicate that, of adolescents who requested contraceptive services, a high percentage (63%) stayed in the program for one year and managed contraceptive use effectively. Unplanned pregnancies occurred in only 10% of the enrollment over three years. Furthermore, age alone did not affect continuation in the contraceptive program. Younger girls (14-15 at enrollment) were as likely to continue in the program as were older girls (16-18 at enrollment).

Contraceptive use involves a learning process which engages several psychological dimensions. The user must be aware of the techniques involved in contraception. She must accept herself as a sexually active person and recognize that pregnancy is a likely result of her sexual activity. Finally, she must be able to decide whether or not she wants a pregnancy.

The cognitive demands of contraceptive use often conflict with other pressures. Students may realize that they need contraceptives, but may find them difficult to obtain. They may experience sexual activity, but may have limited information concerning the likelihood of pregnancy. Misinformation about "safe" times and misunderstanding of consistent contraceptive use were among the most common problems reported by girls who became pregnant.[7] The reality of teenage sexual activity may conflict with moral pressures against extramarital intercourse. A common psychological mechanism to defend against such conflict is denial of the consequence — in this situation, pregnancy. Many teenagers think pregnancy is not a real possibility. Finally, teenagers may identify with the maternal role, but few are prepared to bear the economic, psychological, and social consequences of parenthood. Their milieu, however, may romanticize maternity and obscure the problems of, and alternatives to, early child-bearing.

Our data do not support the idea that teenagers become pregnant because they choose to become pregnant. Most teenage pregnancies probably are truly unwanted. But simply dispensing contraceptives is not enough. Contraceptive use involves conflicting social, emotional, parental, and peer pressures which affect utilization and continuation of contraception.

There is no clear mandate for teenagers to be responsible for their bodies and health, and this affects physicians' services, programs, and the teenagers' use of contractive and/or other health services. It is our belief that teenagers moving into sexual activity deserve the opportunity to protect themselves from unwanted pregnancy, and that the best way to provide this is through the educational and emotional support that teaching-oriented health care services can offer.

In our program at the University of Pennsylvania, we strive to provide initial and continuing guidance concerning all aspects of sexual activity. We are attempting to move beyond the simple dispensing of contraceptives and the brief sex education talks at school, to develop the foundations of self-management in all areas of health care. Such an approach reduces the cost of health care as compared to costs of prenatal and delivery care for a pregnant teenager, pediatric care for an unwanted child, and the obvious difficulties of self-support, self-respect, and life prospects for a teenage mother.

The program concerning self-management of reproductive health care is now under the direction of the newly-established Stuart and Emily B. H. Mudd Professorship of Human Behavior and Reproduction. This professorship, with joint appointments in obstetrics/gynecology and psychiatry, seeks to identify ways that social, psychological, and behavioral factors relate to reproductive problems. It is hoped that this information will be the basis for improving treatment and prevention of teen pregnancies. In the Teen Program, the work reported here is currently being extended through a study of multiple factors influencing contraceptive use and through "rap" sessions for teens during clinic visits. Such sessions provide increased information and emotional support. In addition to the teenage years, during which sexual activity begins, contraceptive use is limited, and the problems surrounding unintended pregnancies are greatest; two other aspects of women's reproductive lives are now being investigated:

1. The adult reproductive years, when problems of depression, anxiety, or other psychosocial factors affect successful contraceptive use.
2. The problems of infertility encountered when couples find they cannot achieve desired pregnancies.

The Teen Program is a vital link in this span of human behavior and reproduction that we are seeking to better understand.

REFERENCES

1. Baldwin, W.H., "Adolescent Pregnancy and Childbearing – Growing Concerns for Americans." *Population Bulletin.* Washington, D.C.: Population Reference Bureau, pp. 31–32, 1976.
2. Dickens, H.O., Mudd, E.H., and Huggins, G.R., "One Hundred Pregnant Adolescents: Treatment Approaches in a University Hospital," *American Journal of Public Health* **63**, 9:794–800, 1973; and Dickens, H.O. *et al.*, "Teenagers, Contraception and Pregnancy," *Journal of Marriage and Family Counseling* **1**, 2:175–181, 1976.
3. Sear, A.M., "Clinic Discontinuation and Contraceptive Need," *Family Planning Perspectives* **5**, 2:80–88, 1973.
4. Grimes, D. and Romm, F., "Fertility and Family Planning among White Teenagers in Metropolitan Atlanta," *American Journal of Public Health* **64**, 7:700–707, 1975.
5. Hambridge, W.R., "Teen Clinics," *Obstetrics and Gynecology* **43**, 3:458–460, 1974.
6. Derogatis, L.R., Lipman, R.S., Rickels, K., Uhlenhuth, E.H., and Covi, L., "The Hopkins Symptom Checklist (HSC): A Self-report Inventory," *Behavioral Science* **19**:1–15, 1974; and Rickels, K., Garcia, C.-R., Lipman, R.S., Derogatis, L.R., and Fisher, E.L., "The Hopkins Checklist: Assessing Emotional Distress in Obstetric-gynecologic Practice," *Primary Care* **3**, 4:751–764.
7. The Alan Guttmacher Institute, *11 Million Teenagers.* New York: Planned Parenthood Federation of America, 1976.

22

Employee Fitness in Today's Workplace

W. Brent Arnold

Xerox International Center
For Training and Management Development

American Association of Fitness
Directors in Business and Industry

A few years ago, no corporate president or executive officer would even think of implementing physical fitness programs for the well-being of the company's employees. Now, almost everywhere one looks one sees physical fitness in some form. Management realizes that regular exercise improves the health and morale of employees, increases productivity, reduces absenteeism due to illness, and relieves a wide range of problems associated with physical inactivity. Private industry is also aware of paying in two ways when the nation's work force is physically unfit: 1) through increased taxes to support federal health care programs, and 2) through increased health insurance premiums for employee health benefits. Many corporate executives, therefore, now believe good health is good business.

Why is there this surge of employee physical fitness today? One only has to look at the health statistics of today's industrial society: $25 billion is lost annually due to premature death; $3 billion is lost due to illness; heart attacks alone cost industry close to 132 million work days every year, 4% of the gross national product in direct cost; and the common backache is responsible for an estimated $1 billion in lost goods and services to industry, plus another $225 million in workmen's compensation.[1]

General Motors, for example, spends approximately $825 million per year for its employee health plan, more than it spends to purchase steel from U.S. Steel, its principal supplier. In 1975, health benefits added $175 to the price of every vehicle manufactured by General Motors.[2]

Other examples of rising health care costs have occurred in the U.S. government. The rate of disability retirements has risen 170% since 1955. Absenteeism in the executive branch alone costs the government $1.34 billion and accounts for more than 25 million sick days a year.[3]

In the U.S., the President's Council on Physical Fitness and Sports has been assisting business and industry, government, and labor organizations to develop physical fitness programs to elevate employee health and reduce the financial and human costs resulting from physical inactivity. The Canadian government also puts a high priority on improving the quality of the work environment. The Department of National Health and Welfare in Canada, for example, has taken several steps to initiate preventive health programs.

Recently, many corporations have been implementing preventive medicine programs to curb spiraling health and medical costs. Management realizes that the employee is the single most important resource. Without the employee there is no productivity. The ultimate goal, then, is to provide optimum fitness and mental well-being for all employees.

Today, people in our society accept diseases — such as heart disease and lung cancer — "by choice." People smoke, drink, eat fatty foods, become obese, lack exercise, and are careless on the highway. Health and fitness professionals are now studying lifestyle, behavior, and the environment, as well as the medical sciences. Behavior problems with medical consequences cannot be cured with medicine alone. In the Public Health Services Forward Plan for 1978-1981, it is maintained that it is more productive to focus attention on the underlying and antecedent causes of preventable diseases than to concentrate on the diseases themselves.

Corporations, therefore, are introducing employee fitness programs as a preventive medicine technique. They are aware of the cardiovascular risk factors associated with poor fitness levels, as well as what physical fitness does medically for employees enrolled in a regular exercise program (the heart rate, blood pressure, and triglyceride levels drop proportionately, participants feel better, and the cardiovascular system becomes more efficient).

Management also realizes that employee fitness programs are not only a form of preventive medicine, but that such programs are also cost-effective. Management is becoming aware of the correlation between improved employee fitness and an increase in productivity and morale, as well as a decrease in absenteeism and employee turnover. It also sees the dollar value placed on the cost of replacing management personnel who may fall victim to heart attacks and other health crises associated with poor fitness. Take, for example, an executive who makes $100,000 per year and works for a corporation which provides its people with good pensions, insurance, profit-sharing, and other benefits. If this executive dies from a heart attack, the corporation will lose not only the wealth of knowledge he or she has gained, but it will also lose between $500,000 and $1 million. This expense includes not only previous management training, salary, and benefits, but also the cost of locating and training another executive.

Abroad, we can look at two countries that have been utilizing industrial fitness for a number of years, Sweden and the Soviet Union. The Swedes stress the preventive medical value of sports and physical fitness. The government devotes the largest single part of its budget to health and education, and if physical fitness programs can keep people well and fit, this is not only good in itself, but it is good economy. As a result, government agencies, primarily within the administration for health, welfare, and education, work closely with the Swedish sports federation, the national association for intercompany sports, and other groups, to provide the maximum possible physical fitness opportunities for the most people — young, old, men, women, children, and the handicapped. The aim is to get the body doing what it is built for: activity, not rest. This is probably why the Swedish male heart pumps 5.3 years longer than the average American male heart.[4]

Some of the most extensive research has been carried out in the Soviet Union, long the world leader in exercise physiology and sports medicine. Russian experts have repeatedly documented the economic benefits of exercise. They have found that working people who exercise regularly produce more, visit the doctor less frequently, and are far less prone to industrial accidents. According to Dr. Professor V. Pravosudov of Leningrad, regular exercise can reduce absenteeism from three to five days per year per person.[5] At a Goodyear plant in Norrkoping, Sweden, researchers have found that absenteeism is nearly 50% lower for those who exercise regularly.[6]

Quantitative research in the field of employee fitness as it relates to productivity, absenteeism, employee turnover, and morale is almost non-existent in the U.S., today. Objective studies must be done to demonstrate the effects of increased exercise on job performance. Several agencies and corporations are conducting research in these areas at the present time; however, only a few studies have been performed to date.

In 1968, the National Aeronautics and Space Administration (NASA), in cooperation with the Heart Disease and Stroke Control Program of the Public Health Service, provided a thrice-weekly exercise program for 259 executives, men aged 35-55. After a year, the participants completed questionnaires and underwent thorough medical examinations. The results were most impressive. Half the regular participants reported improvement in job performance and better attitudes toward their work. Twelve percent of the sporadic participants reported similar performance and attitude improvement. Nearly all the regular participants reported that they felt better; 89% reported improved stamina; and nearly half said they felt less stress and tension. More than 60% lost weight, and half that number reported sounder sleep. Many participants quit smoking or cut down, and nearly half said they were paying more attention to their diets. Significantly, one fifth of all participants reported that their colleagues had urged them to take part. Most important, there was a "highly consistent and positive relationship" between the perceived benefits of the program and the results of medical tests. Those who reported improved stamina showed marked improvements in cardiovascular performance, as measured by treadmill tests.[7]

One recent study, entitled "A Program of Heart Disease Intervention for Public Employees: A Five Year Report," by Larry A. Bjurstrom, Ph.D., and Nicholas Alexiou, provided interesting results. The five-year experience involving 847 employees resulted in favorable modifications in risk factors, amelioration of health problems, and reductions in employee absenteeism. Similar programs should be implemented to facilitate self-health principles and practices and encourage modifications of self-imposed risks.[8]

The U.S. Department of Justice has instituted a Health Prevention Program which includes an exercise testing program. A total of 23 people have been identified with advanced coronary heart disease, and another 350 people were identified as high coronary risks. All of these people are presently being treated for their conditions. Every employee who has a heart attack and goes to the hospital costs the government $11,000.

These studies, however, substantiate that more quantitative research is necessary concerning industrial fitness to show the importance of fitness within the workplace. Many corporate presidents will not initiate employee fitness programs for their corporations until they can see a definite link between fitness and increasing productivity and decreasing absenteeism.

In past years, there were very few resources available to corporations interested in developing physical fitness facilities for their employees. Today, corporate representatives can seek advice from physical fitness personnel at the local Young Men's/Young Women's Christian Association, Christian Youth Centers, Jewish Community Centers, Park and Recreation Centers, high schools, and universities. The American Heart Association, the American Cancer Association, and other non-profit associations can also be contacted. Several states have recently organized governor's councils. Nationally, the President's Council on Physical Fitness and Sports and the American Association of Fitness Directors in Business and Industry can be called upon for assistance.

One of the major questions that management has to answer if it decides to have an employee fitness program is whether or not the fitness facility should be located in-house. If the fitness program is located outside the business office, then employee participation will be cut by at least one-half. This factor in itself can make or break the program. Many of the above-listed resources have ongoing fitness programs on a cost fee basis. There are also many health and fitness consultants available. However, if a corporation wishes to seek the assistance of a consultant, the consultant's references should be thoroughly checked.

Control and accessibility are the main assets of an in-house employee fitness program. Prior to organizing and implementing such a program, management should consider the following:

1. Goals and objectives
2. Manpower (supervision)
3. Public relations — education
4. Budget (participant fees, etc.)
5. Liability
6. Program content
7. Equipment, materials, and facility layout
8. Hours of operation
9. Participant eligibility
10. Program evaluation and follow-up.

Proper motivation and leadership also play important roles in the success of any employee fitness program.

The planning of any fitness program must include provisions for personnel and supervision. These elements, in turn, depend not only on budget considerations, but also on the variety of people to be served. Will they be executives only, or will middle management be included? Will employee's families be eligible to participate? These are all decisions that must be made before the program is opened to the employees.

In regard to administration, there will be several questions for consideration. Who is going to make the selection of the physical fitness specialist or exercise physiologist? In whose department will this person work? Will the fitness leader be a trained professional, a recreation staff person, or a volunteer?

Will fitness activities be supervised? Will the fitness program be organized or will it be casual and individually directed? Some corporations simply provide a fitness room, often with equipment and no supervision. Others provide a room and equipment with a supervised, personalized program for all participants. It must be determined which approach will work, at least initially, in the organization.

A fitness specialist should be consulted prior to the planning of *any* fitness facility. He or she can help make the best use of whatever space and budget are available. Even a small space can be converted to a fitness facility. Showers, as well as a circuit trainer and a treadmill, can be installed. Most employee fitness programs are cardiovascular in nature and utilize aerobic exercises, such as walking, jogging, cycling, and swimming. Other areas of concentration include flexibility and muscle strength and tone.

The program's hours of operation will depend on the fitness staff and the company's work hours. It must be decided whether the fitness facility should be open before, during, or after work. Operation during noon hours, weekends, and holidays must also be considered.

Xerox Corporation is an excellent example of a company that has several in-house programs. There are four employee fitness facilities in Rochester, New York, and one in each of the following cities: Leesburg, Virginia; Stamford, and Greenich, Connecticut; Dallas, Texas; El Segundo, California; and London, England. In the Xerox Corporation's employee fitness programs in New York, employees may work out either at noon or after work, depending on their work schedules. In the Rochester executive fitness program, participants work out at times during the work day which are convenient to both the executives and the fitness specialists. Students and staff at the Xerox International Center for Training and Management Development in Leesburg work out at noon, during the evenings, and on weekends. All programs are cardiovascularly oriented to the four aerobic exercises previously mentioned, and each location has mechanical treadmills and/or indoor and outdoor running tracks. Each location has a fitness specialist who develops personalized fitness programs for each of the participants. The Rochester location has been ongoing since 1965.

Is the corporation going to subsidize the fitness program in part or altogether? If the employees are going to pay a fee, what will it be? In Rochester, Xerox employees enrolled in the employee fitness program pay $20.00 per quarter to cover registration costs and towel fees. The executive fitness program participants at Xerox Square, also in Rochester, are charged $200 per year for their regimen, which includes personalized programs as well as cardiovascular exercise tests.

It must be remembered that having the best financed facility does not necessarily mean having a good program. Success depends wholly on the professionals who are running the program.

When the physical fitness program is operating, its success must be reviewed on a regular basis. After such reviews, fitness personnel can build on the strengths of the program and incorporate new ideas. If the objectives are not being met, the program must be reevaluated and its weaknesses corrected. Once the program is solidly established, it will contribute significantly to the overall health of the organization and participating employees.

What do some of the more prevalent trends indicate? One has to understand that the unprecedented concern over health evidenced in the past 25 years has created the second largest and fastest growing industry in the U.S., employing 6% of the nation's workers, amounting to approximately 9% of the gross national product, and billing 1500% more than it did in 1950, while serving only 43% more people.[9] Approximately 13¢ of every federal dollar goes to the health industry.

Health care has grown at an extraordinary pace. Today, U.S. corporations are leaders in preventive medicine. In order for business and industry to cut costs, corporations are not only providing physical fitness facilities, but are running health screening programs and health education modules as well. Companies are now investing in these programs even though a lot of the research is subjective in nature and the results may not be available for several years. In fact, over 400 companies in the U.S. today have employed full-time physical fitness directors.

Recently, one study of more than 50 corporations showed that even though 97% of the fitness programs were cardiovascular in nature, other health evaluation modules in diet, smoking, alcohol, drugs, and stress management were offered. The same study also noted that most of these corporations were recording body weight, cardiovascular status, body composition, flexibility, and body strength. In most of these categories, more than 50% of the fitness directors used these measurements for follow-up, and reported improvement in more than 75% of their participants.

Other new trends that can be seen as a result of employee fitness programs are discussed below.

The American Association of Fitness Directors in Business and Industry (AAFDBI), an affiliate of The President's Council on Physical Fitness and Sports, was established by a group of industrial fitness directors who realized a need to develop their own professional organization. To date, the association has increased its membership by 1200% and the total membership now exceeds 1,500 members. The purpose and objectives of the AAFDBI are as follows:[10]

1. To provide a professional organization to support and assist the development of quality physical fitness programs in business and industry.
2. To create an increased awareness of the importance of initiating and maintaining a high level of physical, emotional, and mental health among employees.
3. To cooperate in national programs of physical fitness and sports with the President's Council on Physical Fitness and Sports and other groups with similar purposes and objectives.
4. To recommend qualifications and professional standards for fitness directors and other professional personnel in business and industry.
5. To encourage and provide support for in-service training activities and programs of continuing education for fitness directors and other professional personnel in business and industry.
6. To stimulate active research and compile and disseminate research information regarding the effects of physical fitness programs.
7. To provide leadership in physical fitness and health for the professional.
8. To serve as a clearinghouse for information and services pertaining to physical fitness programs.
9. To develop operation, administration, and education material for physical fitness programs in business and industry.

Governors' councils on physical fitness and sports are now established in most states. These are composed of citizens concerned about the health, fitness, and well-being of today's society. The Oklahoma Industrial Recreation and Fitness Council, for example, is a statewide effort to promote employer/employee fitness and recreation programs.

Government agencies, such as the National Aeronautics Space Administration, the Environmental Protection Agency, the U.S. Departments of Transportation, Interior and Justice, and the State Department, have instituted fitness programs. Other federal agencies are in the planning stages of developing similar programs.

Insurance companies, including Travelers, Blue Cross/ Blue Shield, Connecticut Mutual Life Insurance Co., and others, have launched nationwide employee health awareness programs for not only their policy-holders, but for the chiefs of police and for firemen throughout the U.S., as well as for interested citizens.

Senate hearings are presently ongoing concerning exercise and aging. Testimony is being presented by noted cardiologists and medical doctors in gerontology about the benefits of exercise for older Americans. The special advisors on physical fitness in business and industry to the President's Council on Physical Fitness and Sports have made statements urging establishment of exercise programs for older Americans. The advisors also urge all school districts to require physical education for children and youth for grades K-12.

Legislation by the Senate Subcommittees on Health and Scientific Research to establish an office for physical fitness and sports medicine indicates congressional concern with this issue. This office, if established, would conduct research, support projects, and disseminate information about physical fitness and sports medicine. This legislation is of obvious significance because it shows the government's concern for physical fitness and fully addresses the potential of physical fitness to reduce the human and financial losses associated with physical degeneration. (In 1976, Frederick Swartz, M.D., speaking on behalf of the American Medical Association, told a Senate subcommittee that poor fitness is the country's greatest health problem"Exercise," he went on to say, "could have a tremendous impact on grim morbidity and mortality rates – at minimal cost."[11] In the same year, Roger Egeberg, M.D., special assistant to Secretary Matthews for health policy, told a White House gathering that "proper fitness could contribute as much to the nation's health as immunization and sanitation advances have done in the past. We sometimes forget that progress in public health has owed more to preventives like sanitation, nutrition, and immunization than to the treatment of disease.")[12]

The increase of employee health and fitness programs has seen a large number of industrial fitness workshops, seminars, and conferences develop around the country. The purpose of these meetings is to present to management of corporations an awareness and understanding of employee health and fitness in the workplace.

Awareness of health education is not a new concept, but it is being integrated into physical fitness programs as well as being presented in modules to employees and to management development sessions. Examples of specific topics for such modules include stress management, obesity, nutrition, drugs and alcohol, smoking, and hypertension. Xerox Corporation has recently developed a program entitled "The Xerox Health Management Program" (XHMP). Its main purpose is to present an awareness of health and fitness to all employees, especially those in Xerox field locations that do not have in-house fitness facilities. This program is of major importance because 99% of the corporations that have employee fitness programs do not have an awareness program established for all employees. This type of program brings an awareness to Xerox employees and is divided into the following topic divisions:

1. What is fitness?
2. Evaluating your health and fitness.
3. Personal medical history looking at medical guidelines.
4. Risk factor estimate.
5. Daily fitness scoresheet.
6. Fitness self-tests.
7. Flexibility and back development exercises.
8. Modules on stress management, obesity and nutrition, alcoholism and drugs, and smoking.

Xerox employees are given the XHMP literature for three reasons: 1) to make employees aware of their fitness and health; 2) to encourage those employees not in an ongoing fitness program to start one of their own, following XHMP guidelines and their personal physician's advice; and 3) to encourage family participation.

There has been more exposure through television, radio, newspapers, and magazines regarding the importance of exercise and health. The President's Council on Physical Fitness and Sports has launched a nationwide campaign to advertise fitness. The following excerpts are from periodicals: "I couldn't believe that just walking could be such a good exercise. But it's true." "Productivity is up ten percent to twenty percent." "Lower absenteeism." "We can identify savings."

Colleges and universities are realizing the need to develop curricula for students desiring to pursue employee health and fitness as a career. Curricula include not only anatomy, physiology, and physical education courses, but also preparation in exercise physiology, finance, business management (including organization and administration), human relations, and communication skills.

It is obvious from these trends that there is an awareness of employee health and physical fitness in today's society. It is also obvious that several groups, as well as individuals, are trying to do something about our nation and the health and fitness of our people.

The President's Council on Physical Fitness and Sports has noted that America's fitness attitudes and practices have changed dramatically since 1976. These changes, listed below, play an important role in our occupational setting today, either directly or indirectly.[14]

Physicians routinely prescribe exercise as a means of maintaining and enhancing health, and exercise is accepted therapy for many heart patients and the victims of other degenerative diseases.

America is in the midst of a *genuine participant sports boom.* We are buying more bicycles than automobiles; sports fashion and athletic footwear have become major industries; and the number of skiers and tennis players has tripled.

Joggers, back-packers, and bicycling commuters, once sources of amusement or amazement, are commonplace in most communities. *There are 10 million joggers, 15 million regular cyclists, and 15 million serious swimmers among America's 110 million adults.*

The number of young women participating in interscholastic and intercollegiate sports has quadrupled in a decade.

Fifteen million boys and girls try out for the Presidential Physical Fitness Award each school year.

Ninety percent of the Americans questioned in a national survey say we should have physical education programs in our elementary and secondary schools.

The U.S. Department of Health, Education, and Welfare (HEW) is encouraging the development of health promotion programs in occupational settings. In January 1979, HEW hosted a working conference in Washington, D.C. to explore the feasibility of implementing such programs in various occupational settings throughout the country. The objectives of this conference were as follows:[15]

1. Develop a set of guidelines for the implementation of health promotion programs at the worksite.
2. Identify the resources needed and available to implement these programs.
3. Identify the public and private sector roles in health promotion programs.
4. Recommend appropriate follow-up measures.

This conference was significant in that this was the first time representatives from the federal government, unions, industry, insurance carriers, and the scientific community had come together to meet concerning health promotion programs in the occupational setting. Equally important was that the employee physical fitness programs were definitely recognized as being one of the health promotion programs in business and industry today.

Conclusion

The average working person spends one-third of each day at his or her job. This person's employer can play an important role in developing the employee's health, both from a physiological and a psychological point of view. Employers, through utilizing the proper resources, could provide preventive medicine and health programs which would help develop their employees to their fullest potential. Business and industry are now starting to realize the importance of providing such programs for the good of both the employee and the employer.

Employee physical fitness can make — and is making — a contribution to our nation's society and its health. More quantitative research is needed to further show that there is definitely a direct correlation between improved physical fitness and productivity, morale, absenteeism, and employee turnover. Funding is needed to conduct such research in both industrial and governmental settings. To date, no such study demonstrating an increase in productivity as a result of exercise program participation has been conducted in the U.S.[16] In the future, it is hoped that all business and industry will be able to provide employee fitness programs to make our society more healthy and fit. The famous Swedish naturalist, Carl Von Linne, stated in 1783: "It is not God, but people themselves who shorten their lives by not keeping physically fit." His thesis is more alive than ever today.[17]

REFERENCES

1. President's Council on Physical Fitness and Sports, *Physical Fitness in Business and Industry*. Washington, D.C., 1976, p. 2.
2. Keelor, O., "Address to 1976 Blue Shield Annual Program Conference." Chicago, Illinois, October 4, 1976, p. 5.
3. Gladis, S., "Running is Good for Business," *Runner's World*, September 1977, p. 54.
4. Brattnas, B. and Gullers, K.W., *Fit for Fun*. Stockholm, 1973, p. 4.
5. Pravosudov, V. "The Effect of Physical Exercises on Health and Economic Efficiency." Paper presented at the International Congress of Physical Activity Sciences, Quebec, July 1976, p. 6.
6. Keelor, R. O., Testimony to the U.S. Council on Wage and Price Stability Hearings on Health Care Costs. Chicago, Illinois, July 1976.
7. Keelor, R.O., "Address to 1976 Blue Shield Annual Program Conference." Chicago, Illinois, October 4, 1976, pp. 8-9.
8. Bjurstrom, A. and Alexiou, N.G., "A Program of Heart Disease Intervention for Public Employees," *Journal of Occupational Medicine* 20, 8:521, August, 1978.
9. "Unhealthy Costs of Health Care (Special Report)," *Business Week*, September 4, 1978, p. 58.
10. American Association of Fitness Directors in Business and Industry, *Purpose and Objectives*. Washington, D.C., 1975.
11. Swartz, F.C., Testimony to the Senate Subcommittee on Aging. Washington, D.C., 1975.
12. Keelor, R.O., "Address to 1976 Blue Shield Annual Program Conference." Chicago, Illinois, October 4, 1976, p. 5.
13. President's Council on Physical Fitness and Sports, Nationwide Advertisement. Washington, D.C., 1978.
14. President's Council on Physical Fitness and Sports, "Organization, Objectives, Programs and Situation Report." Washington, D.C., 1978.
15. Department of Health, Education, and Welfare, "National Conference on Health Promotion Programs in Occupational Settings." Washington, D.C., January 17-19, 1979.

16. Haskell, W.L. and Blair, S.N., "The Physical Activity Component of Health Promotion Programs in Occupational Settings," *National Conference on Health Promotion Programs in Occupational Settings,* January 1979, p. 8.
17. Brattnas and Gullers, *op. cit.*

BIBLIOGRAPY

American Association of Fitness Directors in Business and Industry, *Purpose and Objectives.* Washington, D.C., 1975.

Arnold, W.B., "Before You Start a Fitness Program . . . Take Time to Analyze Your Approach," *Recreation Management*, July 1976, p. 10.

Arnold, W.B., "Cardiovascular Health Program," *Recreation Management,* April 1973, p. 21.

Arnold, W.B., "Organization Profile: Xerox International Center for Training and Management Development," *Recreation Management*, January 1978, pp. 30–32.

Arnold, W.B., "Program and Administration," *Employee Physical Fitness in Canada, Proceedings on the National Conference on Employee Fitness, Ottawa (1974).* Information Canada, 1975, pp. 55–59.

Arnold, W.B., "The Physical Treatment of A Company of Good Minds," *Recreation Management,* November 1974, pp. 6–8.

Boller, C. and Park, F. (Eds.), "Putting Their Hearts Into It," *Xerox World* 20:2, December 1975.

Boston University, "A Layman's Guide to Cardiovascular Disease," *Bostonia,* Winter 1978.

Brattnas, B. and Gullers, K.W., *Fit for Fun.* Stockholm, 1973, p. 4.

Bjurstrom, L.A. and Alexiou, N.G., "A Program of Heart Disease Intervention for Public Employees," *Journal of Occupational Medicine* 20 8:521, August 1978.

Cage, T., "Fitness: An Exercise in Good Business," *Oilways* 5:2–7, 1978.

Collis, M.L., *Employee Fitness.* Ottawa: Minister of State for Fitness and Amateur Sport, 1977.

Condon, J., "Executive Sweat," *Women Sports*, October 1977, pp. 20–23.

Conrad, C., "Why Your Organization Should Consider Starting A Physical Fitness Program," *Training/HRD,* February 1979, pp. 28–31.

Department of Health, Education, and Welfare, "National Conference on Health Promotion Programs in Occupational Settings." Washington, D.C., January 17–19, 1979.

"Fitness Movement Seen Curbing High Cost of Illness to U.S. Industry," Commerce Today, February 3, 1975.

Fogle, K.R. and Verdessa, A.S., "The Cardiovascular Conditioning Effects of a Supervised Exercise Program," *Journal of Occupational Medicine* 17, 4:240–246.

Geannette, G., "Inside the Corporate Gymnasium," *American Way* 12, 1:21–23, January 1979.

Gladis, S., "Running Is Good for Business," *Runner's World,* September 1977, p. 54.

Gunn, R.R., "An Analysis of the Beliefs and Policies of Companies, Businessmen and Medical Experts with Respect to Physical Fitness." Unpublished Master's Thesis, Salt Lake City, Utah 1970.

Haskell, W.L. and Blair, S.N., "The Physical Activity Component of Health Programs in Occupational Settings," *National Conference on Health Promotion Programs in Occupational Settings*, January 1979, pp. 1–26.

Heinzelmann, F. and Durbeck, D.C., "Personal Benefits of a Health, Evaluation and Enhancement Program." Report given at the Annual Conference of NASA. Cambridge, Massachusetts, October 13, 1970.

Howe, G., "Employee Physical Fitness Programs: Protecting the Companies Investment." Unpublished Master's Thesis, Clemson, South Carolina, April 1978.

Judge, J.F., "Business Moves, Government Lags," *Government Executive,* April 1974.

Keelor, R.O., "Address to 1976 Blue Shield Annual Program Conference." Chicago, Illinois, October 4, 1976, p. 5.

Keelor, R.O., Testimony to the Joint Hearing on Health and Long-term Care, Federal, State and Community Relations, Select Committee on Aging, "The Role of Physical Fitness in Reducing Health and Long-Term Care of the Elderly." April 1976.

Keelor, R.O., Testimony to the U.S. Council on Wage and Price Stability Hearings on Health Care Costs. Chicago, Illinois, July 1976.

"Keeping Fit in the Company Gym," *Fortune*, October 1975, pp. 136–143.

Knitter, B. (Director of Occupational Health Program at Department of Justice), Interview, Washington, D.C., May 1977.

Koerner, D.R., "Cardiovascular Benefits from an Industrial Physical Fitness Program," *Journal of Occupational Medicine* 15, 9:700, September 1973.

Kreitner, R., "Employee Physical Fitness: Protecting an Investment in Human Resources," *Personnel Journal* 55, 7:340, July 1976.

Lalonde, M., *A New Prospective on the Health of Canadians.* Ottawa: National Health and Welfare, 1974.

Martin, J., "Corporate Health: A Result of Employee Fitness," *Physician and Sports Medicine,* March 1978, pp. 135–137.

Martin, J., "The New Business Boom – Employee Fitness," *Nation's Business* , February 1978, pp. 68–73.

Oklahoma Industrial Recreation and Fitness Council, *Life Style*, Summer 1977.

Oppenheim, C., "Physical Conditioning Fits Right in with Business Ideas," *Chicago Tribune,* September 24, 1978.

Pravosudov, V., "The Effect of Physical Exercises on Health and Economic Efficiency." Paper presented at the International Congress of Physical Activity Sciences, Quebec, July 1976, p. 6.

President's Council on Physical Fitness and Sports, Nationwide Advertisement. Washington, D.C., 1978.

President's Council on Physical Fitness and Sports, "Organization Objectives, Programs and Situation Report." Washington, D.C., 1978.

President's Council on Physical Fitness and Sports. *Physical Fitness in Business and Industry.* Washington, D.C., 1976, p. 2.

Pyle, R.L., "Corporate Fitness Programs – How Do They Shape Up," *Personnel Magazine,* January/February 1979, pp. 58–67.

Schwab, S., "Xerox Corporation an Original Approach to training," *The Northern Virginian,* September 1978, pp. 27–31.

Swartz, F.C., Testimony to the Senate Subcommittee on Aging. Washington, D.C., 1975.

"The New RX for Better Health," *Business Week,* January 5, 1974.

"Unhealthy Costs of Health Care (Special Report)," *Business Week.* September 4, 1978, p. 58.

Wanzel, R.S., "determination of Attitudes of Employees and Management of Canadian Corporations toward Company Sponsored Physical Activity Facilities and Programs." Unpublished Doctoral Thesis, Edmonton, Alberta, 1974.

Welch, R., "Ontario strives for Fitness," *Pools, Parks and Rinks*, Summer 1977, pp. 8-14.

Yarvote, P., McDonagh, J.J., Goldman, M.E., and Zuckerman, J., "Organization and Evaluation of a Physical Fitness Program in Industry," *Journal of Occupational Medicine* **16**, *9*:589–598, September 1974.

Zaleski, H. K., "Shaping Your In-House Physical Fitness Program," *Industry Week,* September 18, 1978, pp. 121–124.

Zohman, L., *Run for Life.* Hartford, Connecticut: Connecticut Mutual Life Insurance Company, 1978.

23

The Promotion of Physical Activity and Healthy Lifestyle Behavior

Richard R. J. Lauzon, Ph.D.
Sandy C. A. Keir, Ph.D.

Fitness and Amateur Sport
Government of Canada

A concise definition of health promotion continues to elude health workers as they attempt to rationalize their program activities according to the preventive health ethic. In its most inclusive sense, health promotion might be characterized by the implementation of flexible working hours which allow employees to engage in noon-hour fitness programs; in its simplest manifestation, health promotion may signify the mass distribution of illustrative pamphlets on exercise to high school students. The common object of all such actions is their ultimate beneficial influence upon personal health.

As a result of the wide array of influences which may affect one's health both positively and negatively, a logical strategy demands the application of a comprehensive approach to the solution of personal health problems. Many of the health promotion activities of the past were oriented to cause-specific information dissemination, such as anti-smoking appeals, venereal disease warnings, planned-parenthood promotions, and physical fitness campaigns, among others. Unfortunately, these efforts were limited to the mere presentation of facts directed toward the individual in the belief that the transmission and subsequent acquisition of such knowledge would stimulate salutary living habits by eliminating a negative influence. The natural limitations of information-oriented programs upon health practices have been widely recognized.[1] Furthermore, intensive behavioral efforts have, for the most part, produced less spectacular results than anticipated.[2]

A comprehensive strategy is dictated also by the multi-faceted contributing characteristics of major causes of death and ill health. We have been sensitized to the relationship of cigarette smoking, blood lipid levels, blood pressure, and physical inactivity as modifiable precursors to cardiovascular disease processes.[3] Similarly, licit and illicit drug use, environmental and social factors, abuse of health services, iatrogenic conditions, and many other factors have been impli-

Table 23-1.

Epidemiological Component	Target	Selected Influence Activities
Host	Sedentary Active Vigorous	Education Advertising Testing Behavior modification
Agent	Automation	Engineering Regulation Legislation
Environment	Physical Sociocultural Economic Mass media	Facilities Sanction Incentives

cated as among the major causes of death.[4] Purposeful intervention programs would generate a highly complex and varied litany of tactical responses in combating these threats to health and social well-being. There is much to be gained by adopting a strategy which consolidates many of the program responses to date, and which may be used to elicit complementary influence activities.

This chapter will present an epidemiological approach to improving the physical activity participation rate within the sedentary North American population. Lauzon[5] has previously described a health promotion model based upon the epidemiological paradigm. This model recognized the need to adopt a comprehensive perspective in the modification of maladaptive lifestyle behavior, and suggested a taxonomy of activities designed to influence health-related behavior (Table 23-1). The model is modified herein to portray the case for physical activity.

Each epidemiological component will be discussed in the context of the relevant targets and selected influence activities noted in Table 23-1. Other internal subdivisions of the host-agent-environment trilogy are no doubt possible. The divisions identified by the authors are the ones most personally meaningful at this time. Furthermore, the list of selected influence activities has been consciously abridged because of limitations of space. The fundamental principle integral to the application of the model is the reliance upon a systematic review of the particular problem (or agent), and the need to engage in influence activities on many fronts in order to optimize the synergistic potential of complementary activities where the resultant effect of two problem-specific programs may be greater than the sum of both alone.[6]

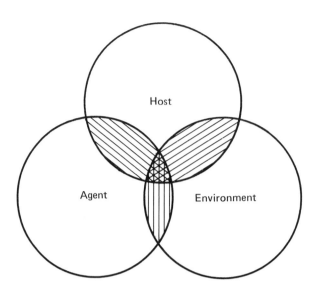

Figure 23-1. Modified characterization of the epidemiological model.

Basic to the employment of the systems-like strategy of the epidemiological approach is the recognition of the reinforcing impact which the program action in one sphere (for example, the host) has upon the other related epidemiological components (for example, the agent and the environment), as illustrated in the simple Venn diagram of Figure 23-1. This representation suggests that some influence activities are peculiar to individual epidemiological components, while other activities may gain their optimal influence through the interdependence of two or more component-related actions, implied by the interfaces between and among components. For example, a program to legislate compulsory motor vehicle seat-belt use may require an intensive advertising program pointing out the advantages of such action in order to "drum up" the necessary public and political support for the proposed legislation. The advertising campaign could be developed to increase the public's awareness of the need to employ seat-belts, to improve the level of knowledge about the advantages of seat-belt use, and to inoculate the public against arguments used by opponents of compulsory seat-belt legislation.

With regard to the sections relating to selected health promotion activities, the authors will describe some of the products and services sponsored by the Fitness Canada of Fitness and Amateur Sport, Canada within the context of the epidemiological model. Almost all example activities have been rationalized to conform with the proposed epidemiological strategy to support the tenet that a systematic approach such as the one proposed accommodates current activities and may be useful in determining program priorities for the future.

Host-Oriented Activities

The host component of the model is concerned with the people to whom the particular health promotion program is aimed. The simple classification of target groups in Table 23-1 takes into consideration the potential mediating effects of selective perception where the health-message recipients may "misinterpret or distort a communication so that it will be more compatible with their own attitudes, habits or opinions."[7]

Selected Influence Activities: Host. The first fundamental strategy of the traditional epidemiological model is to decrease the vulnerability of the host to the agent. Thus, alerting the population to the potential dangers of inactivity, emphasizing the personal benefits of physical activity and demonstrating appropriate behavioral responses are the types of programs which respond to the host's needs. It is felt that physical activity messages should be planned to appeal as appropriately as possible to the particular personal, cultural, and social motivations inherent within any target group.

The three-way classification also underscores the necessity to include messages for each group. Oftentimes, behavior change programs overlook the long-term reinforcement efforts critical to the maintenance of continuous healthy lifestyle habits.[8] Messages to the "converted" are worthwhile and ensure long-term support for health promotion programs. This might be compared somewhat to maintaining a large immune population for various communicable disseases within a given community.

Greater message-specificity could be obtained by different subdivisions of the target groups. For example, if one is trying to persuade business or industry to approve the adoption of an employee fitness program, slightly different messages would be planned for a group of senior executives than for union personnel. The more precise the description of the target audience, the greater the chance of success with the message.

Education. Education tactics have a fundamental role to play in any health promotion strategy. Educational activities sponsored by Canada's federal fitness agency provide an informed awareness about the role of physical activity, as in the *Health and Fitness* booklet, or through state-of-the-art documents such as *Employee Fitness*, which describes the administrative and logistical considerations important in the development of an employee fitness program.[9] Unfortunately, many politicians and much of the public have inflated expectations of educational approaches. Contrary to popular belief, there are no simple linear relationships among knowledge, attitudes, and behavior. Similarly, an appreciation of the diffusion of innovation concept helps the health promotion practitioner to apply educational tactics at appropriate places in the encouragement of some target health practice.[10]

Advertising. The maintenance of a continuous awareness of the importance of physical activity demands an advertising program. In Canada, PARTICIPaction is a private, non-profit corporation funded by the government to promote physical activity.[11] PARTICIPaction creates and produces mass media commercials, which are then offered on a gratuitous basis to broadcast and print media outlets. In addition to its national mass media efforts, the corporation has joined with various community-wide fitness consortia to promote physical fitness activity intensively on a local level. These community demonstration projects have been quite successful in encouraging impressive changes in physical activity participation rates, when integrated with existing programs offered by public, private, and institutional fitness and physical recreation agencies.[12]

Testing. The Canadian Home Fitness Test (CHFT) is a two-stage, double step of cardio-respiratory fitness developed as a self-administered testing tool.[13] When the pulse rate is measured reliably, and when combined with other factors in a multiple regression formula, the resultant index provides a relatively sophisticated analysis of one's aerobic fitness status.[14]

To date, the CHFT has been used in numerous displays at professional meetings, as a promotional tool in soliciting recruits to employee fitness programs, and in many shopping malls and county fairs. It appears that the testing experience stimulates a much more interested discussion of the relationship between fitness and health than one could expect with other non-activity-oriented displays.   The resultant interaction between the test administrator and the participant produces a more meaningful context to discuss healthy lifestyle behavior.

In general, test results poses a very personalized message for the individual, but should be treated with caution when used as a health promotion influence mechanism, especially in a "mass" situation. Although the application of such testing has great public appeal, the test administrators must be wary of potential dysfunctional consequences related to the testing program. These problems result when the sensitivity and specificity of the test protocol have not been determined. Furthermore, follow-up information and services should be reasonably capable of assisting test participants to improve upon poor test results.[15]

Behavior Modification. The Fit-Kit is a comprehensive fitness testing and information package intended to convey some insight to users about their personal fitness status, to provide information about fitness and health in general, to suggest attractive fitness-enhancing acitivites, and to assist individuals in evaluating their progress.[16] Its theoretical bases are awareness, education, personal solutions, and reinforcement, stages similar to those of the Health Belief Model.[17] Behavior modification techniques, such as establishing a base-line fitness status, identifying minimum physical activity standards, self-recording, physiological feedback success criteria, and other positive reinforcement features, were integrated into the Fit-Kit design.

Fitness Canada has discovered that its most successful programs involve the provision of some activity, product, or service that appeals to the target group. As a follow-up to the initial interest, it is possible to elicit repeatedly greater involvement in physical activity programs.

This "foot-in-the-door" approach has been applied successfully with individuals, professionals, and public and private agencies, and in various industrial and institutional settings.[18] It has been observed also that the participation in physical activity programs often stimulates changes in other health-related lifestyles.[19] Physical activity program directors should strive to include as much information as possible on related lifestyle topics in their activity sessions. Similarly, health promotion personnel active in these other areas should investigate the possibility of incorporating some form of physical activity element within the context of their own programs.

Agent-Oriented Activities

The agent component of the model may be considered as the target problem. Although physical inactivity is the traditional culprit, the authors have chosen to present automation as the causal agent responsible for our sedentary popu-Actually, any home influence, occupational endeavor, or in-service training program whose byproduct is physical inactivity presents a legitimate target problem. The evolution of Western society's economy from an agricultural to an industrial — and now to a post-industrial or a services-based — economy has produced a sedentary population. In much the same way, our overburdened school curricula compel children to a sedentary educational experience strangely similar to the sedentary occupations awaiting them upon graduation. Homo sapiens who thrived biologically with habitual physical activity is evolving at an accelerated pace into homo sedentarus — who shuns any physical activity opportunity.

Selected Influence Activities: Agent. The general "agent" strategy in the traditional epidemiological model is the consideration of mechanisms to decrease the toxicity of the agent. Thus, the general objective would be the implementation of actions intended to re-introduce physical activity into various settings in order to minimize the ill effects of sedentary living.

Engineering. Engineering refers here to a modification or improvement in the design of structures, machines, products, systems, and processes.[20] With regard to the agent, automation, the Exercise Break Package and employee fitness programs have been promoted by Fitness Canada to counteract sedentary work patterns. The exercise break presents a light series of exercises performed to music over a seven-minute period during the mid-morning or mid-afternoon break as a form of active relaxation.[21] Although not intended to significantly improve one's physical fitness status, the exercises provide a short interlude of movement to music in order to stimulate circulation, improve posture, relax tense muscles, and counteract boredom and fatigue.

On the other hand, employee fitness programs are geared toward the improvement and/or the maintenance of adequate personal fitness levels. Experience indicates that successful employee fitness programs do not require elaborate facilities or major time commitments on the part of the personnel involved. Experienced leaders and a facility which is reasonably accessible appear to be the most crucial requirements.[22] In addition to the usual physiological and psychological benefits, and the secondary effects upon other health-related lifestyles, the employer can expect a favorable influence upon productivity, absenteeism, and job satisfaction.[23]

Regulation. Often, very significant long-term behavioral changes are engendered by regulatory controls. When accompanied by sound, humanistic reasons for such forced compliance, the regulations may yield important health benefits. For example, minimum standards for physical fitness have been required for certain occupational groups: selected armed forces personnel, policemen, firemen, and airline pilots, among others. Similarly, flexible working hours may provide an opportunity to incorporate an activity program into the work day or in transit to the workplace.

Although the following regulations mentioned are not in force, it is felt that their adoption would facilitate a greater degree and variety of work-related physical activity. It is proposed that the Canada Building Code require the developers of high-rise office buildings to include adequate shower and change room facilities within their structures. Moreover, some basement space – a minimum of 40 by 40 feet square – should be included in the basement area for use as an employee fitness facility. The former would accommodate those workers who wish to cycle or jog to and from work, or during the lunch hour, whereas the latter would house an in-building employee fitness program. Each of these facilities could be self-supporting through the application of a user fee. Such regulations would have a profound impact upon employee fitness. Furthermore, similar regulations adopted for apartment and condominium complexes by urban developers could stimulate the development of community programs.

Legislation. Mandatory daily physical education classes for students attending elementary and secondary schools should be implemented. Parents become concerned about the academic success of their children when more time is devoted to physical activity. Numerous studies have demonstrated that no deleterious academic events materialized; moreover, children exposed to large amounts of time on physical activities were equal not only in terms of academic success, but psychologically were more adjusted, happier, and posed fewer discipline problems.[24] It is unfortunate that physical activity programs and related field study experiences are regarded as frills. The fathers of our existing educational philosophies never intended that students would be shackled to the sedentary lifestyle common in classrooms today.

Environment-Oriented Activities

The environment component is identified as the place in which the host and agent interact. In addition to the usual environment subdivisions encountered — physical, sociocultural, and economic — the mass media have been added to reflect the pervasive influence of the print and broadcast media in our daily lives.

Selected Influence Activities: Environment. The third general strategy postulated by the traditional epidemiological model is the creation of barriers within the environment to prevent the agent from reaching the host. Rather than proposing only inhibitory measures, it may be more conducive, in the application of the model within the context of health promotion, to suggest facilitative influence initiatives or the elimination of barriers which would promote physical activity. This is especially relevant when one considers that the objective is to *add* physical activity to one's lifestyle, as opposed to eliminating or reducing some maladaptive behavioral response.

Facilities. Physical facilities conducive to conducting formal fitness programs are obvious advantages in establishing sound physical activity programs. Similarly, community cycling and cross-country ski trails by their existence facilitate physical activity. It must be recognized, however, that the resurgent social fad surrounding physical fitness and outdoor recreation has contributed significantly to the use of such facilities. In Ottawa, the National Capital Commission, a federal agency, in attempting to revitalize the downtown area, plowed off the snow and flooded five miles of the Rideau Canal for ice skating, creating what is billed as the world's longest ice rink. The original intention was not health related, but the tens of thousands who skate regularly on the canal have a new winter recreation, with its attendant physiological and psycholocal byproducts.

Coupled with the availability of such a facility, there is the chance of seeing the Prime Minister, a Deputy Minister, or even one's own boss skating, which reinforces the possibility of most government officials who work in Ottawa donning the blades from time to time to see and be seen. A winter season in Ottawa is incomplete without going skating on the Canal at least once.

Often, individuals are simply unaware of the options available to them to re-introduce physical activity into their daily lives. Mass transit advertising emphasizing the door-to-door convenience of its subway and bus routes unconsciously advocates a more sedentary population.   Similarly, the profusion of high-speed elevators subliminally deny activity to their passengers.   The individual must be made aware that he or she should not default in daily decisions to seize opportunities for physical activity.   In some instances, such decisions are financially rewarding.   The use of parking lots two or three blocks further from the office are often less expensive than those closer to the central city core.

Sanction.   The pursuit of physical fitness has gained approval in the corporate boardrooms of the nation.   In fact, the role model of the successful senior executive often demands a fit executive.   As employee fitness programs gain acceptance, support for the idea of physically fit employees may be formalized to such a degree that standards would be adopted regarding minimum fitness levels.   Many large companies have numerous recreational sport opportunities for employees through house and industrial leagues.

As the physical activity or fitness boom continues to gain momentum, more and more people are influenced by their friends to participate in some form of outdoor recreation.   The rational messages which have always been directed toward such audiences must take a backseat to the social motivations, which themselves ironically become rationalized by such remarks as, "It will surely be good for my health to participate."

Women have traditionally been denied the social approval to engage in fitness activities until relatively recently.   Even today, it is not uncommon to hear people heckle women joggers as they pursue their interest.   It has been suggested that participation by women in fitness-enhancing activity sometimes appears to be motivated by the desire for social contact, whereas males exercise primarily for health reasons.[25]

As another form of sanction, the necessity of seeking physician approval often acts as a barrier to participation in physical activity.   This medicalization of exercise is a phenomenon peculiar to North America, because of the emphasis on the risks as opposed to the benefits of habitual physical exercise.   In Canada, the Physical Activity Readiness Questionnaire (PAR-Q) is being utilized increasingly as a reasonable first step to take prior to initiating fitness programs or participating in a fitness test.[26]   The seven-item questionnaire alows each individual to determine for him/herself whether or not it is prudent to do some exercise without a physician's consultation.

Incentives.   Incentives could be a combination of intrinsic and extrinsic rewards, monetary or non-monetary.   Many people have suggested tax incentives from the federal government to stimulate personal involvement in fitness classes or the pursuit of various physical recreation activities.   Such a step, however, would be plagued by determining the nature of activities qualifying for tax incentives, the unequitable treatment of physically and mentally disabled citizens, and the monitoring problems associated with ensuring that abuses of the tax credit were kept to a minimum. It may be that insurance companies will reduce premiums for fitter clients when more definitive mortality information becomes available regarding exercise and longevity.

Some employers currently support partially or fully the participation of company personnel, usually upper and middle level management, in community and/ or privately administered fitness programs. The Canadian Broadcasting Corporation in Montreal assists company personnel financially to attend private fitness programs if the individuals attend a given percentage of classes. Others contribute company space and time to employee fitness activities. Whereas the latter are employee incentives, the potentially increased productivity, decreased absenteeism, and increased job satisfaction are recognized as desirable corporate incentives.

The Canada Fitness Awards constitute an incentive program for Canadian youth 7–17 years of age. Teachers and youth group leaders administer the tests, and all who achieve certain standards of performance on the six tests qualify for Bronze, Silver, Gold, or Award of Excellence crests. Over five million awards have been earned during the eight years the program has been operating.[27] The Young Olympians program is a similar incentive program based upon participation in a series of physical recreation experiences.[28]

Holistic View of the Model

In its basic form, the epidemiological model developed about the theme of physical activity presents a somewhat simplistic and incomplete taxonomy of influence activities. In order to optimize the strategic advantage of adopting the model, the health promotion practitioner must seriously consider the relative trade-off of engaging in various influence activities with regard to money, manpower, time, public and political acceptance, and perceived effectiveness.

Cost-effectiveness considerations such as the above are necessary in determining the proper allocation of resources. Similarly, the sequence of influence activities is very important. For example, although a regulatory strategy might produce a greater and longer-lasting compliance to a given target behavior, the intended program recipients should have sufficient and appropriate information prior to the attempted regulatory stratagem in order that its successful adoption is not defeated by uninformed opposition. Furthermore, a sound educational strategy in advance of the regulatory controls would ensure a more committed degree of compliance with the regulations afterwards. Kotler and Zaltman[29] have addressed the issue of systematic program coordination very well in their article on social marketing.

The epidemiological model emphasizes the tremendous synergistic potential of related influence activities. Rather than each program acting in a vacuum, the messages of one activity, both verbal and non-verbal, complement and supplement one another. Moreover, if the target problem is broken down into more manageable sub-problems, the additive and multiplicative effect of incremental program activities soon presents an amazing response to the problem's solution. Thus, solutions to physical inactivity as perceived within various settings – the home, the school, and the workplace – as well as in transit to these settings, require slightly different approaches by a variety of change agents, including the individual him/herself.

The role of the health promotion practitioner is the identification of the targets and their subdivisions; the selection of appropriate influence activities; and the determination of the most effective sequence in the application of program activities. The skillful elaboration of the model allows the health promotion practitioner to conceptualize all of the physical activity programs within the community and to recognize possible gaps in programming, as well as to suggest timely strategies to achieve further gains.

Summary

The problem of physical inactivity was confronted using a modification of the traditional epidemiological model. The selected influence activities identified in the model were exemplified by products, services, and activities associated with the Fitness Division of the Fitness and Amateur Sport Branch, an agency of the Canadian federal health department.

REFERENCES

1. Sackett, D.L., Gibson, E.S., Taylor, D.W., Haynes, R.B., Hackett, B.C., Roberts, R.S., and Johnson, A.L., "Randomized Clinical Trial of Strategies for Improving Medication Compliance in Primary Hypertension," *Lancet*, May 18, 1975, p. 1205; Somers, A.R., *Preventive Medicine U.S.A., Health Promotion and Consumer Health Education*. New York: Prodist, 1976; Bradshaw, P.Q., "The Problem of Cigarette Smoking and Its Control," *International Journal of the Addictions* 8:353–371, 1973; and Richards, N.D., "Methods and Effectiveness of Health Education: The Past, Present and Future of Social Scientific Involvement," *Social Science and Medicine* 9:141–156, 1975.

2. Bernstein, D.A., "Modification of Smoking Behavior: An Evaluative Review," *Psychological Bulletin* 71:418–440, 1969; and Pomerleau, O., Bass, F., and Crown, V., "Role of Behavior Modification in Preventive Medicine," *New England Journal of Medicine* 292:1277–1282, June 12, 1975.

3. Kannel, W.B. *et al.*, Precursors of Sudden Coronary Death: Factors Related to the Incidence of Sudden Death," *Circulation* 51: 606–612, April 1975.

4. Lalonde, M., *A New Perspective on the Health of Canadians.* Ottawa: Government of Canada, 1974.

5. Lauzon, R.R.J., "An Epidemiological Approach to Health Promotion," *Canadian Journal of Public Health* 68:311–317, July/August 1977.

6. Bogart, L., *Strategy in Advertising*. New York: Harcourt, Brace and World, 1967.
7. Cox, D.F., "Clues for Advertising Strategists," in *People, Society and Mass Communications*, edited by Dexter, L.A. and White, D.N. (Eds). New York: The Free Press, 1964, pp. 359–394.
8. Zifferblatt, S.M. and Wilbur, C.S., "Maintaining a Healthy Heart: Guidelines for a Feasible Goal," *Preventive Medicine* 6:514–525, December 1977.
9. Astrand, P.O., *Health and Fitness*. Ottawa: Recreation Canada, 1974; and Collis, M., *Employee Fitness*. Ottawa: Department of Supplies and Services, 1977.
10. Rogers, E.M. and Shoemaker, F.F., *Communication of Innovations: A Cross-Cultural Approach*. London: Collier-MacMillan, 1971.
11. PARTICIPaction. (For more information, contact the following office: 80 Richmond Street West, Suite 805, Toronto, Ontario. M5H 2A4.)
12. Jackson, J.J., "Diffusion of an Innovation: An Exploratory Study of the Consequences of Sport Participation: Canada's Campaign at Saskatoon." Doctoral Dissertation, University of Alberta, 1975.
13. Shephard, R.J., Bailey, D.A., and Mirwald, R.L., "Development of the Canadian Home Fitness Test," *Canadian Medical Association Journal* 114:675–679, April 17, 1976.
14. Jetté, M., "The Canadian Home Fitness Test as a Predictor of Aerobic Capacity," *Canadian Medical Association Journal* 114:680–682, April 17, 1976.
14a. Jetté, Maurice, "A Comparison Between the Predicted VO_2 max from the Åstrand Procedure and The Canadian Home Fitness Test," *Canadian Journal of Applied Sport Sciences* 4: 214–218, 1979.
15. World Health Organization, *Mass Health Examinations*, Public Health Papers No. 45. Geneva: World Health Organization, 1968.
16. Lauzon, R.R.J., "Fit-Kit for Fat Cats?" *Canadian Journal of Public Health* 67:95–100, March/April 1976.
17. Rosenstock, I.M., "Historical Origins of the Health Belief Model," *Health Education Monographs* 2:328–335, Winter 1974.
18. Freedman, J.L. and Fraser, Scott, C., "Compliance Without Pressure: The Foot-in-the-Door Technique," *Journal of Personality and Social Psychology* 4:195–202, 1966.
19. Durbeck, D.C., "The National Aeronautics and Space Administration U.S. Public Health Service Health Evaluation and Enhancement Program," *American Journal of Cardiology* 30:784–790, November 1972.
20. Lauzon, "An Epidemiological Approach to Health Promotion," *op. cit.*
21. Peepre, M., *Exercise Break*. Ottawa: Fitness and Recreation Canada, 1978.
22. Cox, *op. cit.*
23. Donoghue, S., "The Correlation Between Physical Fitness, Absenteeism and Work Performance," *Canadian Journal of Public Health* 68:201–203, May/June 1977.
    Shephard, Roy J. and Cox, Michael H. Toronto Employee Fitness and Lifestyle Project. A Report to Fitness Canada, Ottawa, 1980.
24. MacKenzie, J., "The Vanves Experiment in Education." Mimeographed Report, Regina Board of Education; and Mironuck, E.M. and MacKenzie, N.J., *Sherwood School Project*. Mimeographed Report, Regina Board of Education.
25. Bannister, R., "Sport, Physical Recreation, and the National Health," *British Medical Journal* 4:711–714, December 23, 1972.
26. Chisholm, D.M., "Physical Activity readiness," *British Columbia Medical Journal* 17: 375–378, November 1976.
27. *Canada Fitness Awards*. Ottawa: Fitness and Amateur Sport Branch, 1970.
28. *Young Olympians of Canada*. Canadian Olympic Association Program Ottawa.
29. Kotler, P. and Zaltman, G., "Social Marketing: An Approach to Planned Social Change," *Journal of Marketing* 35:3–12, 1971.

24

Corporate Mental Health
Programs and Policies

James S. J. Manuso, Ph.D.

Employee Health Services Department
Equitable Life Assurance Society of the U.S.

Introduction

In our increasingly secular society, we come into contact with organizational life
at every step along the developmental road. As a result, we are subject to those
facets of the organizational structure which both enhance and detract from the
quality of life. The organization has evolved into a site for the delivery of a multitude of human services, previously in the exclusive domain of government. Modern American corporations, perhaps the best examples of highly developed organizational structures, are increasingly finding themselves in the position of mental
health care providers. The corporate experience is demonstrating that preventive
services are the most cost-effective and viable in an institutional setting. In the
future, more corporate mental health programs and policies will reflect this
discovery.

Large organizations, in an effort to maximize their incrementally decreasing
return on investments in human resources, have recognized their role as a stressor
to their citizens. Because large organizations are dynamic, the stressors they
generate are frequent, intense, and sustained over time, creating an environment
conducive to the development of stress-related disorders. In turn, such disorders
bring about significant deficits in the application of employees' social, intellectual,
and learned skills, which are particularly important in organizational life. Moreover, these deficits are communicable in a social environment, bringing about
measurable productivity declines. Since this means a measurable net loss to the
employing organization, the selfishly altruistic need to correct the problem in a
cost-effective manner consistent with sound business practice becomes paramount. This is fortunate for the mental health industry, which needs to become
more cost-effective and preventive in its applications.

There are other social, legal, and economic reasons for a growing cottage industry of corporate mental health policies and programs at this time in our history. American society has become increasingly complex, demanding rapid

change, both interpersonally and institutionally. Previously avoidable confrontations with the full emancipation of women and minorities; with job changes, new sex roles, social alienation, divorce, relocation, and greater competition; and with new technologies and management systems are no longer avoidable. It should come as no surprise that the President's Commission on Mental Health[1] suggests that 25% of all Americans are suffering severe emotional stress, that the majority of Americans are dying from stress-related disorders, primarily through heart attack and associated hypertension and coronary artery disease, and that one-third to one-half of all general practice patients, including those seen in corporate medical departments, have stress-related problems. Americans, feeling more health-conscious and seeking a higher quality of life, are recognizing the importance of assisted behavioral change. Psychological health care is becoming less of a stigma and more popularly accepted; people feel that they need not be "sick" in order to get better, and are more preventive in their approaches to personal health care. Employees, corporations, and unions are all being educated as to the benefits of preventive mental health measures. The "new breed" of employees, the younger, more politically and socially sensitized group, is more insistent on the corporation's demonstration of social responsibility and its associated services.

From a legal perspective, with the advent of Affirmative Action and Equal Employment Opportunity come the corporation's responsibilities for ensuring the success and development of women, minorities, and the disabled in the organization. Thus, the vast problems of inner-city minorities, who have historically received the least of the worst mental health care, become the problems of the employing corporation. People cannot be fired — nor can hiring be denied — for health-related problems which affect an employee's overall performance. The maintenance of confidentiality with respect to employee health records has encouraged employees to make use of corporate mental health programs. And corporations continue to eschew governmental mandate, preferring to act before being acted upon.

From a purely economic perspective, profit-minded corporations can no longer afford to close their eyes to the stress-related genesis of costly employee lateness and absenteeism, poor decisions, terminations, dissension in work groups, lost sales, lowered worker morale, overtime costs, disciplinary actions, grievances, and the like. And the corporate bill for our nation's health care costs and employee benefits (now one-third of salary and increasing) is emerging more and more on the balance sheet. On the services end, there are more mental health practitioners available, practitioners trained in interventions that are typically short in duration, making use of drugs and new technologies, and which are more effective and less expensive. Finally, because most corporations already sponsor employee medical departments, it becomes a relatively inexpensive task to integrate a mental health program into an already existing health service.

In the pages that follow, occupational stressors peculiar to corporations and partially responsible for the causation of the stress-related disorders will be discussed. Using the Equitable Life Assurance Society of the United States as an example, a variety of preventive mental health policies and programs will be examined. Finally, recently completed research regarding the stress management training program, using industry's first in-house biofeedback laboratory, and related cost-benefit data, will be reviewed.

Corporate Stressors and Their Outcomes

For the working population, most of the waking hours are spent traveling to and from work, performing the job at the worksite, and engaging in job-related activities or thoughts at home. Though clerical, executive, and blue-collar employees exhibit roughly equivalent stress levels,[2] and executives are more mentally healthy than the general population, the corporate office setting provides multiple psychological, environmental, and occupational stressors which must be confronted. And it is these very stressor situations, when sustained, that have the capacity to induce the stress response and its accompanying symptomatic expressions.[3]

Many corporations, located in problematic urban areas, subject their employees to the stressors of crowding and noise. Corporate work requires long periods of sedentary confinement, with the frequent outcome of boredom and monotony. With executive jobs come the responsibilities of public speaking, of learning new tasks, of traveling and relocating; these often interfering with recuperative sleep. And, due to the harried interpersonal nature of corporate office work, the emotions of anxiety, fear, depression, and anger are commonly aroused. Hans Selye[4] has collected research identifying the foregoing characteristics of corporate life as effective in eliciting typical non-specific stress manifestations, which may ultimately generate symptoms.

In a more direct demonstration of the relationship between corporate stressors and stress, Weiman[5] studied 1540 managerial employees and found that four job factors were positively correlated with heavy smoking, hypertriglyceridemia, essential hypertension, arteriosclerotic heart disease, hypercholesterolemia, exogenous obesity, and peptic ulcer. The four factors were too much or too little to do, extreme ambiguity or extreme rigidity in relation to one's tasks, extreme role conflict or little conflict, and extreme amounts of responsibility (especially for people) or little responsibility. Another study[6] reported two additional commonly occurring occupational stressors — low social support from supervisors and from others at work, and a high amount of unwanted overtime, along with a subjective sense of quantitative work overload.

Job changes, including promotions, terminations, and the introduction of new mangement and work techniques, when they require considerable adaptation and usurp from the employee his or her traditional avenues of self-esteem, can result in stressor states, such as anxiety, depression, and anger and in stress-related symptomatology. One study[7] reported on a group of office employees' visits to the corporate health center for stress-related presenting problems three months before and three months after their management and work methods were changed precipitously. A 716% increase in such visits was observed. In decreasing order of incidence, the majority of visits were for exacerbation of hypertension, functional gastrointestinal disorders, anxiety, and muscular tension. Another study[8] found significant increases in norepinephrine excretion and in serums creatine, uric acid, and cholesterol, all indicative of the stress response, in employees whose jobs were abolished. The transmission of depressive thoughts and attitudes and acute depression requiring treatment have also been reported attendant to job abolishment.[9]

When 699 manager-members of the American Management Association were queried, they most frequently identified a lack of consideration for others, a need for recognition and approval, greed for power, envy, and a fear of criticism as those factors which led to the frequent phenomenon of damaging competitiveness at work.[10] " Damaging competitiveness," an unhealthy one-upmanship, involving the denegration of another's achievements, was reported to characterize nearly all of the managers' organizations.

Maccoby,[11] through a series of in-depth interviews with 250 executives from 12 of the largest U.S. manufacturing corporations, reported that half of his subjects admitted to a tendency to blame themselves, anxiety, uncertainty about what they wanted, and depression, which he traced to careerism. Thus, in a paradoxical fashion, corporate-encouraged careerism appears to develop those qualities least conducive to effective leadership.

The job site, a social situation as well, combines the subleties and complexities of social interactions within a hierarchically structured environment.[12] There are work role, normative, social, economic, and cultural expectations on the part of the company and its employees. At once the corporation excites emotional arousal, yet simultaneously imposes inherent limits on the expression of feelings both in peer relationships and in power relationships within the organization, thereby fostering the development of psychological defense mechanisms and a template for the development of stress-related disorders. The corporation, for its own survival, encourages its employees to define their egos in terms of the organization and to depend upon it. In this way, however, any work-related problem becomes more central and engrossing, and the dependency generates a stress-inducing sequence of hostilities, which must be suppressed.

On a smaller scale, it must be appreciated that corporate office life requires hourly, if not more frequent, adaptation to stressor situations, however minute. For example, in the course of a given work day, a corporate employee might be delayed enroute to work, miss an elevator, arrive late at an important meeting, lose a dime in the coffee machine, disagree with the boss, etc. These regular, intermittent excitations of the stress response ultimately cause some systemic wear and tear.

Thus, the very nature of the corporate setting creates multiple, daily stressors to which employees must adapt. If there is no adaptation, or if adaptation is slow and uncertain, stress may result and find expression through the development of stress-related disorders. And, as with any epidemic, unless stress carriers, who convey stressful affect and arousal levels throughout the social fabric of the organization, are recognized and treated, then the conditions for a threat to the institution itself are being satisfied. It will subsequently be shown that the cost to the employing corporation of unchecked stress overloads are tremendous.

The Corporation's Reponse To Its Mental Health Needs

In the previous section, it was established that any corporation is a stressor to its employees. Therefore, corporations may be distinguished from one another not in terms of the presence or absence of stressors, but in terms of their response (or lack thereof) to the problem. It appears that the corporation's central objectives are to maximize profits in a competitive market and to thereby perpetuate itself, its growth, and its power, through the management of employees by way of rational and authoritarian organizational structures and systems. It is clear that corporations are not in the business of curative mental health. However, mental health promotion and preventive policies and programs are wholly consistent with corporate goals, and in fact enhance their achievement, as some corporations are learning.

At Equitable, it is corporate policy to provide a program of health care for employees during the working day and to assist management in handling problems in which the physical or emotional well-being of an employee may be involved. The overall employee health program is the responsibility of the Employee Health Services Department at the New York Home Office. The Emotional Health Program of the Employee Health Services Department is dedicated to the detection, prevention, education, treatment, referral, and follow-up of troubled employees. All services are completely confidential, free of charge, and on company time. Indeed, employee health problems are recognized as treatable and are not to jeopardize one's job. The Emotional Health Program is physically housed in the Employee Health Services Department, thereby enabling the delivery of multi-modality (psychological and medical) services. Company physicians and nurses work closely with emotional health program staff. Emotional health program staff size varies from one practitioner for every 2000 employees during times of "business as usual, " and one for every 1000 employees during times of major organizational change.[13]

The Emotional Health Program offers a variety of optional and confidential services to employees. Short-term psychological treatment (i.e., 10 sessions or less) for anxiety and depression, the stress-related disorders, phobias, sexual dysfunction, and related non-psychotic problems is offered through two major modalities: conventional insight-oriented and cognitive-behavioral psychotherapy, and through the Stress Management Training Program utilizing industry's first biofeedback laboratory, wherein clients are neuromuscularly re-educated, or taught to achieve and maintain low levels of psychological and physical arousal. Psychological diagnostic testing is offered, but not for purposes of employee selection. In the Substance Abuse Program for self-referred or otherwise identified alcoholic and other drug abusers, clients are offered the option of treatment with followup or of facing the administrative consequences of their drug-induced behavior. The overwhelming majority of identified substance abusers opt for treatment. Emotional Health Program staff members are always on immediate call for acute crisis situations involving, for example, suicidal or homicidal threats, psychotic episodes, and aggressive behavior. The Managerial Training Program offers presentations to managers and supervisors regarding the recognition, proper handling, and appropriate referral of troubled employees. Advisory and consultative services are available to management for assistance in solving social and psychological problems encountered in their work. Employees requiring or requesting longer-term or highly specialized care are referred to the proper outside agency, institution, or practitioner. And, whenever a common problem, such as job abolishment, is shared by a large number of employees, some form of group intervention may be undertaken.

Though not formally a part of the Emotional Health Program, there exists a significant number of additional corporate programs which are ultimately preventive in their mental health impacts. For example, the Equal Employment Opportunity Office assists women and minorities with job-related difficulties, serving as advocate, educator, and negotiator on their behalf. An upward communications program facilitates employees' airing of their job-related concerns, when they feel they have been inappropriately dealt with by the corporation. On a regular basis, the Chief Executive Officer hosts advisory panels in order to maintain contact with employee morale, concerns, and attitudes. Other programs assist managers and supervisors in appropriately exercising their responsibility for others who report to them. The Personal Concerns Program, a hot-line and referral service, is intended to assist employees and their family members throughout the U.S. Whenever legal or financial problems affect an employee, consults are arranged with in-house professionals. In addition, a Pre-retirement Counseling Program offers employees age 55–65 the opportunity to discover alternatives which they may consider in their retirement years. Finally, a Career Counseling Program is available to employees who are considering changes in their careers.

The experience of the Emotional Health Program shows that the vast majority of troubled employees report not job-related problems, but personal, situational, or interpersonal problems. In decreasing order of frequency, the problems seen are anxiety disorders, 25%; depression, 20%; stress-related disorders (including headache, generalized tension, and myalgia), 15%; substance abuse, 15%; situational problems, such as a death in the family or financial dilemmas, 10%; and all others, 15%.[14] Although males and females use the services of the Program in equal proportions, males require more sessions of treatment than do females. This is because males tend to minimize or ignore the warning signals of emotional problems, whereas women respond quickly to emotional disequilibrium and seek out the proper care sooner, thereby not allowing symptoms to progress. The Program's experience demonstrates that the group reporting the most severe problems was composed of white or hispanic males in their twenties or thirties, married, with five or more years of service, working in pre-supervisory and pre-managerial jobs. It is at this point during the take-off phase for one's family and career lives, that the occupational stressors outlined earlier and others have their greatest additive impact.

A recent study indicated that 60% of all employees who received mental health services stated that these services were very helpful in terms of positive changes in the initial problem, their life in general, attendance, and job performance and satisfaction; 30% said the services were somewhat helpful; 8% said they were not helpful; and 2% did not respond. Therefore, 90% of Emotional Health Program services are found to be concretely helpful on the part of employees. Thus, it has been demonstrated that employees suffering mental health problems may be effectively treated at their worksite, this being a form of prevention.[15]

In a more general sense, emotional health programs such as the one at Equitable tend to evolve in specific directions over time. There is a tendency to move from a curative (that is, disability-oriented) stance to one of prevention and health enhancement. There is a movement away from addressing only the most severe problems with gross consequences to recognizing the importance of working with milder problems that nonetheless evidence significant hidden costs. There is a tendency to refer out less and offer more in-house, short-term treatment to employees. From a one-on-one orientation in intervention, there develops a willingness to work with groups of employees simultaneously. As such programs grow, they become more powerful in the host institution, establishing more liaisons with external resources, particularly with universities. Internship programs develop and research begins to emanate from the programs. As a critical mass of practitioners is achieved, a more aggressive marketing of the program to employees takes place.

Walter Wriston,[16] the Chairman of Citicorp, has indicated that "it is a business problem to set up sensitive Emotional Health Programs. An economic reality necessitates this rational and legitimate business decision." In the next section, by examining Equitable's Stress Management Training Program and its cost-benefits, an attempt will be made to validate this statement.

A Preventive Stress Management Training Program For Employees

One of the more forward-looking components of the Equitable's Emotional Health Program for Employees is the Stress Management Training Program. This Program is intended to assist people with stress-related disorders, and uses muscle and temperature biofeedback. The Program is intended to identify and train in the practice of anti-stress techniques those employees who evidence some suffering from the symptoms of stress overloads. This section will describe recently completed research[17] on the Stress Management Training Program.

There are four stages of the Stress Management Training Program. The first is a two-week intake phase, wherein the employee with a chronic stress-related disorder is referred by him/herself or by a physician in the Health Center. Usually, presenting problems are tension or vascular headache, generalized anxiety, or myalgia. In some instances, hypertension, pain, dermatitis, general intestinal dysfunctions, and the like are treated. There is a screen via medical evaluation, a neurological work-up, a psychological evaluation, a level of symptom activity (a composite of intensity and frequency of the symptom) at least in the moderate to severe range, and, finally, a determination that the patient is "motivated" for treatment.

In the second, baseline phase, also lasting two weeks, the employee comes to the Biofeedback Laboratory once a week, where forehead tension and hand temperature baseline measures are taken during a "stress state" and during a "relaxed state." In the baseline phase, employees also fill out two weeks of a daily log of symptom activity and behavior. This instrument also taps into their symptoms' interference with their functioning in the world.

The third phase constitutes treatment lasting five weeks. During this time, employees come to the Biofeedback Lab for deep relaxation training two to three times weekly. They receive primarily forehead muscle tension feedback with both audio and visual components in the first week. In subsequent weeks, feedback is primarily audio. Each laboratory session lasts approximately 20 minutes, with 10 1-minute trials measured for the subjects. There is a post-session questionnaire inquiring as to the nature of the subject's twilight state mentation, interfering thought processes (which typically refer back to a person's daily work problems), physical sensations during the session, and method of achieving relaxation.

To assist subjects in their development of stress awareness and control, they receive a cassette relaxation program,[18] an article on biofeedback training,[19] a list of self-hypnotic, autogenic phrases,[20] and verbal instructions for the twice-daily practice for deep relaxation in periods lasting from 5 to 15 minutes. The subjects are also taught a series of behavior modification, isometric, and breathing exercises in order to enhance their learning and application of the anti-stress response. Toward the end of treatment, subjects are weaned from the biofeedback machinery, and from dependency on feedback. This is accomplished by initially interspersing trials of feedback with no feedback, and, ultimately, a whole series of no feedback sessions. Immediately following treatment are three months of no contact whatsoever with the subject. They do not fill out the daily log and are given no special instructions other than to continue practicing what they have learned.

In the fourth and final phase, the follow-up, lasting two weeks, baseline measurements are again taken, subjects fill out the daily log, and they are medically and psychologically evaluated. Subsequent to the first follow-up, there are six-month and annual follow-ups.

The results of research on 30 subjects, 15 headache subjects and 15 anxiety subjects, who had been in this program from intake to first follow-up, show that subjects learned to decrease the absolute value of their forehead tension levels by approximately 50%, and that the within-session variation or variability of such tension decreased by approximately 600%. Thus, their tension levels were at a lower level and were more consistent. Symptom activity decreased from the high-moderate level to the low range. The interference of symptoms with subjects' ongoing activities decreased from 9% per hour to 1.5% per hour and, at work, from approximately 18% to 4%. The interference of symptoms at work is considerably higher than that in general, before and after treatment, because most of the stressors that people mention as having the greatest impact in terms of bringing about symptoms relate to their work environments. The subjects' weekly medication intake decreased from seven pills to two pills per week ("pills" may be Fiorinal or Percodan for headache patients and Valium or Librium for anxiety patients). Subjects' monthly visits to the Health Center for stress-related and other symptoms also decreased, from two visits per month to less than one-half visit per month following treatment. Their twilight state mental imagery reported during deep relaxation increased from non per session at baseline to approximately 0.6, nearly one image per session for all subjects, at follow-up. The interfering thoughts that were reported during deep relaxation decreased from approximately three to slightly less than one per session at follow-up. Most of the interfering thought content experienced related to the work environment of the subjects. And, finally, the number of physical sensations of relaxation, or "proprioceptive awareness," that people developed in the course of training increased from 0.22 per session at he outset to approximately 2.33 at follow-up.

Analyses of variance over all phases of the Program showed that there were no significant differences between headache and anxiety subjects on all measures but the number of interfering thoughts and twilight state images reported, thereby suggesting that a unitary dimension of dysfunction is shared by both of these stress-related disorders. It appears that anxiety subjects, who were much more prone to experiencing interfering thought patterns, had more difficulty in relaxing to the point where twilight state mental imagery would begin to occur.

The *additional* weekly pre-treatment costs to the corporation of employing one person (average salary, $270.00) with chronic headache or anxiety amounted to $70. This cost derived from three major categories. First, visits to the Health Center. Second, the interference of one's symptoms with his or her capacity to work. Finally, "meta-interference," or the effect of one person's anxiety on a co-worker, a boss, and a subordinate. This represents the "stress carrier" potential of employees suffering from the chronic stress-related disorders. Thus, the total additional pre-treatment costs to the corporation of employing individuals with stress-related disorders are not, as may have been suspected, related to lateness and absenteeism. The costs are hidden. The employees experiencing stress-related disorders typically work very hard, are not late, or are putting in extra hours. But the effectiveness of their time is less than what it could be in the absence of interfering symptoms.

After treatment, the additional costs of employing a subject with stress-related symptoms dropped dramatically to $15.00 per subject per week. Cumulative cost-benefit ratios demonstrate that, for every dollar invested in such a program, there is a $5.52 return on that investment per person per year. Also on the financial side are the perhaps incidental observations that unchecked stress difficulties pre-dispose employees to a higher-than-average likelihood of being terminated, and that employees suffering stress symptoms who complete the Program are more likely to advance their careers in the corporation at rates higher than the average.

It is evident that the Stress Management Training Program is a preventive and health-enhancing effort consistent with corporate objectives and individual health care concerns. To the corporation, offering stress management enhances productivity and decreased medical costs, while decreasing the number of stress carriers, who would otherwise cause a diffusion of stress throughout the delicate social network of the corporation. For the individual employee, effective stress management frees time and enhances alertness, composure, and relaxation in the absence of interfering symptoms. Both employer and employee gain.

Conclusion

The epoch of preventive health care, of wellness, and of self-regulation of behavior is truly beginning in corporate America. Increasingly, corporate employee health programs are serving as the earliest tier of preventive health service delivery. Government will no doubt encourage this development further, through financial and other incentives and, perhaps, through mandate. The tasks of developing and managing efficient, cost-effective preventive mental health programs will be met by the private sector: corporations must tame their creations for their own survival. Corporations are learning the ultimate in management. They are learning how to manage the stress they — of necessity — engender in their employees.

REFERENCES

1. Manuso, J., "Testimony to the President's Commission on Mental Health, Panel on Costs and Financing," *Report of the President's Commission on Mental Health* **II**, *Appendix.* Washington, D.C.: U.S. Superintendent of Documents, 1978, p. 512.
2. Dunn, J. and Cobb, S., "Frequency of Peptic Ulcer Among Executives, Craftsmen and Foremen," *Journal of Occupational Medicine* 4:343–348, 1962.
3. DiCara, L. (Ed.), *Limbic and Autonomic Nervous Systems Research.* Reading, Massachusetts: 1974.
4. Selye, H., *Stress in Health and Disease.* Reading, Massachusetts: Butterworths, 1976.
5. Weiman, C., "A Study of Occupational Stressor and the Incidence of Disease/Risk," *Journal of Occupational Medicine* **19**, 2:119–122, 1977.
6. Caplan, R., Cobb, S., French, J., Van Harrison, R., and Pinneau, S., *Job Demands and Worker Health: Main Effects and Occupational Differences.* U.S. Department of Health, Education, and Welfare, Publication No. (NIOSH) 75–160, 1975.
7. Manuso, J., "Coping with Job Abolishment," *Journal of Occupational Medicine* **19**, 9:598–602, 1977.
8. Cobb, S., "Physiologic Changes in Men Whose Jobs were Abolished," *Journal of Psychosomatic Research* **18**:245–258, 1974.
9. Manuso, "Coping With Job Abolishment," *op. cit.*
10. McClean, R. and Jillson, R., *The Manager and Self-Respect – A follow-up Survey,* AMACOM, 1977.
11. Maccoby, M., *The Gamesman: The New Corporate Leader.* New York: Simon and Schuster, 1977.
12. Levinson, H., Price, C., Munden, K., Mandle, H., and Solley, C., *Men, Management and Mental Health.* Cambridge, Massachusetts: Harvard University Press, 1962.
13. Manuso, J., *Staffing in a Corporate Emotional Health Program* In press as part of Springer-Verlag's series on Industry and Health Care, Monograph 8.
14. *Ibid.*
15. *Ibid.*
16. Wriston, W., "Opening Remarks, Employee Mental Wellness Conference," Washington, D.C., December 1–2, 1978. Washington Business Group on Health/Boston University Center for Industry and Health Care.
17. Manuso, "Testimony to the President's Commission on Mental Health, Panel on Costs and Financing," *op. cit;* and Manuso, J., "Stress Management Training in Large Corporations." Unpublished manuscript, 1978.
18. Budzynski, T., *CRP-1 Cassette Relaxation Program,* Boulder, Colorado: Biofeedback systems, 1975; and Manuso, J., *A Methodology for Achieving Low States of Psychophysiological Arousal,* cassette tape, 15 minutes, copyrighted, 1975.
19. Green, E., "Biofeedback: What It Is and How It Can Help You," Interview in *U.S. News and World Report,* April 4, 1977, pp. 63–64.
20. Cyborg Corporation, "Relaxation Training Procedure," copyrighted, 1974.

25

Information Cooperatives: Promoting Health Care

John H. Proctor, Ph.D.

Data Solutions Corporation

This chapter is about information cooperatives, "Health LINC," as a way to help change attitudes and procedures and to disseminate information about health care. It suggests ways of linking people together so they can take more active, informed roles in preventing illness and injury. In so doing, they can help link health care providers with one another and with the people they serve. Ways are suggested that health care professionals can open up to share technical information with non-professionals and perhaps even seek participative contracts for health maintenance to minimize the probability of disability and recuperation or dying. Health information cooperatives could work. Much of the communications technology, data storage and retrieval capability, health care information, and media preparation "know-how" are already available. The problem is that we have no designs for information cooperatives; no development and test plans; no implementation schedules, resource budgets, cost-benefit estimates, or management schemes. But perhaps the time has come for such planning. If so, local health information cooperatives can accentuate the promotion of injury and disease prevention and substantially contribute to lower health care costs.

The Problem

Our generation is part of and witness to a swell of interest in personal health care. In homes and schools, from medical personnel and the media, many of us have heard of the rules for living healthier lives, reducing periods of treatment, and dealing with infirmities with dignity. Health professionals throughout the country are discussing ways of reducing medical costs while expanding research toward new treatments and extending health care to those now unable to obtain even minimal assistance. Discussions concern possible incentive issue modifications by insurance companies; the expanding operation of the Health Maintenance Organization (HMO) as an alternative to conventional health care contracts; debates on pending federal health care legislation; and the acceptance of the President's voluntary cost reduction programs for hospitals. Except for a small minority momentarily addicted to diets, jogging, meditation, and talismans, most Americans lack a focus of orderly learning. We have no sense of personal participation in projects to lower medical costs. That is not to say that most Americans are not informed and concerned about health care issues. I think they are, but not in the way that we, as a nation, participate in a national war on poverty, a moon shot, or saving energy. Citizens and professionals are not working in a partnership to face the anticipated and unanticipated health problems that plague us from before birth until death.

Shifting Attitudes

If prevention of illness and injury, coupled with less expensive, timely, competent medical treatment that results in healthier citizens is a reasonable national goal, three fundamental shifts in attitude must occur in our society:

1. *Individual accountability.* A shift away from the passive, reactive consumption of health services toward an active, involved "self-help" perspective within one's personal physical and mental capabilities is necessary.
2. *Institutional objectives.* A shift away from the health care delivery institutions' efforts to preserve their identities through reaction-based medicine toward a system balanced with preventive medicine is needed.
3. *Information sharing.* A shift away from episodic and haphazard access to health information toward one which shares health information among citizens and health care providers before, during, and after events that shape physical and mental health is necessary.

Current national commitments, institutions, and programs *may* effect these massive shifts within our lifetime, but it is unlikely. The rising interest in personal health during the last decade may only be a prelude to improved health at lower costs. The American health care industry is so massive, and our government is so cumbersome, that to cause even a small discernable redirection requires tremendous, sustained efforts. Prevention needs a "hype." Citizen information cooperatives, with or without the help of government money and guidance, could provide this needed hype. At its best, it would involve all levels of society in sharing health care information geared toward prevention of harm for the individual and reduction of cost for treatment providers.

But what is a hype? Hype is a new word. It doesn't appear in Partridge's book of slang.[1] Webster defines hype as slang for either a hypodermic needle or a narcotics addict![2] It's a show-biz word often used in the magazine *Variety*, referring to the super-charged promotion of a new play, television program, or movie. It means an intensive campaign using pressurized ballyhoo. Such an approach can be used to get people to do something (vote, buy beer) or not to do something (stop smoking, don't drive over 55 mph). Hype covers a type of modern one-way communication designed to persuade, sell, or cause action.

The kind of hype prevention needs is of a different type. It needs vertical communication within multiple levels of the institutions comprising our health care field, as well as communication between households and community treatment resources.

Prevention is the "what" of our goal. An energetic, multi-leveled, participative promotion campaign is the initial "how," and healthier citizens at lower costs is the "why." The big questions are "who" and "when."

Health Activities at the Corporate Level

Prevention of injury and sickness as an integral part of health care is being promoted in a variety of ways. Several American Association for The Advancement of Science panels;[3] the conference on "Future Directions in Health Care: A New Public Policy," convened jointly by the Institute of Medicine of the Rockefeller Foundation, University of California Health Policy Program, and the Blue Cross Association;[4] the "Incentives for Health" conference conducted through the Health Promotion Project of the World Man Fund;[5] and other meetings have addressed this issue. Agendas of professional meetings such as those of the American Medical Association, the American Psychological Association, the American Hospital Association, and the World Health Organization indicate that prevention issues are appearing with increasing frequency.

Government. Government is legislating, studying, and proposing. The National Health Planning and Resources Development Act of 1974 (Public Law 93-641) clearly mandates that federal health systems include preventive measures. The Health Maintenance Organization Act of 1973 (Public Law 93-222 and 1976 amendments) encourages new ways of lowering medical costs through prevention. The National Consumer Health Information and Health Promotion Act of 1976 (Public Law 93-317) charges the Secretary of the U.S. Department of Health, Education, and Welfare with developing national goals and strategies concerning health information and health promotion. Eight different pieces of health-related legislation are before the Congress.

The U.S. Veterans Administration (V.A.) recently completed a multi-million dollar study of V.A. hospitals and health care delivery systems and is currently studying medical school affiliation with V.A. hospitals. "Blue Ribbon" panels are studying military hospital systems.

Efforts by the federal government to promote prevention of illness and prevention of injury at the workplace are relatively new additions to labor laws. The Occupational Safety and Health Administration of the U.S. Department of Labor is setting health standards, inspecting the workplace, and enforcing compliance. The U.S. Department of Labor's Employment Standards Administration, Office of Workers' Compensation Programs, is starting to pilot-test medical standards for work-related diseases concerning heart, lung, back, and psychiatric areas for federal employees. In addition to day-to-day prevention of illness and injury, the President's Reorganization Plan No. 3 for federal emergency management and assistance is designed to support state and local emergency organizations and resources in times of calamity. Couple all this with federal, state, and local safety and disease prevention programs for vehicles, firearms, drugs, water, food, housing, and consumer products, and a massively expensive promotional effort toward healthier, more productive citizens begins to emerge.

Unions and Other Organizations. Government efforts may be only a small part of our society's expression of concern for human health and safety. The International Brotherhood of Teamsters, Chauffeurs, Warehousemen and Helpers (Teamsters), the American Federation of Labor/Congress of Industrial Organizations (AFL/CIO), the United Mine Workers (UMW), and the United Auto Workers (UAW) have pressed long and hard to establish and maintain contract provisions covering worker health and safety.

Most secondary schools, the military services, trade schools, and apprentice programs teach courses about personal hygiene and ways to prevent accidents. Fraternal organizations, the American Red Cross, the Boy Scouts, the Girl Scouts, Future Farmers of America, and civic organizations educate and reinforce practices that contribute to safer and healthier lifestyles. Charitable, non-profit organizations have nationwide fund-raising promotions for education, research, and service delivery in the prevention and treatment of all types of injuries and diseases. Churches of every denomination have national and local programs for preventing and coping with mental and physical problems, and provide assistance to individuals and families in all age groups and circumstances. Several philanthropic foundations are specifically chartered to channel funds to health-related projects.

Business and Industry. Business and industry, long involved in employee health and safety programs, find innovation in this area popular. The International Business Machine Corporation (IBM), Johns Mansville, the Aluminum Corporation of America (ALCOA), Gates Rubber Company, Blue Cross in Rhode Island, and Hawaii's Blue Shield are reported to be trying out ways to reduce skyrocketing costs and promote self-care and early medical diagnosis of difficulties.[6] Most small businesses have annual medical checkups for key personnel and provide time and financial support for community health, safety, and recreation activities. Pharmacies and food stores advertise, explain, and sell home remedies. Hardware, paint, sporting goods, and hobby shops provide pamphlets and explanations for the safe operation and storage of the products they sell.

Health Care Professionals. Finally, to all these trillions of words poured out on the subject, to the millions of paid and volunteer hours of work, and the billions of dollars, must be added the cornerstone contributions of the professional and para-professonal health care community of hospitals, clinics, nursing homes, pharmacies, medical equipment manufacturers and suppliers, group and private practices, and medical, dental, graduate, and technical schools. A bewildering array of medical, psychological, and health-related technical specialties results. Much of this activity is reported to us by the press, advertised by word and picture, and dramatized on paper, in plays, and on film. We may be the most well-informed, if not the healthiest, people in history.

The Crossroads

While all of these activities are produced in generally the same moral, legal, and economic environment, they do not add up to form a single system responsive to commands of a single power group. The system was not designed and developed, it just grew. In far too many ways, some of the institutions and activities mentioned above do not exhibit efficiency and effectiveness. Compared to the health of other peoples of the world, however, or to the prospects of healthy living enjoyed by Americans of earlier times, only a few of today's Americans would wish to change places with any other group of people. Our riches and talents have produced wonders. Few would dismantle key elements of our health care community, but many want improved health at lower costs for more people.

But the objective of improving health at lower cost puts us at a crossroad. One road sign is labeled, "Leave things alone. It will work out." Another sign reads, "Force health and safety organizations to be more responsive." One more sign reads, "Shift your premises and get the people involved." I prefer the third route.

Many persons would argue that a single monolithic system is definitely not desirable no matter how orderly or efficient it might be. Variety is the pattern to be sought for effectiveness, they believe (and with reasonably sound motives). People and groups should be left to march to their own drummer with minimum legislative constraints and governmental interference, they suggest.

To improve health at lower costs, the three required fundamental shifts in point of view (individual accountability, institutional objectives, and information sharing) can, in my judgment, be accelerated, and gains can be sustained, by using a prevention "hype."

Information sharing may be an absolute necessity for prevention hype. But I do not only urge greater information sharing. Each information transfer or transform costs money that is ultimately paid by the patient and/or the taxpayer. Medical costs are too high now and people are less willing to let the "experts" be in charge. New knowledge and new technology exist that suggests the old one-way linkage of the healing professions to the healed is not only breaking up but a new link forming: a two-way link, drawing the previous "clients" into the process as partners in health maintenance and illness/injury prevention. The probability of such a partnership improving health, as well as causing lower costs, would be greater if information cooperatives were involved.

Information Cooperatives

Farm and neighborhood cooperatives for food, equipment, consumer products, transportation, and child care have been around for years on the local level, and within the cooperative lifestyles of some churches and political groups. The kind of prevention hype I have in mind calls for medical information cooperatives at the local level. Individuals and families would be linked to all community mental and physical health services through an information cooperative. The information cooperative is the local pool of information on what and who is available where and when, under emergency, as well as under normal conditions. Such a local health and safety directory could also become a local health information center. It could answer members' questions and help resolve difficulties between members and health care organizations. It could become a lending library for audio and video tapes and equipment for self-improvement of health. It could arrange meetings, seminars, speakers, and home health care. The objective would be to pull together volunteer and para-professional community resources to augment the established health care services provided by hospitals, clinics, and medical and psychological practitioners, with prevention and health maintenance activities. Such health information cooperatives could remain small entities located conveniently and servicing no more than 10–15 thousand people. It would be important for the link between the individual and the health information cooperative to be open and personal 24 hours a day, all year round.

Mini-computers.   A key feature of the local health information cooperative would be the mini-computer and the decentralized information processing networks that are now possible.

This new approach promises a de-emphasis of, and a departure from, the currently prevalent, centralized computer operations. Such systems would be replaced in favor of decentralization and delegation of function to the component elements of a system of dispersed computers. Such decentralized systems are frequently referred to as distributed or federated systems. Less expensive mini-computers became available in the early 1970's. Offsprings of the space program, these new computers revolutionized computing by making information processing technology available to a much larger number of potential users, in larger quantities, at greatly lower costs. Some mini-computers have been mass-produced since 1978 and are retailed for under $1000.

Mini-computer hardware is one of two innovations to permit escape from the massive, centralized complexity of the computerized world. The second is a way of breaking down the single centralized system into a *system of systems* to reduce that complexity. With the advent of switching capability, this is now possible. At least as significant is the fact that the complexity of computer programs can now be overcome: a number of relatively simple programs can take the place of a single, massive, hierarchically structured program.[7]

Some Possible Objectives. As I see it, the local health information cooperative would extend the ability of a family to discuss health matters at home, would allow neighbors to chat with one another about health maintenance, and would assist with the logistics of providing treatment. The local health information cooperative would remove some of the pressure from health care providing organizations by answering questions before, during, and after treatment, and by reducing the demand for treatment. Information exchange within the local cooperative could be accomplished face to face, in writing, by telephone, through videotape replay, or by radio and television broadcasts. The short distance citizens band (CB) radio and longer range amateur radio, now used in rural and remote areas, could be utilized. Information sharing between computers via commercial or dedicated phone lines could also be facilitated. In short, the imagination and commitment of the local people would determine the extent of their health cooperative.

Local cooperatives could be linked into a network at the community level and linked again at a regional level. The kinds of system architectures and procedures discussed by cyberneticians[8] could be applied to such health information federations. This would reduce costs and increase responsiveness.[9]

I believe health information sharing at the individual family level is the key to larger combinations of information cooperatives. In my view, the one-way communication of mass media to consumer results in an under-utilization of the abilities of the consumer.

I share the view that, despite our information-intensive society, people are less linked to their major institutions than they should be. Health information cooperatives could be established at almost no cost as part of existing or planned neighborhood facilities. Incentives could be business and industry sponsorship, lower insurance premiums, lower health plan membership fees, and government tax credits.

If health maintenance and avoiding disease and injury are considered economic matters, health information sharing would be a local political matter of redistribution of access to available information sources. Health information cooperatives as part of a community's public safety network, supported by tax dollars, would open up the community's health resources to individuals of low income, of various ethnic and age groups, situated in both rural and inner city locations. Health information cooperatives should also reduce the unreasonable individual and community demands upon treatment resources by accentuating prevention.

The prevention "hype" could be sustained through local relationships in everyday health matters, and would utilize in-place channels to mobilize the community against large disasters as well.

Getting Started

These thoughts concerning information cooperatives to promote prevention are compatible with the intriguing proposal of Drs. Lorenz K.Y. Ng, Devra Lee Davis, and Ronald W. Manderscheid[11] for health promotion organizations:

> We propose the establishment of voluntary community-based health promotion organizations (HPO's) that will a) reward healthy lifestyles by teaching people to take greater responsibility for their own health, and b) create incentives for health promotion and disease prevention by stimulating a closer working relationship among government, business, labor, and the health care system.

Health information cooperatives could be part of HPO's. Cooperatives could spring up like daisies in a field. Their form, sponsorship, services provided, and capabilities would depend on local circumstances. "Health Local Information Network Cooperative" (LINC) pilot projects, in which the people in a selected area are connected to health care institutions through a health information cooperation, are possible now with private or government seed funds. The need is clear; the technology is here.

Health care professionals have worked diligently to revise their conceptual frame of reference regarding how to deliver both services and knowledge about services and preventive measures. Nothing new is being said here about the art and science of mental and physical medicine, but there are forces at work, other than rising medical costs, prompting this stand. Among the deepest and most fundamental human desires are to postpone death and to ease pain. Dissatisfaction with health care — real or imagined — has been, and will continue to be, part of daily life. Health information sharing would not or should not be confined to public and private groups walled off from one another and the individual citizen by rigidly defined roles. Their goals should not include protecting the *status quo*. Such action would only earn either inordinant government controls or implosion of the health care community of interests.

As we look toward the future, one of the brightest prospects is that, perhaps for the first time, Americans have the freedom and resources to combine their own traditional wisdom with the expertise of science and technology to provide affordable solutions to the problems of health care.

REFERENCES

1. Partridge, E. (Ed.), *Dictionary of Slang and Unconventional English, 7th Edition.* New York: MacMillan, 1970.
2. *6000 Words, Supplement to Webster's 3rd New International Dictionary.* Springfield, Massachusetts: G & C Merriam, 1976, p. 94.
3. Proctor, J.H. and Papier, L.D., "Sense and Non-sense In Health Service Delivery to Families," a paper delivered at the 21st Annual North American Meeting of the Society for General Systems Research with the American Association for the Advancement of Science. Denver, Colorado, February 21–25, 1977; and the panel, "Health Enhancement: Prevention and Promotion." Houston, Texas, January 3–8, 1979.
4. Ng, L.K.Y., Davis, D.L., and Manderschied, R.W., "The Health Promotion Organization: A Practical Intervention Assigned to Promote Healthy Living," *Public Health Reports* 93, 5, September/October 1978.
5. "Report of a Working Conference on 'Incentives For Health'." Bethesda, Maryland: World Man Fund, February 1977.
6. Ng, *et. al., op. cit.*
7. Data Solutions Corporation, "Alternatives for the Development of U.S. Navy Requirements for Distributed Data Base Technology," a report prepared for the Office of Naval Research under Contract NOOO14-77-C-0626, September 12, 1977.
8. Ackoff, R.L., *Redesigning the Future: A Systems Approach to Societal Problems.* New York: John Wiley & Sons, 1974.
9. Proctor, J.H., "A Value Sensitive General Systems Approach to Organization Design and Improvement," in press.
10. Beer, S., *Platform for Change: A Message from Stafford Beer.* London: John Wiley & Sons, 1975.
11. Ng *et al., op. cit.*, p. 450.

26

Kaiser-Permanente: Preventive Medicine and Health Promotion

H. Frank Newman, M.D.

Health Maintenance Organization Program
Department of Health, Education, and Welfare, Region 10

Preventive Medicine, Public Health, and Health Promotion

There is increasing interest in our society in preventing illness and in maintaining and promoting health through personal activities and changes in individual lifestyle.[1] Such personal preventive medicine should be distinguished from public health measures which seek to immunize susceptible populations or to remove pathogens or carcinogens from our environment. I am not referring to public health measures initiated by governments or by industries at the insistence of governments. I am referring to actions initiated by the individual to change his or her behavior or lifestyle with the hope of promoting health. Such actions may involve use of tobacco, alcohol, or drugs, nutrition or diet, exercise, and handling of stress — factors which are controlled by the individual and can be modified by appropriate health care services.

Health professionals are expected to encourage good health habits in their patients, whenever appropriate, as a part of good health care delivery. Personal preventive services should include disease prevention, disease detection, health maintenance, and health promotion.[2] The problem has been to develop an environment with emphasis on preventive measures rather than on curative medicine: an environment where preventive measures can be easily introduced, where monitoring of health status can be done, where diseases can be detected early, and where health promotion activities, such as improvements in lifestyle, are encouraged. To do this, both the patient and the health care provider should be rewarded for keeping the patient healthy.

I would like to describe a health care delivery system that provides this type of environment — one which rewards the physician for keeping the patient as healthy as possible, not one based on "fee for illness" treatment. The health care delivery system is based on payments to providers, and is what the government calls a health maintenance organization (HMO).

The HMO — An Effective Health Care Delivery System

Prepaid group practice is an idea whose time has come. Recognition by the government of this concept accelerated in the early 1970's when the U.S. Department of Health, Education, and Welfare (HEW), singled out prepaid group practice organizations (renamed health maintenance organizations) as the administration's chosen instruments for effecting a rational reorganization of the delivery of health services.[3] Since that time, Congress has passed the HMO Act of 1973 to provide grants, loans, and loan guarantees to developing HMO's and to require most employers of more than 25 persons to offer HMO's as a choice for their employees.

HMO's continue to interest Congress and the administration, primarily because of concern about the cost of health care and bringing these costs under control. HMO's have a proven record of providing quality health care in a cost-effective manner. For example, studies done by the Research and Statistics branch of the Social Security Administration indicate savings of 20-25%, in providing care to Medicare beneficiaries.[4] (I will discuss some of the reasons for this cost-effectiveness later.)

The current popularity of group practice prepayment HMO's represents a remarkable change from the preceding four decades, when both organized medicine and government fought the fledgling organizations with numerous potent weapons: state laws outlawing "lay controlled" medical plans; invocation of the common law rule against the "corporate practice of medicine"; professional boycotts; expulsion of associated doctors from medical societies; refusal of hospital privileges to associated physicians; and refusal to make available Hill-Burton funds and other government assistance to such plans.

Landmarks in this evolutionary development include a series of Federal and State Supreme Court decisions finding medical societies guilty of restraint of trade and ordering them to stop boycotting the maverick organiziations; a New York law specifically prohibiting denial of hospital privileges because of affiliation with a group practice plan; the 1959 Report of the American Medical Association Commission on Medical Care Plans, which was adopted by the House of Delegates of the AMA affirming the patient's right to a free choice of medical plans as well as individual doctors; provisions permitting prepaid group practice plans to participate in the Federal Employees Health Benefits Act, in 1959; and the laudatory endorsement of prepaid group practice by the President's National Advisory Commission on Health Manpower, in 1967.

Today, if all HMO-type plans are counted, there are approximately 230 in existence, covering some 6.5 million persons. Development of new plans, plus expansion of the existing ones, has been facilitated by increased interest and aid from business, insurance companies, organized labor, and government. Plans are being developed with federal aid and through use of private resources. We in HEW are interested in seeing all types and forms of programs developed. We are particularly interested in promoting an interaction between business and industry and the health professionals to form new plans. We would like to see programs develop in the Midwest, the South, and the Southwest, where few now exist.

It may seem reasonable to ask why group practice prepayment HMO's have *not* grown faster. Many of the legal and professional barriers mentioned earlier still remain in areas where new programs are attempting to start. They may be in more covert form, but they are there. Furthermore, the building of a prepaid group practice is a difficult and costly job, since you are, in effect, building an entire medical care system. Money is needed for facilities and equipment. Skilled managerial talent is needed, and health care professionals must be recruited. Such difficulties have led to the development of a second form of HMO, the "foundation type" or independent practice association (IPA). Easier and less costly to put together, an IPA permits doctors in solo practice who are paid on a fee-for-service basis to form a network of participating doctors.

Let's digress for a moment and examine the origin of the term HMO and define it. The originator of the term "health maintenance organization" was Dr. Paul M. Ellwood, a physician and health policy researcher who saw the need for reorganizing the medical care delivery system of the U.S. and saw prepaid group practice plans and medical care foundations (IPA's) as potential instruments to achieve this and to help control the cost of health care.[5]

Ellwood defined an HMO as "an organization which delivers comprehensive care — including preventive services, ambulatory and inpatient physician services, hospital services, laboratory and x-ray services and indemnity coverage for out-of-area emergency services — to voluntarily enrolled consumers, on the basis of fixed price contracts.[11] By its contract, the HMO guarantees the availability of quality health care services to its enrollees for a prepaid monthly premium that the individual, business, union trust fund, or government unit can budget for and be assured that the consumer will have relatively small additional charges.

Prepaid group practice plans can qualify for federal certification as HMO's by meeting the requirements of the Health Maintenance Organization Act of 1973 as amended in 1976 and 1978.

Prepaid group practices can be hospital-based. For example, five of the Kaiser-Permanente Program's six Regions are hospital-based, with the hospitals owned and operated as an integral part of the program. Most prepaid groups are not hospital-based, and operrate like the Colorado Region of the Kaiser-Permanente Program — where community hospitals are used.

The HMO Act also recognizes IPA's where individuals or groups of physicians join a foundation type plan.

How can the public be assured that an HMO is a quality program capable of delivering what it contracts to do? This concern is reflected in the HMO Act, which sets forth a strict set of guidelines and regulations that a plan must meet in order to be qualified. HMO qualification requires a demonstration of quality and performance. In addition, the Civil Service Commission certifies HMO's to participate in the Federal Employees' Health Benefits Program.

Group practice prepayment plans have a national organization, GHAA, which will not grant full membership to a plan unless it has met the standards established by GHAA and has had an on-site inspection. Medical groups associated with HMO's may belong to the American Group Practice Association if they have met a set of quality standards established by AGPA. These qualifications, plus state licensing, certification to participate in Medicare by the Social Security Administration, and the use of hospitals accredited by the Joint Commission on Accreditation of Hospitals, are factors to look for when enrolling or entering into a contract with an HMO.

HMO's do not offer a panacea to all the problems of health care delivery in the U.S. Many people do not like the idea of getting care from a structured organized system. HMO's are difficult to set up in rural and sparsely populated areas — although some versions of plans show promise.

In spite of these problems, interest in HMO's continues, and HEW projects 442 HMO's by 1988.

HMO's of the prepaid, group practice variety follow six basic principles, the so-called "genetic code" orginally described by Dr. Ernest Saward when he was medical director of the Permanente Medical Group of the Oregon Kaiser-Permanente Medical Care Program. The principles are as follows:

1. *Group practice.* Each Permanente Medical Group is a multi-specialty group, with the physicians practicing as a team together with their supporting personnel.
2. *Prepayment with community rating.* Prepaid rates applied on a community-rated basis cover a majority of the plan's financial requirements. Prepayment requires careful budgeting, and community rating helps achieve financial stability.
3. *Organized facilities and services.* Health care services are provided at specified facilities by specialized groups of physicians. Health care resources are integrated to maximize efficiency and the options available to the physician and thus aid physicians in selecting the most appropriate care for the patient.
4. *Voluntary enrollment.* Enrollment in the program is voluntary. No group is enrolled unless at least one other choice of health benefits coverage is available and subscribers have the option of changing plans periodically.

5. *Preventive services.* Preventive medicine and early diagnosis and treatment are emphasized and are part of the prepaid coverage.
6. *Role of physicians.* Their interest and responsibility are not limited to those health services that they provide directly. They also participate in the allocation of resources and in the planning and direction of the total program.

Note that preventive medicine is part of this "genetic code." Let us look at recent developments in preventive medicine and health promotion and briefly describe observations made by Drs. Morris Collen and Sidney Garfield, pioneer Kaiser-Permanente Medical Care Program physicians, in development of a "systems approach" to personal preventive health care services in a prepaid group practice environment.

The Kaiser-Permanente Medical Care Program

In 1933, Dr. Sidney Garfield started a prepaid group practice plan at Desert Center in southern California to care for the industrial injuries and illnesses of workmen constructing the aqueduct from the Colorado River to Los Angeles. Dr. Garfield discovered that a large number of workmen were coming to him with puncture wounds in their feet. On some afternoons, the waiting room seemed to be filled with men, each with one boot removed, exposing bloody socks torn by stepping on nails. Under the prepaid capitation system, the treatment of what Dr. Garfield considered avoidable injuries was costing him time and money and he decided to do something about it. He and a colleague spent their few free hours removing dangerous nail-bearing scrap wood from the walkways in the work areas and asked that in the future such walkways be kept clean. Since a healthy, uninjured worker was an asset, accident prevention and preventive care become a regular part of Dr. Garfield's professional practice. His tiny prepaid group practice lead to the formation of the Kaiser-Permanente Medical Care Program. Today, the Kaiser-Permanente Medical Care Program accepts the responsibility for organizing and delivering medical and hospital services to 3,500,000 members in California, Oregon, Washington, Hawaii, Colorado, and Ohio. It is the nation's largest prepaid group practice and is used as a prototype example of a health maintenance organization both by government and by students of health care delivery.

The mission of the program is to provide quality care at a reasonable and affordable cost to subscriber-members on a prepaid basis. The program, which operates on a decentralized basis in six geographic regions, consists of three separate but closely cooperating organizations,[1] the Kaiser Foundation Health Plan, Inc. (Health Plan) which contracts with[2] Kaiser Foundation Hospitals, and[3] the Permanente Medical Groups, to provide the services needed by the health plan members.

A Systems Approach to Preventive Health Services

Given the state of the art and the fact that society has been oriented toward treatment rather than toward the prevention of disease, what has the Kaiser-Permanente Medical Care program learned about provision of preventive services to an enrolled population?

1. *Disease prevention.* Disease prevention for the individual includes periodic immunizations, with particular emphasis on childhood immunizations for communicable diseases. A comprehensive health history, describing an individual's lifestyle, occupations, and hobbies, and identifying exposure to environmental factors which are health hazards, is taken, and attempts to control or remove such hazards are made. Individuals who, because of heredity, occupation, or other predisposing factors, are high risks for specific diseases are identified and programs are instituted to either prevent or forestall disease in the best manner possible, thus preventing complications such as blindness, cardiovascular disease, circulatory, or skin complications, etc.

2. *Disease detection.* Disease detection usually involves health status check-ups and includes tests for specific conditions as an attempt to identify abnormalities early enough to postpone or prevent disability or death. Breast and pelvic examinations in women and rectal examinations in men are examples of productive activities for disease detection. A variety of processes are available to provide the above, including traditional periodic checkups, periodic multiphase health testing,[6] and a recently proposed lifetime health monitoring program.[7]

3. *Health maintenance.* Health maintenance uses periodic monitoring of health status to retain one's health and prevent or postpone the effects of previously identified health hazards or risk factors.

4. *Health promotion.* Health promotion really transfers the responsibility to the individual and employs education and counseling to convince the individual to obtain health status through improved lifestyle, diet, exercise, etc.

To implement the preventive health measures in traditional medical practice, tests are generally selected and arranged for by each physician for each patient on some periodic basis. In the Kaiser-Permanente Medical Care Program, the system has been set up so that either the physician or the patient may initiate the process.

Through the work of Morris Collen, M.D., a Permanente Medical Group physician, considerable evidence has been developed which shows that if a program of prevention is to be cost-effective, it should be based on the individual patient's age, sex, and specific risk factors. In other words, a health care provider should prescribe a set of tests tailored to information gathered regarding the individual's age, sex, health history, occupation, and lifestyle. Risk factors should be identified and a cost-effective set of tests given, with reexamination done using the time intervals determined appropriate for that individual's risk category.

Dr. Collen, working with Dr. Sidney Garfield, the founding physician for the Kaiser-Permanente Medical Care Program, advocates a systems approach to personal preventive health care services. In contrast to the care of the sick, the care of the well is easily adapted to a "systems approach." The system assumes that:

1. Most people in the community are well.
2. "Sick care" is the exception rather than the usual situation for individuals. Sick care is less susceptible to programming and protocols and, thus, is best obtained on an individual basis from physicians.
3. Preventive care or "well care" can be a routine, repetitive process, programmable for almost everyone.
4. Well care is adaptable to application of protocols, automation, and a systems approach, using allied health personnel trained in specific skills.
5. A well-organized system, based on repetitive encounters, tends to exploit economies of scale and the efficiency potential of automation, and lends itself to assurance of quality through control process monitoring.
6. The potential is there to reduce cost while improving service and quality through developing a systems approach.

Building on these precepts, Dr. Collen built a multiphasic health checkup[8] system to provide an efficient solution to periodic health examinations. He has some 25 years experience in this systemized approach. The system is not based on a universal procedure for all people, but classifies individuals by age, sex, and health status. The type of test done, the frequency of tests, and the follow-up by physician or other health care providers, varies dependent on age and test results.

The system employs automated laboratory procedures and specially trained allied health personnel who collect data concerning a patient's medical history, and clinical, X-ray, and other physiological test measurements in a programmed sequence.

The result is a Multiphasic Health Checkup (MHC), provided by using Multiphasic Health Testing (MHT), followed by a physical examination and a physician's determining if the patient is well or sick. Appropriate recommendations for follow-up care are then made. The system has been expanded to use Automated Multiphasic Health Testing (AMHT), which employs automated equipment and computerized decision rules to sort out those who have disease. Further expansion of the system to Multiphasic Health Testing Programs (either manual or automated) includes health care delivery systems to provide adjunctive services such as entry triage, health counseling, health education, and preventive health maintenance.

Kaiser-Permanente's experience with MHC indicates that adults find such checkups to be very acceptable, and that a substantial percentage of adults voluntarily avail themselves of periodic health checkups. Studies[9] show that this approach is very effective for early disease detection and health maintenance. By the appropriate selection of tests, the checkup process can be very cost-effective. Studies also show that such a systemized approach not only decreases the cost of the initial health status evaluation, but decreases significantly the total cost of care for at least one year (by about 20%), compared with the traditional mode of the patient-doctor encounter.[10]

Dr. Collen also showed that promotion of periodic multiphasic checkups decreased significantly the mortality for people over age 35 for some conditions that could potentially be postponed to which the checkup was directed (by as much as 50%). Also, he was able to demonstrate a lower mortality rate from all causes for those who elected to come in for checkups as compared to those who did not. There were also decreases in disability, and increases in average net earnings for middle-aged men.[11]

In summary then, the Kaiser-Permanente Medical Care Program has attempted to develop a cost-effective system of disease prevention, early disease detection, health insurance, and health promotion. Systemized health checkups such as MHT, MHC, and MHTS can effectively identify each person's health needs and arrange for appropriate services to meet those needs. The process, which uses tests tailored to the individual's characteristics and health risks, selects out the high-risk persons and those who have early asymptomatic illness. It then refers the sick to sick care services and the well to health education and health counseling services, to further improve their current health status. Using this approach provides an efficient entry mode to health care, and provides each individual the opportunity for assistance with categorical and lifestyle problems such as control of obesity and stop-smoking programs. Although the efficiency of health checkups has not been demonstrated to everyone's satisfaction, checkups are for the majority of Americans a "part of life."

Since in a health maintenance organization such as Kaiser-Permanente, these services and costs are included and promoted as integral parts of the health care delivery system, the system sought out a cost-effective manner to provide them. By doing this, the system satisfies its membership and enables itself to compete successfully with other health care providers. If the government and the public choose to encourage provision of preventive health services, both also should support the systemized approach.

REFERENCES

1. *Task Force Reports, Preventive Medicine, U.S.A.* New York: Prodist, 1976; and *Conference on Health Promotion and Disease Prevention*, Institute of Medicine, National Academy of Sciences, February 1978.
2. Nightingale, E.O., Cureton, M., Kalamar, V., and Trudeau, M., "Perspectives on Health Promotion and Disease Prevention in the U.S.," a Staff Paper, Institute of Medicine, National Academy of Sciences, January, 1978.
3. Department of Health, Education, and Welfare, "Toward a Comprehensive Health Policy for the 1970's: A White Paper." Washington, D.C.: Government Printing Office, pp. 31–32.
4. Corbin, M. and Krute, A., "Some Aspects of Medicare Experience with Group Practice Prepayment Plans," *Social Security Bulletin* **39**:3, 1976; and Gaus, C.R., Cooper, B.S., and Herschman, C.G., "Contrasts in HMO and Fee-For-Service Performance," *Social Security Bulletin* **39**:3, 1976.
5. Ellwood, P.M., "Testimony before the Subcommittee on Health, Committee on Labor and Public Welfare," U.S. Senate, 1971.
6. Collen, M.F., "A Case Study of Multiphasic Health Testing in Medical Technology and the Health Care System: A Study of Equipment Embodied Technologies by the National Research Council's Committee on Technology and Health Care," National Research Council's Committee on Technology and Health Care. Washington, D.C.: National Academy of Sciences, 1978.
7. Collen, M.F., "Cost Analysis of Alternative Health Examination Modes," *Archives of Internal Medicine* **147**:73-79, 1977.
8. Breslow, L. and Somers, A.R., "A Lifetime Health-Monitoring Program," *New England Journal of Medicine* **296**:601–608, 1977.
9. Collen, "A Case Study . . . ", *op. cit.*
10. Collen, M.F., Feldman, R., Soghikian, K., Richart, R.H., and Duncan, J.H., "Evaluation of an Ambulatory Medical-Care Delivery System," *New England Journal of Medicine* **294**:426–431, 1976.
11. Collen, "A Case Study . . . ", *op. cit.*
12. Corben and Krute, *op. cit.*; Breslow and Somers, *op. cit.*; and Collen *et al., op. cit.*

Index